D0228904

'This book is an impressive indictment of the changes made recently by the Government to the National Health Service. The damage these changes have inflicted on the people of Suffolk, especially the elderly and other vulnerable people, is documented in damning and relentless detail. Sadly Suffolk isn't the only place where promises are being broken, the principles of the NHS abandoned, the needs of communities ignored and financial targets ruthlessly pursued regardless of the consequences.

Michael Mandelstam's analysis is unanswerable and his criticisms robust. His book should be studied by everyone concerned with how health care is delivered in Britain. If any of the politicians, civil servants or administrators who devised or implemented these changes have the nerve to read it they should hang their heads in shame and resign at once.

The author has been generous in the book about the contributions other people, including myself, have made to fighting these changes and exposing their consequences. The truth is that the person who has done the most in this respect is Michael Mandelstam himself. His tireless work, persistence in the face of all kinds of bureaucratic and other obstructions and his considerable expert knowledge of health and social service issues have made him an inspiration to the whole community. I am privileged to have him as one of my constituents.'

– *Tim Yeo, MP for South Suffolk and former Health Minister*

'Michael Mandelstam has vividly illustrated and authenticated his grand theme – the warranted collapse of public trust in NHS Trusts – by a blow-by-blow account of hospital closures, in Suffolk particularly. In the course of it he tells of public consultations of shameless insincerity and of almost Orwellian "mantras, euphemism, and doublethink". Above all, his is a cautionary tale of our times – of ideological centralisation out of touch with local realities.'

– *Lord Phillips of Sudbury, life peer and lawyer*

Betraying the NHS

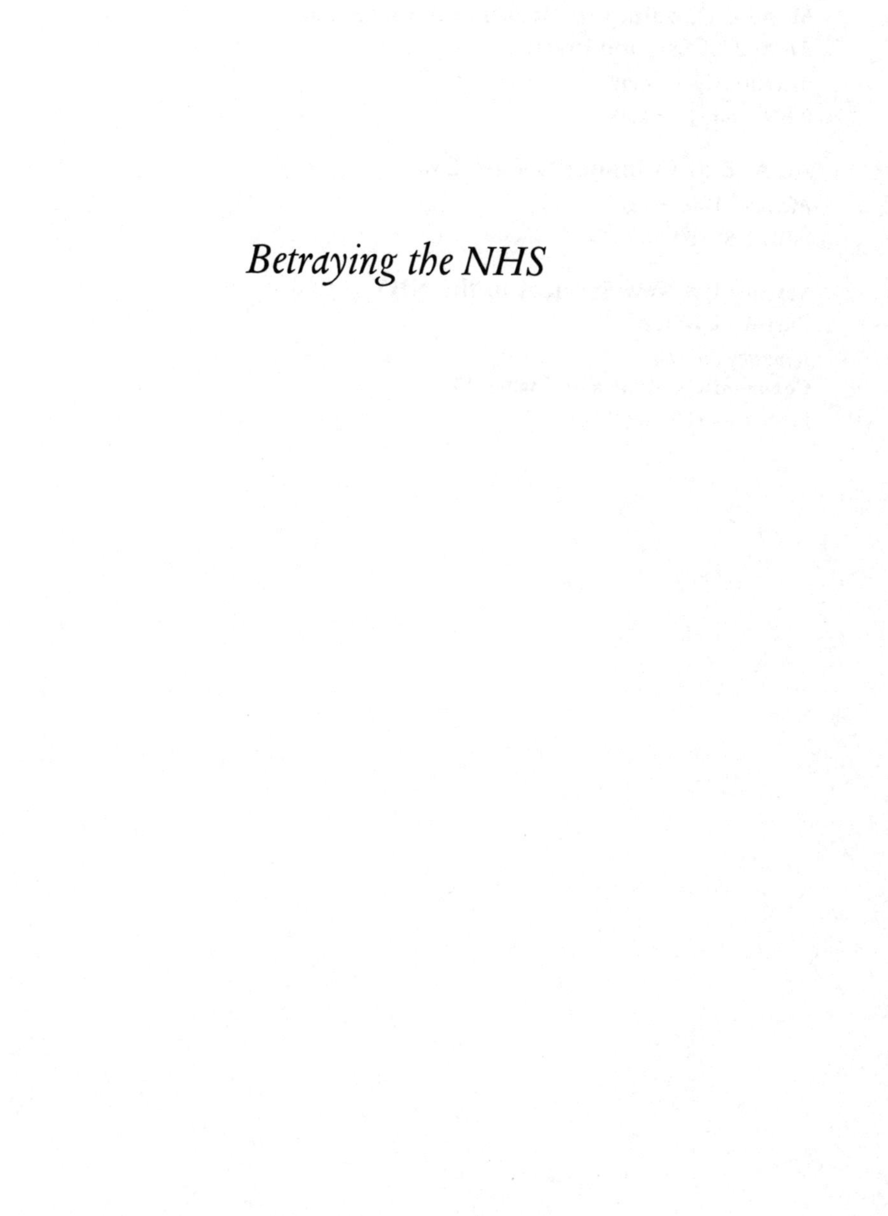

of related interest

Community Care Practice and the Law
Third Edition
Michael Mandelstam
ISBN 1 84310 233 1

Manual Handling in Health and Social Care
An A–Z of Law and Practice
Michael Mandelstam
ISBN 1 84310 041 X

An A–Z of Community Care Law
Michael Mandelstam
ISBN 1 85302 560 7

Setting Up New Services in the NHS
'Just Add Water!'
Kingsley Norton
Community, Culture and Change 13
ISBN 1 84310 162 9

Betraying the NHS

Health Abandoned

Michael Mandelstam

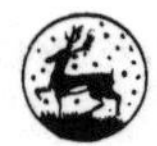

Jessica Kingsley Publishers
London and Philadelphia

First published in 2007
by Jessica Kingsley Publishers
116 Pentonville Road
London N1 9JB, UK
and
400 Market Street, Suite 400
Philadelphia, PA 19106, USA

www.jkp.com

Library of Congress Cataloging in Publication Data

Mandelstam, Michael, 1956-

Betraying the NHS : health abandoned / Michael Mandelstam.

p. ; cm.

Includes bibliographical references and index.

ISBN-13: 978-1-84310-482-7 (hardback : alk. paper)

ISBN-10: 1-84310-482-2 (hardback : alk. paper)

1. National health services--Great Britain. 2. Health services administration--Great Britain. 3. Medical policy--Great Britain. I. Title.

[DNLM: 1. Great Britain. National Health Service. 2. State Medicine--organization & administration--Great Britain. 3. Delivery of Health Care--Great Britain. 4. Health Care Reform --Great Britain. 5. Health Policy--Great Britain. W 225 FA1 M271b 2007]

RA395.G6M364 2007

362.10941--dc22

2006025130

British Library Cataloguing in Publication Data

A CIP catalogue record for this book is available from the British Library

ISBN-13: 978 184310 482 7

ISBN-10: 1 84310 482 2

Printed and bound in Great Britain by
Athenaeum Press, Gateshead, Tyne and Wear

Contents

Author's Note

My mother, Dorothy Mandelstam, worked in health and social care most of her life. She began in rehabilitation units during the Second World War. She ended up pioneering incontinence advice services – at a time when people talked about incontinence even less than they do now. She died shortly before Tony Blair was elected in May 1997. Like so many other people, she believed that the health service she had worked for all those years would be safe if New Labour were to gain power. She had always voted for the Labour party. How appalled – but how approving I hope – she would have been that her son felt driven to write this book.

I lay no claim to the omniscience apparently claimed by the Secretary of State for Health and her local NHS trusts and primary care trusts about what is best for us all. I simply have done my best to describe policies and decision-making in the NHS that seemed, on their very face, to be harmful. In particular, it seemed that people with the greatest needs, and especially older people, people with learning disabilities and people with mental health problems, were the ones being targeted. Nonetheless, the wider population at large also stood to lose, as local services affecting people of all ages and health status – for instance, maternity services, minor injuries units, and accident and emergency departments to name but a few – came under threat up and down the country. This was being achieved through decision-making characterised by a singular lack of transparency, high-handedness and lack of evidence. In principle, such decision-making characteristics lead to poor outcomes.

In addition, this was happening at a time when the government seemed to be pushing through surreptitiously a largely concealed agenda to fragment and dismantle the NHS. This was in order to open up provision to the private sector in a competitive marketplace. Increasingly, financial and performance targets were driving the NHS towards a business model. The way in which the ground was being cleared to achieve this did not augur well for the more vulnerable groups of patients, especially older people – that is, all of us, sooner or later.

Many senior, highly experienced clinicians, managers and other health and social care professionals – together with patients and their carers – have taken a lot of time and trouble explaining to me just why the issues are so important for older (but also some younger) people with complex needs, disabilities or chronic conditions and illness. A large number of these clinicians, managers and professionals were from within Suffolk. I have mentioned none of their names, because they are afraid of the repercussions. Of the many outside of Suffolk, I would like to thank in particular Dr Rory O'Connor, Consultant in Rehabilitation Medicine. Likewise Helen Tucker, for opening up the world of community hospitals. In a strange way, there are thanks also to the indirect encouragement of those members of the Suffolk West PCT Board who, privately, were prepared to express their dismay at the PCT's proposals – even though, publicly, they felt compelled to go along with them.

This book is not an attack on any individuals. It is an analysis of a system of decision-making undertaken by public bodies. These range from the Department of Health and Secretary of State for Health and strategic health authorities, right down to NHS primary care trusts, NHS trusts and local councils. However, because local events are set out, individuals are sometimes identifiable, explicitly and implicitly. This is inevitable and also right because decisions do not, self-reflexively, take and implement themselves. I see the decisions – and all the paraphernalia surrounding them – as flowing from public bodies. When NHS senior managers and the board members take decisions and make statements they are doing so as representatives of a public body.

This needs emphasising because events in Suffolk and elsewhere became very heated indeed during 2005 and 2006. And, when local conflicts break out, there is always the danger that they might become personalised, thus deflecting focus away from the real issues, which are in fact systemic. By definition, therefore, the book is not attacking the good faith, abilities or competence of any particular individuals. It would defeat the entire object of the book to do so.

I have no party political axe to grind. There are, however, other interests to which I should draw attention. I was and am a member of the Walnuttree Hospital Action Committee in Sudbury, Suffolk (but the book reflects my own views and not necessarily those of the committee). My wife, Halcyon Mandelstam, works at the Walnuttree Hospital. She is a senior and skilled physiotherapist (with nearly 20 years' experience) providing rehabilitation for older patients with more complex problems. Sudbury is her home town. Unchivalrously, I must own that the campaigning and the writing of this book are not to do with saving her employment. I understand and hope that, one way or another, it is not directly in jeopardy. I should make it clear, and in particular to her employers, that she has had nothing whatsoever to do with the writing of this book.

Nonetheless, I have watched how, for six years in Sudbury, she has struggled to run a grossly under-resourced service. Her conscientiousness and dedication – like that of so many other staff – mean that she has been systematically exploited in terms of inestimable amounts of unpaid overtime. Appreciated it seems by grateful patients rather than the PCT Board, she (together with many of her clinical colleagues) sees a bleak future for older and disabled people requiring more complex and slower stream rehabilitation. To all appearances, it would seem that in many areas, including Suffolk, the NHS is behaving as if such patients are just too awkward and too expensive. Perhaps this is because they are perceived not to deliver quick and easy returns. Consequently she and countless others are now weighing up whether they have a future in the NHS at all.

In addition, under 'Agenda for Change' (pay reform for NHS staff), her reward is that she has just been effectively downgraded. It appears that staff members such as she are being measured against a series of tick boxes related more to organisational and management process or structure than to patient outcomes. Overall, there is a real risk that such skilled staff, together with the patients they treat, are being driven away. We will be the losers. And, those in Whitehall – who believe that modernisation comes in the form of computers – may be interested to know that she still has no reliable access to a computer.

Many years ago, I was also very fortunate to spend a great deal of time with a Welsh consultant obstetrician of immense insight, known to his friends and colleagues only as Ap Rosser. Starting out in medicine in the 1920s and 1930s, he was there at the inception of the NHS. Many years ago, when in retirement and at his inimitable hearthside, he told me, through countless stories and personal experiences, about just why the NHS was so important.

The overall reason for writing the book is to put on record what is happening. Ultimately the book stands or falls on the evidence. In my view, this is overwhelming. Despite all the extra money and New Labour's repeated claims that it is improving our health care, something has gone terribly wrong. The NHS is being increasingly betrayed with every day that goes by.

Note. There are a few organisational abbreviations that are used throughout the book, although the full names of the organisations are used as well. This inter-changeability is simply for the sake of variety. They are:

NHS – National Health Service.

PCTs – Primary care trusts (local NHS bodies responsible for commissioning a wide range of local services, including acute hospital and general practitioner services; also, they directly provide community health services, but probably not for much longer).

NHS trusts – (local NHS bodies running acute hospital services).

SHAs – Strategic health authorities (regional NHS bodies with financial and performance oversight of local primary care trusts and NHS trusts).

WHAC – Walnuttree Hospital Action Committee (local committee).

Reference to local social services authorities is to those local councils with responsibility for providing social care services.

Lastly, the book has only seen the light of day at all because of Jessica Kingsley's great support and encouragement – and the immensely hard work of all her staff involved with the book, especially Jessica Stevens.

The author would like to thank all the publications and individuals who have granted permission to quote from their articles and letters.

1

Introduction: the Death Throes of a Health Service

This book was written against the backdrop of fundamental changes being made to the National Health Service (NHS) in England during 2005 and 2006. They were being achieved by a number of linked policies driven by the New Labour government.

These policies included significant financial investment in the NHS, giving patients more choice, keeping health services local, involving local communities in reconfiguration to local health services, transferring NHS provision to the private sector, creating a competitive marketplace for improved NHS services, and introducing a new system called payment by results.

In addition, other policies were put in place specifically to ensure that potentially vulnerable groups were not sidelined. These groups included older people, people with learning disabilities, and people with mental health problems. Even better, it seemed, central government was committed to something called 'joint working'. This envisaged closer cooperation and sometimes a degree of integration between 'health care' services provided by the NHS, and 'social care' services provided by local councils. This was to iron out the gaps and misunderstandings that sometimes occurred between the NHS and councils.

Overall, the government stated itself still to be committed fully to the fundamental principles of the NHS dating back to 1948. These were universality, comprehensiveness and, by and large, health services free of charge to the patient. If the government was to be believed, everything in the health garden was rosy and set to become even more so.

The acid test of policy is how it actually affects individual local people and communities. Chiefly, this book sets out this range of national policies and then considers empirically, step by step, the direct effect they had on local communities during 2005 and 2006. Examples are taken from all over the country. However, in order to show close-up the effects on the ground, the county of Suffolk, and in particular West Suffolk, are the focus. This in no way renders the book merely local in scope or relevance. The same issues were being played out across the country. West Suffolk was not a little local difficulty; in many ways it epitomised a widespread pattern. The local detail spelt out from Suffolk and many other places is by way of evidence that it really was all happening and was affecting real people in real localities.

Therefore, as well as setting out the national picture, the book contains local detail. Much of this is described through local voices, including patients, relatives, voluntary organisations, clinicians, councillors and MPs. This is to emphasise the effects on real people and local communities. It is also to hear from these people inherent common sense and wisdom about health care. Unfortunately, despite all the lip service paid to 'patient choice', and to the empowerment of frontline clinicians, central government and local NHS senior managers seem to pass by on the other side.

As central government policy played out in West Suffolk and other locations, the implications became apparent. Instead of health service improvements and expansion, it was severe cutbacks that came to the fore. Ward closures, bed and job losses and community hospital closures were being reported, it seemed, from every quarter. Rehabilitation services for older people seemed to be in the process of being strangled in some areas. Both wards and day services for people with mental health problems were likewise being targeted. And the NHS strove still harder to reduce its provision for people with learning disabilities. More generally, and affecting the population at large of all ages and health status, were cuts to maternity services, accident and emergency departments, minor injuries units and a range of other services. Local health services generally, both rural and urban, were under assault. Increasing numbers of NHS Trusts and PCTs were reported to be in significant deficit.

The government's reaction to this apparent bonfire of health services was inadequate and lacked transparency. First, it would generally ignore and play it down. Then it would focus on those local NHS bodies with the more spectacular deficits and attempt to portray the problem as affecting just a very few areas. It ignored the fact that a large number had financial problems.

It also seemed that measuring the 'crisis' in terms of financial deficits was only half the picture. This was because it appeared that significant numbers of NHS Trusts and PCTs were in financial balance only through having already made substantial cuts to services. In effect, the government seemed to be concerned less with patients losing services, and more about those NHS Trusts and PCTs that had failed to make sufficiently drastic cuts.

Second, the government's response, namely that each local NHS Trust and PCT in deficit had to 'live within its means', was incoherent. This was because it meant that, through no fault of their own, local communities would be forced to pay – with their own health – for the mistakes, mismanagement or miscalculations of senior NHS decision-makers at both local and national level. Given that we are all tax payers, who contribute to a national health service, such an approach is self-evidently unfair. The Secretary of State's office opined that the NHS must 'experience pain locally'. This was, no doubt unintentionally, a sadistic-sounding statement. But it was not, in substance, far off the mark; only it would be patients who would be punished and suffer that pain (literally), not NHS chief executives, chairmen and their Boards.

Third, the government would ritually respond that waiting times had improved, with, for example, cancer and cardiology services particularly benefiting. But this seemed to miss the point. The achievement of targets is not meant to bring the rest of the organisation to its knees. Yet this is what seemed to be happening. It was as if the Secretary of State fiddled to the tune of her targets, while other parts of the NHS burned. There seems to be little doubt that in various ways, both directly and indirectly, patients have suffered as a consequence of the obsession with targets, both clinical and financial.

The cost to patients has sometimes been high and very direct. None more so than when, at one major hospital (Stoke Mandeville), nearly forty patients died during two major outbreaks of *Clostridium difficile* – and hundreds of others were infected. The Healthcare Commission investigated and published its findings in July 2006. It concluded that, despite having been well advised by its infection control team, the NHS Trust Board had other priorities, on which it would not compromise. Infection control advice was disregarded, even after the first outbreak of infection. Even with the advent of the second outbreak, the Trust only changed its priorities when the story was leaked to the national media.

The priorities, to which the Board so doggedly stuck, comprised waiting list targets, financial control and reconfiguration of services. Right across the NHS, such pressures arising from these priorities daily lead to all manner of shortcut being taken with people's care – particularly that of older people. And so it happened in Buckinghamshire. It just came to national attention because of the extreme and lethal consequences. It might be tempting to hope or assume that the behaviour of the NHS Trust was an aberration, a statistical outlier. But we should make no such assumption. Nor did the Healthcare Commission. It concluded that the pressures, which led to the Trust running off the rails, exist for all acute NHS trusts in England. These pressures stem from the uncompromising demands of central government, levelled at local NHS Trusts, via strategic health authorities.

On a different tack altogether, 'joint working' between the NHS and local authorities was all the rage – but would frequently seem to be a cover for moving people away inappropriately from NHS health care to local council social care. Health services could then be re-labelled or not provided at all. A lack of appropriate health-care rehabilitation will leave people more disabled and requiring social care services they might not otherwise have needed. Social care can be charged for, whereas NHS services mostly cannot. This creates an added incentive to shunt people and services over to local councils. People may have to use their savings to pay for services and even sell their home. That is, if local councils have the resources to provide social care services for them at all. Increasingly they do not and, year by year, they are rationing provision according to ever-stricter criteria. Fewer and fewer people are eligible for their services.

This means that even in those circumstances where this shift from health care to social care is appropriate (which it sometimes is) – local councils are in any case hamstrung in terms of finance and resources. It is not then a case of an orderly and beneficial transfer of responsibility and of an enlightened approach to meeting people's needs. Instead it can degenerate into an unseemly and detrimental pushing of people from pillar to post – from a shoulder shrugging NHS to the overburdened but increasingly flinty, and financially rapacious, arms of local councils.

Once within the orbit of social care, people are also deluged with the politically correct language of 'choice', 'control' and 'independence'. All highly laudable and important principles. Central government's favoured method of achieving of these is to pressurise local councils into not providing services directly, but instead contracting them out to the private sector. If possible, the government wants people to purchase, or at least direct the purchase of, services through things called 'direct payments' or 'individual budgets'. The money can then be spent on the private sector.

While these payments or budgets do have the potential genuinely to give people more control and independence, the signs are that, once they are given in larger numbers, this may not happen. They are likely instead to be used by councils to cap expenditure and force vulnerable people to fend more for themselves – even when this is inappropriate and the required services are either not available or not affordable. Direct payments and individual budgets may be the flavour of the month among policy makers and beneficial for some users of services; but potentially they also constitute a Trojan Horse by which council social care services will be finally dismantled – whether or not this is in the interests of all users of services.

Overall, these government policies were having harmful effects. People with complex, longstanding health-care needs were being victimised and excluded from NHS provision in order to save money. Patients were being increasingly treated like financial and business units, as NHS trusts sought at all costs – both financial and human – to meet targets and save money. It became increasingly evident that New Labour was attempting to dismantle the NHS by privatising the provision of its services and throwing it open to market forces.

Universality and comprehensiveness were being eroded. Change, it seemed, was being achieved particularly at the expense of vulnerable groups, including older people with more complex needs, younger adults with disabilities, people with learning disabilities and people with mental health problems. In other words, perversely, those with the greatest needs were losing out. Allied to this was the loss, or further erosion, of what for want of a better term we might refer to as 'good, basic care'. That is, treating people as people and not as business units, outstaying their allotted welcome by blocking beds or 'frequently flying' in and out of hospital. Real care, for instance, involves making sure that older people are treated with dignity and respect, treated in a non-discriminatory fashion, assisted to eat their daily nourishment, assisted to avoid pressure sores, are not unnecessarily written off as incontinent, are not discharged from hospital prematurely, and so on.

At Stoke Mandeville Hospital, for instance, the Healthcare Commission uncovered just such shortcuts in care, stemming from concentration on targets and not people. These shortcuts – which are entirely unacceptable even had they not resulted in a lethal outbreak of infection – included the following. Side rooms were not used for isolation of infected patients but for non-emergency surgery cases (to meet targets) thus putting other patients at serious risk of infection. People were frequently moved from ward to ward for reasons of capacity rather than clinical reasons. They would end up on the 'wrong' type of ward, where staff would be less knowledgeable about their condition. Doctors would then be unable to find their patients. Low levels of staffing and an effective recruitment freeze meant that staff might have no time to assist patients to the toilet in time (or to change the sheets when patients didn't make it in time), write up care plans, wash hands, wear appropriate aprons and gloves, ensure that faeces were not coating bed rails, give patients their food supplements, give therapists the information they needed, and so on.

All such basic, humane care might be unglamorous in the supposedly bright new world of the NHS, but it is fundamental to us all. The pressure on acute hospitals is increasing, although it could be relieved cost effectively in part by community hospital beds. Yet nearly 30 per cent of community hospitals in England are faced with cutbacks (particularly of beds) or closure altogether. This is despite the fact that community hospitals across the country are viewed by many as an invaluable bastion of care in its real sense.

Furthermore, the ill effects were not confined to the more vulnerable among us. Accident and emergency services, maternity services, children's services – in fact a whole range of local beds, clinics and services affecting people of all ages – were being removed all over the country.

As the picture became clearer, the worse it looked. This was not just because of the apparent harm being done. A chasm was opening up between government policy and local practice. Change was occurring with a lack of transparency. Decision-making at all levels seemed increasingly to be characterised by the deployment of emotive language, mantras, euphemism, doublethink, and the use of red herrings to achieve concealed aims. Casualties along the wayside typically included evidence, logic and genuinely participative and democratic decision-making.

Instead of working with the local community, local NHS bodies would try to impose change by diktat and confrontation. They would break assurances and promises without notice, often without convincing explanation or apology. Transparency was notable – but only for its general absence. Breathtaking statements were made about how the severe cuts taking place would have no detrimental effects on patients. The more severe the cuts, the more NHS chief executives and chairmen protested that it was all for the best. It was, we were told, about 'changing for the better', modernisation and improvement, or a service fit for the future. 'Less' truly had become 'more'. In some instances, the statements and explanation emanating from the NHS were so absurd that in any other context they would have been taken for outright parody.

In the same vein, the more trumpeted a government policy – such as keeping health services local and involving local communities – the greater the departure from it in practice. Local services were melting away. The ensuing reasoned objections and protests of local communities were mostly disregarded. The engagement between communities and their PCTs was not of the cooperative and enlightened type portrayed in government policy. Instead, all too often, it involved fierce and bitter conflict, driven by fear and anger.

The crucial point is not that there should be no change. But importantly, there needs to be a sensible transition between the old and the new. People are likely to be supportive of change if an effective, well evidenced, fair and comparable alternative is in place. However, instead, throughout 2005 and 2006, the country was treated to closures and cutbacks bearing all the hallmarks of panic, chaos and mismanagement. In many cases, it would prove impossible to detect a decision-making process that could in any sense be described as well evidenced, planned, communicated, organised or implemented. As for adequate – let alone improved – replacement services, they appeared in many instances to be so many figments of the imagination.

The policy of having specialist regional services (to which people would have to travel further) might have made sense – if the basic range of services were made more local, just as the government said would happen. Thus, it announced a new generation of community hospitals and that it would be keeping the NHS local and providing 'care closer to home'. But in reality, local services were being scythed down indiscriminately in both town and countryside. Both basic and more specialist services were set to become more distant than they had been. Existing community hospitals (old or new build) – beacons of local NHS care (in the true sense of the word) and treatment – were threatened by the score. District general hospitals were starting to be closed – or downgraded and rebadged as community hospitals. And care closer to, or in, people's own homes? This seemed – through lack of resources, staff and proper planning – to be more about leaving people to fend themselves or forcing family members to look after them, than about providing reliable NHS care and treatment. In sum, the policy about local services smacked of a confidence trick. Services were in fact moving further away from, not closer to, people – if they were not disappearing altogether.

In addition, it seemed that NHS trusts and primary care trusts were prepared to proceed by ignoring – or referring highly selectively to – relevant evidence. Logic and facts would sometimes be apparently abandoned in equal measure, wholesale if necessary. Policies, reasonable on the surface, would be hijacked and used for quite different purposes. In such a way, the world could be turned upside down with impunity. A 'model of care', all the rage one day, could without rhyme or reason be abandoned the next. Anybody querying this would run the risk of being labelled sentimental, emotional or just plain reactionary.

For instance, one of the central battlegrounds was over something called 'intermediate care', a policy aimed mainly, but not only, at older people. It was designed mainly to avoid unnecessary stays in acute hospitals. On its face it was a sensible policy. But like so many central government policies, it lent itself to distortion and misuse. Local NHS bodies, seemingly unable to help themselves in the face of severe pressure from central government, would hijack the policy. Sometimes this could lead to justification of proposals to implement severe and seemingly unevidenced cuts to health services for vulnerable people. Intermediate care was in principle designed originally to complement and add to all-important rehabilitation and recuperation services. Now it was in more danger of being perversely misused as a cover for the NHS to do quite the opposite – actually to run down rehabilitation services.

Above all, local NHS bodies were perceived to be riding roughshod over the unprecedented objections of local communities. Across Suffolk (and in many other parts of the country) public meetings, marches and petitions would abound but bear no real fruit. People would take to the roads, the waterways, the buses, bicycles, chartered trains, boats, vintage cars, Harley Davidson motor bikes, tractors – and to Whitehall. Skeletons and grim reapers would stalk the streets. Physical protests would routinely run into thousands. Local people expressing opposition to local closures would regularly number tens of thousands. It all seemed to make little or no difference.

Desperate local campaigns would be run by local committees, drawing together expertise and support from all corners of the community. Patients and their relatives, the people who really knew first hand about the importance of rehabilitation and recuperation, would express their views. In

Suffolk alone, they protested in their tens of thousands, but would be all but ignored. Military metaphor is used to describe one of these campaigns towards the end of the book, for the good reason that it was a conflict and it ran deep. Local communities soon discovered the nature of the beast they were up against. They had to try to work with PCTs and NHS Trusts, but at the same time many had swiftly to learn not to take these NHS bodies, or their ritual reassurances and deceptive promises, at face value. They also had to grasp that the NHS does not speak the language used by the rest of us. Skilled interpretation is often required.

Dire warnings from their own clinicians would be downplayed by NHS primary care trusts, the clinicians sometimes dismissed as suffering from a lack of understanding. From the small parish council to the county council, and through every council in between, local government would let its concerns be known. The protests of the churches and the NHS Patient and Public Involvement Forums (to whom NHS bodies are meant to listen) fell on stony ground. Regional medical associations would present letters in vain, and the unions would appear powerless.

The consequences in Suffolk and many other areas would be disastrous. Fear, anger and distress took hold across the country. In turn, local NHS trusts and primary care trusts, professing bemusement at the hostility they had excited, retreated into their bunker. This was to protect themselves from criticism and also to maintain the integrity of the make-believe world they increasingly inhabited. Abstract models of care would be dreamt up, as well as imaginary armies of health-care workers who would be delivering the new scattered 'care in the community'. To local communities looking on aghast, these NHS bodies adopted what seemed to be an ever more obdurate, uncompromising and detached approach. Even so, as the NHS trusts and primary care trusts scurried underground, so it became clear that they too were in part hapless victims – caught in the crossfire of contradictory demands being made by central government.

Under competing pressure to deliver on all manner of target and policy, local NHS trusts and primary care trusts had come under intense pressure to make financial savings very quickly. In some parts of the country (including Suffolk), huge deficits had to be reined in. The perversity of such sudden, uncompromising demands was highlighted by the fact that many of the deficits were not new. They had been in existence for some years, not only tolerated but also even encouraged by central government, so that vote-winning NHS performance targets would be met. The explanation for a sudden change in approach appeared to be wholly political. It occurred immediately after New Labour's general election victory in May 2005.

Worse still was the lack of accountability. This led to frustration and exasperation in local communities seeking explanation and dialogue. None was to be had. They searched in vain for a true decision-maker but simply could not find one. Local NHS trusts and primary care trusts would quietly concede that their hand was being forced by their political masters. Yet central government would flatly deny responsibility for local decisions. And the intermediaries, the strategic health authorities, lying between local NHS bodies and central government? They had simply donned cloaks of invisibility.

Even so, behind the smokescreen, the hand of central government seemed to loom ever greater. Perhaps the most damaging cue provided, and taken up by local NHS bodies, was the hasty imposition by diktat of ill-thought-out policies, themselves based on unclear aims and ambiguous motives. In this respect, the arrogance and contempt with which local communities felt they were being treated would arguably amount to an abuse of power. All this would be exacerbated by the various concealed agendas apparently being perpetrated by central government, including the exclusion of vulnerable people from, and the dismantling and privatisation of, the NHS.

The scale and nature of local opposition up and down the country was astonishing. Such radical change (and its serious consequences) had not been spelt out plainly by New Labour in its election manifesto. In short, the government clearly had no political mandate for what it was doing. It went ahead all the same.

Local NHS trusts and primary care trusts were being pressurised and told what to do by central government. Schooled in a form of doublethink, which ultimately boiled down to 'less is more', they clearly had convinced themselves that they were acting for the best. But pressurised and rushed decision-making led inevitably to shortcuts being taken.

Pressurised they may have been, but this is not to say that local NHS bodies were victims in the same sense as patients, families and other informal carers. For these, the consequences were very different. They stood to lose in terms of lack of care, respite, rehabilitation, recuperation – leading to greater disability, suffering, pain, distress, stress (physical and mental) on carers and in some cases even avoidable, premature death. For instance, premature death may occur not just through any immediate neglect or omission. It can also flow, quicker or slower, from the all-too-familiar spiral of physical and mental decline attendant on a lack of suitable and timely rehabilitation and recuperation. Local communities were threatened more generally also, as key local services (some involving life and death) for people of all ages and health status – from accident and emergency services to maternity units – were increasingly under threat of closure.

Local NHS primary care trusts would at times be taken aback at the breadth and depth of opposition they faced. They seemed not to realise just how confrontational, aggressive and harmful their actions appeared to be. To local communities, the actions of these 'trusts' spoke far louder than any soothing words offered up by way of unconvincing explanation. Central government's 2006 White Paper had spoken of local communities being fully involved in, and feeling ownership of, decisions about local health services. It was a distant aspiration only. In its place came a fundamental breakdown of communication and trust.

This loss of trust was accompanied by fear. The harm being done (or proposed to be done) to vulnerable people – as well as to people more generally – was perceived to be very real and akin to a policy (whether or not thought through) of the weakest to the wall. It was all made worse because the changes were being implemented so quickly, together with a lack of transparency and of accountability. To take services away from vulnerable people – that is, all of us when we are in need – is bad enough. To do so covertly prevents debate as to whether such a policy is acceptable and, if not, how to ameliorate it. This is unforgivable. But then to add in lack of accountability takes it all beyond the pale. In short, if central government and local NHS bodies wish to remove our local health services generally, abandon certain groups of vulnerable people, undermine the fundamental principles of the NHS, and throw open the doors to privatisation of our health care, they should at least have the courage, political and moral, to say so. Of course it is easy to criticise. But one thing is clear. Answers and solutions may be elusive, but lack of transparency and of accountability will in any event not deliver them.

Perhaps it is summed up by the level-headed, intelligent and well-informed resident of Sudbury in Suffolk who stopped the author in the street. He spoke of the picture he had of NHS decision-makers in Whitehall. This was of people in a darkened room, working out how to cut NHS costs by shuffling older people out of the NHS equation, into social care for which they could be charged and might have to sell their house – and then, if possible, discreetly into a cost-effective early grave. From such a resident this was shocking. Was it all paranoid imagining? The author would like to think so but is not certain any more. As one placard read, during a protest about Suffolk health services: 'The 11th commandment: thou shall not grow old'.[1]

1 Dave Gooderham, 'Health workers step up cuts protest.' *East Anglian Daily Times*, 3 November 2005.

2

Comprehensive, Universal and Free

In order to understand some of what is told in this book, a short background to the National Health Service (NHS) is required. This is to discover the underlying principles and test them against what was happening in Suffolk and many other parts of the country during 2005 and 2006.

When it came to power in 1997, the New Labour government argued that the NHS was safe with it. The implication was that the NHS being saved was the one we all knew and loved – whatever its inherent shortcomings.

The NHS was created politically because of a significant shift in thinking during the Second World War – and legally by means of the National Health Service Act 1946. William Beveridge, the architect of the welfare state, published his report, *Social Insurance and Allied Services*, in 1942. He referred to a:

> national health service for prevention and for cure of disease and disability by medical treatment.

It would be comprehensive, including domiciliary as well as institution-based services. Medical treatment:

> covering all requirements will be provided for all citizens by a national health service organised under the health departments and post-medical rehabilitation treatment will be provided for all persons capable of profiting from it.[1]

1 W. Beveridge (1942) *Social Insurance and Allied Health Services*. Cm 6404. London: HMSO, paras 19xi and 426–7.

This wartime blueprint became a 1944 White Paper. The proposed health service had to be:

> comprehensive in two senses – first, that it is available to all people and, second, that it covers all necessary forms of health care.

It had to 'include ancillary services of nursing, of midwifery and of other things which ought to go with medical care'. There might be temporary exceptions to such comprehensiveness. For instance, full dental and ophthalmology services might not be achieved immediately. However, these were viewed as practical problems to be overcome. They did not cast doubt on the new service's scope and objectives.

The White Paper referred also to the need to develop a full home-nursing service 'to ensure that all who need nursing attention in their own homes will be able to obtain it without charge'; likewise rehabilitation services would have to be developed. As to charges, there should by and large be none:

> as far as individual members of the public are concerned, they will be able to obtain medical advice and treatment of every kind entirely without charge except for the cost of certain appliances.[2]

The consequent National Health Service Act 1946 placed a duty on the Minister for Health to:

> promote the establishment in England and Wales of a comprehensive health service designed to secure improvement in the physical and mental health of the people of England and Wales and the prevention, diagnosis and treatment of illness... The services so provided shall be free of charge, except where any provision of this Act expressly provides for the making and recovery of charges. (s.1)

Thus, in addition to universality and comprehensiveness, a third key principle was that services should by and large be free of charge – other than in the case of a number of specified exceptions. The successor to this 1946 Act, the National Health Service Act 1977, read similarly. It now referred to a duty on the Secretary of State to 'continue' to promote a comprehensive health service – reflecting the past 29 years of endeavour. In 2000, the New Labour government reiterated in its *NHS Plan* that it would remain faithful to

2 Minister of Health (1944) *A National Health Service.* Cm 6502. London: HMSO, pp.9, 41, 46, 57.

all three key principles. It also elaborated on what comprehensiveness and universality should mean in the 21st century. It would be:

> responsive to the needs of different groups and individuals within society, and challenge discrimination on the grounds of age, gender, ethnicity, religion, disability and sexuality. The NHS will treat patients as individuals, with respect for their dignity. Patients and citizens will have a greater say in the NHS, and the provision of services will be centred on patients' needs.[3]

Crucially, central government would increasingly inject a new principle into its policies, namely 'patient choice'. This would:

> mark an irreversible shift from the 1940s 'take it or leave it' top down service. Hospitals will no longer choose patients. Patients will choose hospitals.[4]

Whether this notion of patient choice was compatible with notions of universality, comprehensiveness and even, ultimately, free health care, was however not necessarily clear. This was particularly because of the scale of the changes envisaged. They would be the most:

> fundamental and far reaching reforms the NHS has seen since 1948.[5]

In sum, all three key NHS principles have remained fundamental since the late 1940s. From their inception, they have been subject inevitably to degrees of interpretation. They have sometimes frayed at the edges but remained recognisable. However, although it claimed to be adhering to these principles, the New Labour government would by 2006 appear to be stretching them to their very limit. Some would say to certain destruction, or at least to a totally unrecognisable form:

> The NHS is in transition. Its publicly-funded system of publicly-owned and provided health care is being replaced by a healthcare market, in which providers of services compete with private ones for NHS funds, with legal contracts and external regulation replacing direct political accountability. The pace of the transition is rapid, and the change is

3 Secretary of State for Health (2000) *The NHS Plan: a plan for investment, a plan for reform.* Cm 4818-1. London: HMSO, Preface.

4 Secretary of State for Health (2002) *Delivering the NHS Plan: next steps on investment, next steps on reform.* Cm 5503. London: HMSO, para 5.4.

5 Secretary of State for Health (2000) *The NHS Plan: a plan for investment, a plan for reform.* Cm 4818-1. London: HMSO, Executive summary.

> more far-reaching than is generally recognised. The old structures and organisations are being dismantled and a plethora of new organisations is evolving… But just as steel bedpans have been replaced by disposable grey cardboard, the whole NHS has become in a sense disposable: its hundreds of hospitals and other organisations, transformed into independent market actors, must now increasingly fend for themselves financially. They are becoming answerable to market forces rather than elected ministers…[6]

New NHS policies: modernising the methods of cultivation

New Labour has claimed since 1997 that it is saving the NHS, albeit seeking to modernise it in line with the original, underlying principles. The claim has resonated, because during the 1990s the continuation of a national health service appeared to be in doubt. The policies of the Conservative government of Margaret Thatcher threatened. In fact, radical dismantling did not take place, although significant change was being explored.

On the back of a 1989 White Paper, *Working for Patients*, NHS trusts were created by the NHS and Community Care Act 1990.[7] These new NHS trusts would operate, in theory at least, on a quasi-market and competition principle. A system of 'GP fund-holding' was also introduced. Nevertheless, the market, if that was the right word, was essentially an internal market – that is, the NHS was not yet being thrown open wholesale to private and independent health-care providers.

When the Conservatives were replaced by a New Labour government in 1997, the widespread assumption therefore was that the traditional NHS was safe – even from such tentative tinkering. Certainly, the government played this up for all it was worth. The electorate was reassured. Stealthy erosion of the health service would be halted. The government would 'end the Conservatives' internal market in healthcare'.[8]

In line with its claim to be taking forward the original principles, albeit in a modern and 21st-century context, New Labour launched its grand *NHS Plan*. The main message was about saving, improving, investing in and modernising the health service.[9]

6 Alison Talbot-Smith and Allyson Pollock (2006) *The New NHS: a guide.* Abingdon: Routledge, p.1.

7 Secretary of State for Health (1989) *Working for Patients.* Cm 555. London: HMSO.

8 *New Labour Because Britain Deserves Better.* London: Labour Party, 1997, p.16.

9 Secretary of State for Health (2000) *The NHS Plan: a plan for investment, a plan for reform.* Cm 4818-1. London: HMSO, Preface.

The plan has since been developed and its themes furthered in any number of policy documents. These culminated in repeated slogans during 2005 and 2006 about 'patient choice' and a 'patient-led' health service. The government had by then imposed on the NHS an ambitious series of performance targets. They were to measure whether the health service was delivering to a reasonable standard. The targets included, for example, maximum waiting times of six months for inpatients, of three months for outpatient appointments, and of four hours in accident and emergency departments.[10]

During its time in office, the New Labour government had been stepping up its claims for the NHS. Eventually, after a thrifty approach during its first term between 1997 and 2001, it made a great deal more money available. Its policies would also extol the importance of 'local' services, and of the involvement of local communities in the planning of those services. Involvement of the independent sector was to be welcomed and encouraged – but only where there was spare capacity or in the cause of innovation (provisos that would be subsequently discarded).

Along the way, the New Labour government did not forget to issue fine-sounding guidance and policies on particularly vulnerable or needy groups of people. These included a White Paper called *Valuing People* about people with learning disabilities. A series of 'national service framework' documents covered, for example, older people, people with long-term health conditions and people with mental health problems.[11]

By January 2006, it had issued a further, general White Paper, *Our Health, Our Care, Our Say*, on both health and social care. This stressed the importance of patient choice and local services, including community hospitals.[12] Just in case NHS staff and managers were still standing idle in the face of an endless barrage of directives and new policies, there was more to come. During 2006, NHS primary care trusts and strategic health authorities, having been in existence a mere five years, were subject to large-scale reorganisation. This was, so it was said, to promote greater efficiency and financial savings. All in the cause of improved patient care.

10 *National Standards: Local Action: health and social care standards and planning framework*. London: Department of Health, 2004, Appendix 1.

11 Secretary of State for Health (2001) *Valuing People: a new strategy for learning disability for the 21st century*. Cm 6700. London: HMSO. And *National Service Framework for Older People*. London: Department of Health, 2001. And *National Service Framework for Long Term Conditions*. London: Department of Health, 2005. And *National Service Framework for Mental Health*. London: Department of Health, 1999.

12 Secretary of State for Health (2006) *Our Health, Our Care, Our Say: a new direction for community services*. Cm 6737. London: HMSO.

In addition, from April 2006, the government began to introduce a comprehensive new system called 'payment by results'. This claimed to reward good performance, so that 'money would follow patients' and their choices. Roughly, NHS organisations would only receive money if services were actually delivered within financial tariff limits and according to the number of patients treated – and not simply receive unchanging block payments. The implication was that if local health services did not deliver against both financial and performance targets, and therefore fell foul of both patient and government approval, they might cease to exist.

All this ran hand in hand with an idea of 'contestability' whereby NHS services would be increasingly delivered by independent sector providers. These providers would be in competition with themselves and with 'in-house' NHS services, to the extent that the latter still existed. This was explained as being about raising standards in a health service that would remain free of charge to the patient.

In the meantime, central government had been pursuing investment into the NHS infrastructure by utilisation of the Private Finance Initiative (PFI). The private sector would build new hospitals, and lease them back over long periods of time to the NHS. A parallel scheme for the development of primary care premises, with the private sector leasing them back to GPs, is known as LIFT (Local Improvement Finance Initiative). In addition, new NHS foundation trusts were seeking to unshackle themselves from central government control, and so respond to local needs more flexibly.

All is rosy in the health garden

In sum, taking all the above at face value, the health garden might have looked altogether fragrant and blooming. A government committed to the fundamental principles of the NHS. Universality, comprehensiveness and still a free service. Huge extra sums of extra public money to make improvements. And a whole set of vigorous and modern-sounding policies designed to make it all happen. It surely couldn't get any better. The 2005 New Labour general election manifesto had referred to 'equal access for all' and 'more say for patients in how, where and when they are treated'.[13] Perhaps it was really happening.

Certainly, down in Sudbury, Suffolk, there were many who would have agreed. After some 30 years of attempts to get a new community hospital

13 *Labour Party Manifesto: Britain forward not back.* London: Labour Party, 2005.

built and operational, it had at last been planned and approved, immediately before the general election of May 2005. True, the two old, much-loved hospitals would close in due course, but the local residents were interested in services, not bricks and mortar. West Suffolk was generally a staunchly Conservative voting area. But it seemed that even here, out in the sticks, New Labour's writ ran – in the cause of delivering a modern, universal and comprehensive health service.

Yet the people of Sudbury – and of many other areas of the country – had apparently been deceived. With the general election done, and New Labour re-elected, the garden party was over. By June 2005, a mere two months later, the new community hospital development had been abandoned. The local NHS, in the form of Suffolk West PCT, proposed instead to remove the heart of health service provision from the town, including all inpatient, and many outpatient, services. By November, as the implications sank in, the front-page headlines of the local newspaper said it all:

HEALTH - 'DRIFTING TOWARDS OBLIVION'.[14]

Concerns had been exacerbated when it became apparent during August 2005 that not only were community hospital services under threat but so too was the acute hospital, the West Suffolk NHS Hospitals Trust (at Bury St Edmunds). It was reported to be potentially in line for closure or downgrading as well, as it struggled with a £20 million deficit. This would leave the main hospital for the area in Cambridge, an hour's drive from Sudbury. Bury St Edmunds would be seen as an outpost of Cambridge, much as Sudbury currently was an outpost of Bury.[15]

This report seemed not to be mere scaremongering. By June 2006, West Suffolk Hospital had closed 55 beds and announced 26 more beds to be lost, as well as a reduction of some 260 jobs. Behind the scenes, the strategic health authority had quietly been carrying out a project, looking at which of the district general hospitals in Norfolk, Suffolk and Cambridgeshire might be dispensed with.

Without good local services based in and around Sudbury, there would be real fears that Sudbury would disappear off the NHS map. In fact this was the view of the Chairman of the local Patient and Public Involvement

14 Barbara Eeles, *Suffolk Free Press*, 24 November 2005.

15 Dave Gooderham, 'Hospital bosses play down "merger".' *East Anglian Daily Times*, 13 August 2005.

Forum. This was after it turned out that the Department of Health would not release the 5500 letters and postcards of protest to the PCT:

> It is very undemocratic. Someone in the Department of Health is sat looking at a map of the country and is painting Sudbury and Suffolk out of existence.[16]

By April 2006, the fine words of a year ago had turned to dust:

> PROMISES, April 2005: health chiefs promise Sudbury 32-bed hospital to replace the Walnuttree and St Leonards. PROMISES: health chiefs pledge to axe 32 beds, close two hospitals. New care centre to have no beds.[17]

Events the same or similar to those occurring in Suffolk were being replicated in many other parts of the country. How could it all have happened?

A stony undersoil: less than universality

The neutral observer might have concluded in March 2005 that the NHS would be thriving and delivering a universal service to a high standard. The more seasoned observer might have had reservations.

Beneath the apparently rich topsoil laid by New Labour, a stony undersoil remained. In fairness to central government, this was nothing new. In this sense, the 'good old days' never quite existed. The NHS had always been bedevilled by a lack of resources. Universality and comprehensiveness have never been achieved in any absolute sense.

Shortcomings have always lain there, in one guise or another. They cannot, in principle and origin, be laid at the door of the New Labour government. However, for New Labour, the stakes were undeniably high. From 2001 onwards, it would pour in large investment to the NHS and state that it was reinvigorating the health service in a fashion not seen since its inception. Politically, it would become more difficult for New Labour to admit that these shortcomings were still persisting, and well-nigh impossible to concede that in some respects it was actually exacerbating them.

Naturally, people in West Suffolk generally – just like anywhere else – understand intuitively that universality and comprehensiveness are elusive concepts. Of course, our health services could always be better. However,

16 Paul Holland, '5500 number of letters.' *Suffolk Free Press*, 23 February 2006.

17 *Suffolk Free Press*, 13 April 2006.

what would be so startling in Suffolk and elsewhere is that they were getting worse. New Labour's promises, policies and public financial investment were leading not to improvements, but to a drastic loss of services. An outlook stonier than ever beckoned. Such a mismatch between national boast and local loss would pose a great challenge to the likes of Suffolk West PCT and the Suffolk East PCTs – as well as many other PCTs around the country. They would have to exercise all their ingenuity and display unswerving chutzpah to carry it off.

Large-scale financial savings and cutbacks to services would somehow have to be explained away as improving patient care. A tall order for a new breed of ambitious NHS chief executives and chairmen around the country. But at least their hour had come. Now was the time for them to show their mettle under the gaze of their leader, the Secretary of State for Health.

Enforcing frugality with hard legal implements

The stony undersoil to the NHS is of a distinctly hard, legal variety. It is in contrast to the excessive rhetoric about the NHS that generally emanates all too freely from central government of the day. This is what, legally, makes it relatively easy for the NHS to close, reduce and shed services at will. It is therefore an all-important point to grasp in the context of this book. It means also that of the three original NHS principles, the first two, relating to comprehensiveness and universality, are more by way of political statements than individual legal rights. This makes it relatively easy, through political policies, to change what those principles might mean – without having to debate and to change the legislation.

Central government regularly relies on the knowledge that, legally, NHS provision of services can rarely be enforced by individual patients – especially if the reason for non-provision is purely financial. It doesn't matter how colourful are the claims and promises made for electoral purposes by central government. It knows that most and even all are legally unenforceable. The legal underpinning to the NHS is not generally such as to equip judges to interfere easily.

It might surprise many people to realise that they are not entitled legally to any particular health service at any particular time. The reason for this is chiefly the vagueness of the duties contained in sections 1 and 3 of the NHS Act 1977. They have been repeatedly categorised by the courts as 'general' duties only, and not 'specific' duties owed to, and enforceable by, individual patients.[18]

From the end of the 1970s, a relatively small number of legal cases have been brought to test just what patients are, or are not, entitled to. By and large the answer handed down by the law courts has been unvaried. If the NHS lacks the resources to provide a service to any particular patient (or group of patients) at any particular time, provision cannot be enforced. The patients have been diverse, the answer uniform, the principle resounding. The Human Rights Act 1998 to date has made no significant difference.[19]

The legal cases reveal that this hard edge to health service provision does not just apply to fringe, peripheral or trivial health services. The principle has worked, for example, against babies in need of heart operations, orthopaedic patients facing long waits for much-needed operations in the West Midlands, a ten-year-old girl requiring lifesaving treatment for leukaemia in Cambridgeshire, and a mother requiring help at home to manage day and night her three-year-old child's tracheotomy following the latter's discharge from Great Ormond Street Hospital.[20] In sum, this hard, legal substratum to the NHS can deny even potentially lifesaving treatment to adults and children alike.

Even so, NHS rationing decisions are sometimes susceptible to challenge. This is when a fair decision-making process has not been followed by an NHS body. For instance, it may have not considered all the relevant matters before reaching its decision, including relevant government guidance.[21] In other words, the courts are prepared sometimes to tell the NHS that it has not gone through all the right hoops – in which case the relevant NHS body has to take the decision again. This has given rise to cases being taken against the NHS challenging the lawfulness of the consultation process when decisions are made to close services down. It was on this type of ground that a judicial review was sought in 2006 of Suffolk West PCT's decision to close all community hospital beds in its area.

18 *R v Inner London Education Authority, ex p Ali* [1990] 2 ALR 822, High Court.

19 *R (Watts) v Bedford Primary Care Trust* [2003] EWHC 2401 Admin, High Court.

20 *R v Central Birmingham Health Authority, ex p Walker* [1987] 3 BMLR 32, Court of Appeal; *R v Secretary of State for Social Services, ex p Hincks* [1980] 1 BMLR 93, Court of Appeal; *R v Cambridge Health Authority, ex p B* [1995] 6 MLR 250, Court of Appeal; *R(T) v Haringey London Borough Council* [2005] EWHC 2235 (Admin), High Court.

21 *R v North Derbyshire Health Authority, ex p Fisher* [1998] 8 MLR 327, High Court.

Another ground that sometimes catches the NHS out legally is when it has applied a policy too rigidly or irrationally.[22]

Rarely then do the courts in England find against the NHS. Even then it will be on grounds of process rather than the outcome of the decision. The courts give the NHS a wide discretion to dictate our health and welfare, before they are prepared legally to intervene.

Put yet another way, judicial review against the NHS is generally a blunt, crude and unreliable tool. Notwithstanding this, local communities would be so desperate about threats to local services during 2005 and 2006 that they nevertheless would contemplate the bringing of challenges. In Derbyshire, for example, patients would attempt to prevent United Health, a private sector provider, from taking over GP services.[23] In August 2006, they succeeded in the Court of Appeal, on the grounds that North East Derbyshire Primary Care Trust had not consulted properly. It would now have to do so. The case had been brought by a retired hosiery worker and former Labour councillor. As she pointed out, it was a case of David and Goliath and of patients expressing choice – just as the Secretary of State for Health wished them to. In this case, she explained, local people's choice was that United Health should not take over local health care in order to make profits.[24] And in June 2006 a former nurse in Altrincham, heading the group Health in Trafford, would seek to prevent Trafford Healthcare Trust from closing two rehabilitation wards on the grounds that it also had not consulted on the closure.[25]

In West Suffolk, patients in Sudbury sought also to bring a case, despite the clear difficulty there would be in winning it and the costs that might be incurred. It was a cry for help from a community that had felt itself attacked unfairly by its local PCT. As the local action committee in Sudbury put it:

> What the PCT does not understand is that the legal case is simply a cry for help. It has been brought in desperation because the PCT has not responded to overwhelming local concerns. In fact, we should thank and support these patients. They are acting not just for themselves but for all of us, when we become old, ill or disabled.[26]

22 *R v North West Lancashire Health Authority, ex p G, A, D* (1999) 2 CCLR 419, Court of Appeal; *R (Rogers) v Swindon NHS Primary Care Trust* [2006] EWCA Civ 392, Court of Appeal.

23 'GP contract decision is delayed.' *BBC News*, bbc.co.uk, 7 March 2006.

24 Sarah Hall, 'Pensioner wins court battle to stop US healthcare giant.' *Guardian*, 24 August 2006.

25 Caroline Jack, 'Axed wards win reprieve.' *Manchester Metro News*, 23 June 2006.

26 Walnuttree Hospital Action Committee, 'The state of our health services in Sudbury.' Notice. *Suffolk Free Press*, 8 June 2006.

3

Sowing Financial Seeds: the Great Investment

Nobody would deny that the NHS requires adequate resources. To that end, following its election for a second term in 2001, New Labour made considerable extra resources available.

Nevertheless, it does not follow logically that the universal and comprehensive improvement claimed by central government subsequently occurred. The common refrain from government in 2005 and 2006 – when asked about widespread closures and reductions in service – was simply to deny everything and refer to the extra resources. But this was clearly a non sequitur by way of answer. It was to mistake the input for the output, a basic category error.

A simple example of this, reported by the King's Fund, was that £340 million of extra salary (between 2003 and 2006) for NHS hospital consultants had not delivered – as had been the intention – additional benefits for patients.[1]

Likewise, between 2000 and 2006, the Department of Health had invested considerable resources, time, effort and extra investment into community equipment services. These services are in principle an essential plank in the government's policy of 'care closer to home'. They can be highly effective in enabling people to live more independently. A former civil servant (now working independently), integrally involved with the policy at the Department of Health during this period, wrote a report in

1 Sally Williams and James Buchan (2006) *Assessing the New NHS Consultant Contract: a something for something deal?* London: King's Fund, Summary and p.19.

2006 about what had been achieved. In summary, systems – including joint working between the NHS and local councils – had improved. However, these improvements were now in danger of being lost because of disagreements between PCTs and local councils, triggered by the financial difficulties of the former. Crucially, and irrespective of any such system improvements, things had in any case improved little for those people who needed to use the equipment.[2]

So, this reflex answer about the extra money would not do. During 2005, it became apparent why not. Bit by bit, explanations began to emerge as to why there seemed to be no direct, proportionate connection between the money and improved services. 'BOTCHED OPERATION', crowed the *Daily Telegraph* of 12 March 2006. Underpinning the headline, a King's Fund briefing had found that for the year 2005–6, some 50 per cent of the extra £3.6 billion cash increase had gone on higher pay, and a further 37 per cent on other cost pressures. This apparently left some 1.1 per cent more than in 2004–5 for other developments.[3]

It was reported also that in the space of two years, the salary bill for NHS managers had risen by £578 million.[4] The front page of the *Independent* had already summed it up: 'NHS CRISIS'. Ministers had ordered NHS trusts to cut waiting times at all costs prior to the general election. During this time, there had been 'no Brownie points for balancing your books'.[5] This was scarcely surprising. As one PCT chief executive put it to the House of Commons Health Committee, the setting of priorities was all about 'identifying which targets you are going to be hung for if you don't get it right'.[6] It seemed that targets had been met for political purposes, at all – and as it turned out unsustainable – costs. It had been a case of fire-hosing cash at the NHS without proper reform and then turning the tap off.[7]

The feverish stampede to hit targets had apparently included spending hundreds of millions of pounds, hiring extra staff and using the private sector to treat patients. Now the backlash had occurred, with financial deficits having to be cleared. Realising the financial gravity of the situation,

2 Steve Hards (2006) *Community equipment services in England: are they better now than in 2000?* Online at http://briarwood1000.co.uk/ces_report_steve_hards_june_2006.pdf. Accessed September 2006.

3 John Appleby (2006) *Where's the Money Going?* Briefing. London: King's Fund.

4 Graeme Wilson, 'Wage bill for NHS managers rockets to £2.8 bn.' *Daily Mail*, 2 September 2005.

5 'NHS Crisis.' *Independent*, 18 January 2006.

6 'Waiting times remain NHS priority', *Community Care*, 29 June – 5 July 2006, p.11.

7 Boris Johnson, 'Forget the "porno sirs": the real scandal is going on in the NHS.' *Daily Telegraph*, 19 January 2006.

it appeared that central government ordered strategic health authorities (the regional puppets of central government) to crack down on spending. Turned on with reckless abandon before the election, the financial tap was indeed now being turned off but the targets still had to be hit, as well as other policies and rules adhered to. As Alan Maynard, Chair of an NHS trust and a health economist, put it: there were so many policies, it was akin to a 'wheeze a week'.[8]

The drugs budget was labelled excessive, with the NHS apparently paying more for branded pharmaceuticals than most other European countries.[9] True, it was estimated that an extra 80,000 extra doctors and nurses had been appointed since 2000.[10] Even so, as *The Times* Health Editor commented, it required special skills to engineer a crisis despite an increase in spending of £40 billion.[11]

Another key factor crept out of the woodwork during early 2006. The general practitioner contract that had been agreed back in 2004 had cost £300 million more than expected in the last year. This was because the GPs had, as the Secretary of State for Health put it, 'over achieved'.[12]

Word spread on the health grapevine that severe pruning was to take place as soon as possible – and as far in advance of the next election as possible. However, this proved more difficult than anticipated. The overall NHS debt in England was reported in some quarters as moving inexorably toward £1 billion by early 2006. Nobody seemed to know the actual figure. It was a moving target, because as the financial year-end approached, reported deficits had risen steeply.[13]

More clear was the language of Patricia Hewitt, the Health Secretary. This began to change. Increasingly, she referred to the financial health of the NHS, rather than to patient care. Her spokesmen were even moved to issue sadistic-sounding statements. By November 2005 they were speaking of NHS trusts having to 'experience pain locally' in order to balance the

8 'The NHS blame game.' *Panorama*, BBC 1, 26 March 2006.

9 'NHS Crisis.' *Independent*, 18 January 2006.

10 Jeremy Laurance, 'How did things go so wrong for the NHS?' *Independent*, 9 March 2006.

11 Nigel Hawkes, 'Drive for results was a prescription for disaster.' *The Times*, 24 March 2006.

12 John Carvel, 'Unions plan mass rally over "scorched earth" cuts in NHS jobs and services.' *Guardian*, 19 April 2006.

13 Nic Fleming, 'Problem of NHS deficits far worse than admitted with real debt at £900m.' *Daily Telegraph*, 21 March 2006.

financial books.[14] Richard Taylor, MP, responded that it would of course be patients who felt that pain, not NHS trusts.[15]

Financial whips and local pain: making the countryside smart

This hard-nosed approach, edging out patient care in favour of hastily imposed financial stringency, was not empty gesturing. It would bite hard on the ground. In East Yorkshire, enquiries by the local MP resulted in the following revelation:

> I asked for the brief given to the consultant for each hospital review. In Hornsea's case, he was simply asked to save £500,000 a year and to find a £1 million cash windfall. There was no mention of health improvements, just hard cash.[16]

A clear correlation between community hospital closures and local financial deficits gave the:

> lie to the notion that the exercise is about reconfiguring health care in the interests of local people; it is actually about reconfiguring health service budgets.[17]

Events in Suffolk, too, would continue to reflect accurately the chaos being created and perpetrated by central government. By early 2006, the implications were crystal clear. With local consultation periods concluded, the PCTs were moving inexorably toward their momentous final decisions. Writing in response to the daily reporting of woe across Suffolk, the Walnuttree Hospital Action Committee wrote on New Year's Eve to the *East Anglian Daily Times*:

> your two articles concerning the NHS in Suffolk paint an unseasonably gloomy but accurate picture... Thus have patient outcomes dropped out of the equation. The PCT will indeed make financial savings, to the severe detriment and suffering of elderly, disabled and vulnerable people. Very recently, a spokesman for Patricia Hewitt was reported

14 John Carvel, 'NHS ordered to make £700m winter cuts.' *Guardian*, 17 November 2006.

15 Richard Taylor, MP, 'A high price for winter cuts.' Letter. *Guardian*, 19 November 2006.

16 Graham Stuart, MP. *Hansard*, Westminster Hall, 2 November 2005, column 258WH.

17 Dr Andrew Murrison, MP for Westbury. *Hansard*, Westminster Hall, 2 November 2005, column 278WH.

> nationally as stating that, in order to achieve financial balance, PCTs must 'experience pain locally'. Now the people of Suffolk know what was meant.[18]

It was now evident that the financial injection over the past two years had not led to general improvements across the health service in Suffolk. Even the achievement of the targets, to the extent they had been achieved, had not necessarily been attained cost-effectively. And other services, non-target related, had suffered. The much-vaunted financial fertilisation seemed to have been short-term, ill-planned and unsustainable. The backlash would be equally short-term in outlook. Across Suffolk, this translated into making short-term savings by closing community hospitals or otherwise scaling them down. This, even though they were not the root cause of the recurrent local NHS overspending.

Patricia Hewitt seemed relentlessly to be driving the whole process. In April 2006, she was forthright when she said that Suffolk organisations had to live within budget and do it quickly. Asked about patient care, she was less definite, stating:

> That's a matter for the local NHS. I'm not going to pretend I can sit here in London and make detailed decisions on every part of an organisation. These decisions are much better made locally, where people really know what the needs are.[19]

Asked about cuts to mental health services in Suffolk, she likewise admitted that she didn't know the details; but she was of course 'sure it is what's best for these patients within the available resources'.[19] The implication was that local people's needs were an entirely moveable, resource-driven feast.

Rural neglect: financial dips and hollows

Unlike in Scotland and Northern Ireland, central government's funding formula for the NHS in England takes no account of rurality – even though there is evidence that it results in higher costs of service delivery.[20] Thus, although problems in the NHS were developing in both town and countryside, rural areas had additional difficulties to contend with.

18 Walnuttree Hospital Action Committee, 'NHS savings will be paid for in suffering.' *East Anglian Daily Times*, 31 December 2005.

19 'Hewitt breaks silence over NHS in Suffolk.' *Ipswich Evening Star*, 23 April 2006.

20 Tony Hindle *et al.* (2004) *Review of Evidence on Additional Costs of Delivering Services in Rural Communities.* London: Secta.

This issue would affect West Suffolk. For instance, by late November 2005, it was reported that the average PCT funding per head across England was £1274. In West Suffolk, £223 less per head was spent. Although local funding would be allocated taking account of age in the population and deprivation, rurality was absent as a contributory factor.[21]

Of a total of 300 PCTs, Suffolk West was apparently allocated the 27th lowest level funding. However, it turned out that the actual funding received, even on this arguably inadequate calculation, was 4.5 per cent less than it should have been. The Chairman of the PCT's professional executive committee pointed this out, complainingly.[22] Likewise, over in Waveney, the PCT's director of finance would lament that even by 2008, Waveney would still be receiving 3.5 per cent less than the amount indicated by the 'weighted capitation' formula.[23] Despite this shortfall in funding for Suffolk, the Norfolk, Suffolk and Cambridgeshire Strategic Health Authority confirmed that it had never raised the matter with the Secretary of State, or argued for rectification.[24]

A subsequent study conducted by Suffolk West PCT and published in June 2006 concluded as follows. Trusts in rural areas received less than those in cities on the grounds that the former are healthier. There was however plenty of hidden rural poverty and middle classes expected good medical care. (This is not as odd as it sounds. The government states that it wants people not only to have good healthcare but also to be better informed and to ask for it. In other words, it wants everybody – middle class or otherwise – to exercise consumer choice.) The funding formula did not reflect this. Of NHS trusts in greatest deficit, most serve supposedly affluent areas; but the allocation formula takes no account of the extra costs of providing dispersed services in rural areas. PCTs in deficit received on average £205 less per head of resident population, and £123 less per head of registered population, than PCTs in surplus.[25]

21 Jonathan Barnes, 'Anger over funding for health services.' *East Anglian Daily Times*, 19 November 2005.

22 Dr Andrew Hassan, *The Green Sheet*, 7 July 2005.

23 Chris Bland, 'PCTs will still be below target funding.' Letter. *East Anglian Daily Times*, 23rd November 2005.

24 Lisa Cleverdon, 'Hospitals' fate may be decided by Hewitt.' *East Anglian Daily Times*, 3 March 2006.

25 Padmanabhan Badrinath and others (2006), 'Characteristics of primary care trusts in financial deficit and surplus: a comparative study in the English NHS.' *BMC Health Services Research 6*, 64.

Dust in the eyes: debts, savings and assurances

Beset by financial chaos, and under immense pressure from central government, the NHS would begin to bandy about figures that nobody could follow. The logic was elusive. In the midst of this, PCTs would also attempt to equate financial health with patient well-being, even when it seemed the two were incompatible.

In the West of Suffolk, the PCT's debt stood in 2005 at well over £20 million. During that year, it became clear that short-term savings were to be made by closing community hospitals. The Walnuttree Hospital Action Committee was reliably informed that the Norfolk, Suffolk and Cambridgeshire Strategic Health Authority had, behind closed doors, told the PCTs in Suffolk to sell off community hospitals.

The *East Anglian Daily Times* duly struck a chord in its Saturday edition of 24 September 2005. The headline '£6M SELL-OFF' stretched across photographs of the Hartismere and Bartlet Hospitals.[26] The incentive for the Suffolk East PCTs was not necessarily the capital realised, which might have to go to the strategic health authority, but the saving of £4.8 million of running costs. Even so, concern remained as to whether there really were savings to be made. Redundancy costs could run to a potential £1.8 million. Community services would require £2.8 million in reinvestment, in order to provide the semblance of a service for patients.

For local communities trying to understand how the crisis had occurred, how it was being resolved and the implications for patients, it all became too much. Statements made by local MPs were representative of the frustration. The Suffolk Coastal MP, John Gummer, would refer to the proposals as:

> poorly researched and incompetent...financial jiggery pokery.[27]

Likewise, Michael Lord, MP for Central Suffolk and North Ipswich, dismissed them as:

> piggy-bank economics. You don't just flog off a hospital to cancel debts that have been run up.[27]

Over in the West, the PCT had set aside £2 million to cover some 100 potential redundancies at the Walnuttree and St Leonards Hospitals in

26 Jonathan Barnes, *East Anglian Daily Times*, 24 September 2005.

27 Jonathan Barnes, 'Hopes of raising £6m from sale of hospitals.' *East Anglian Daily Times*, 24 September 2005.

Sudbury.[28] Come April 2006, the PCT announced that up to 90 posts might indeed be lost in cuts to Sudbury's health services.[29]

There were doubts too, in the West, about the evidence base for the savings. The Suffolk West PCT argued for the closure of community hospitals in order to make enduring and recurrent savings, when on its own admission these hospitals appeared not to be the root cause of the recurrent annual overspending.[30] In other words their closure would be a short-term sticking plaster and would not stem the financial haemorrhage in the longer run. This was especially as, in addition, community services, under which the community hospitals came, represented a mere 6.2 per cent of the PCT's spending each year.

Its original consultation document carried concrete detail of savings to be made, but was vague on detail when it came to replacement services and their costings. Subsequent information released provided more information but then still seemed not to explain the evidence base in terms of local population need and how this translated into services, particularly dispersed ones in a rural area.[31] In other words, it looked like service specifications had been squeezed into the available money left over, once the necessary savings had been made.

A report prepared by independent health service experts (including one financial expert) for the Walnuttree Hospital Action Committee expressed doubts about the financial coherence of the PCT's proposals:

> We also conclude that the financial case for the proposal is not made. It is clear the primary driver for these proposals is to reduce costs and make inroads into the financial deficit of the PCT. However, we believe that if demand is to be met, the additional costs that have not been accounted for such as nursing home placements, further additional community based investment, costs to social care, non-inpatients services on the Sudbury site would need to be incorporated into the financial plan. We estimate that the achieved level of cash releasing savings as a result of these changes will be significantly lower in reality than is currently anticipated. We have concerns that not all of the financial implications of the proposal have been taken into account,

28 Dave Gooderham, 'NHS pay-off fund is £2m.' *East Anglian Daily Times*, 21 October 2005.

29 'No escaping job losses with closure.' *Suffolk Free Press*, 13 April 2006.

30 *Modernising Health Care in West Suffolk: consultation, 1 August – 31 October 2005*. Bury St Edmunds: Suffolk West PCT, 2005, p.5.

31 *Modernising Healthcare in West Suffolk: additional information*. Bury St Edmunds: Suffolk West PCT, 2005.

> and that there is insufficient financial allowance made for commissioning or providing of alternative services to replace those that will be lost with the closure of Walnuttree Hospital.
>
> Whilst there is sympathy for the financial position of the PCT, service modernisation should not be used as a cloak for the need to cut cost.
>
> There are still outstanding questions on costs. We are concerned that the PCT may be aiming to release immediate financial savings, at the expense of long term financial prudence. In our opinion the conclusion must be that the financial case for making these changes is not made and as such it would not be possible to support such far-reaching proposals.[32]

In particular, they further pointed out that the underlying causes of the deficit – acute hospital activity, new medical contracts and new legislation – did not appear to be addressed by the PCT's proposals. The cost comparisons employed by the PCT were selective, in that its new community care model was compared only to existing inpatient services – and not to the costs of services in the proposed new community hospital (which the PCT had now abandoned). In other words, the PCT seemed artificially to have restricted the relevant terrain. The report found also that the anticipated savings had not taken account of a range of costs that were likely to be incurred in relation to the replacement services.

It should be noted that the PCT rejected the findings of this independent report in its interim stage, and failed to comment on the final report. It was not acknowledged in the report prepared for the PCT board when it made its final decision about local services in April 2006. The PCT would also not agree to meet with an independent health service finance expert to examine the costings – even though the Walnuttree Hospital Action Committee offered to pay.[33]

The financial never-never land of the NHS

Most worryingly of all, PCTs in Suffolk and elsewhere would make assurances about service provision, even though their financial situation was unclear, shifted from month to month, and they seemed not to know what

32 Helen Tucker and Peter Morgan (2005) *Modernising Healthcare in West Suffolk: response. Prepared by HTA on behalf of Walnuttree Hospital Action Committee (WHAC).* Helen Tucker Associates.

33 'True scale of NHS deficits masked, say's King's Fund.' Press release. London: King's Fund, 7 June 2006.

demands from central government lay just around the corner. To the public, and even to some experts, it all seemed incomprehensible.

The uncertainty itself couldn't be really laid at their door of the PCTs, because it was a national problem. For instance, up to May 2006, an NHS deficit of up to £1 billion had been forecast. It was then announced reassuringly by Patricia Hewitt that it was no more than £512 million. This was immediately dismissed as unreliable by the King's Fund which stated that the figures masked the true scale of the problem. They had been set off against surpluses elsewhere in the NHS system. In fact the gross deficit had increased to £1.27 billion, more NHS organisations were in deficit than predicted, and the net deficits for NHS trusts and primary care trusts were worse than the previous year.[33]

Furthermore, the Chairman of the House of Commons Public Accounts Committee pointed out that with all the burgeoning initiatives from central government, 'parts of the NHS have little idea how much they have spent or are going to spend which makes proper financial management impossible'.[34]

At local level, it did seem bewildering, with debt levels reported to be fluctuating wildly from month to month if not week to week. For instance, in May 2006 it was reported that the debts facing PCTs in Leicestershire had been estimated at £50 million. By June, barely a month later, they had come out at £62 million.[35]

More extraordinarily perhaps, Ipswich Hospital NHS Trust reported a debt of £4.9 million in May 2006. A month later, it had discovered a black hole of £7 million, raising the debt to £11.9 million. Then, by the end of July, it transpired that the auditors had discovered another missing £4.8 million, taking the total to some £16.7 million.[36] In the topsy-turvy world of NHS finance, it got worse. A mere two weeks later, it had become apparent that the NHS Trust had lost a further £2.5 million because it had been treating patients too quickly – rather than forcing them to wait 122 days. As a consequence the Trust was financially penalised by the Suffolk East PCTs, who were responsible for commissioning services from the acute NHS Trust.[37]

34 Graeme Wilson, 'Billions injected but NHS debt hits new high.' *Daily Telegraph*, 8 June 2006.

35 Jenny Hardcastle, 'Jobs at risk under £62m health cuts.' *Leicester Mercury*, 15 June 2006.

36 'Hospital debts rise again'. *Ipswich Evening Star*, 25 July 2006. And: Craig Robinson, 'Hospital's deficit soars to £11.9m.' *East Anglian Daily Times*, 19 May 2006.

37 Mark Bulstrode, 'Surgeon says morale is down at hospital.' *East Anglian Daily Times*, 12 August 2006.

In similar circumstances, the West Suffolk Hospitals NHS Trust – at the time reportedly some £12 million in deficit – also suffered a £200,000 reduction in its funding in August 2006. This was because it had been performing cataract operations too quickly. The Suffolk West PCT had removed the funding, demanding that waiting lists be lengthened to three months for removing cataracts from the first eye and to six months for the second eye. The exasperated local MP, David Ruffley, was reduced to referring to Alice in Wonderland.[38] Barely a month earlier, the Trust had been deprived of a further £2.3 million of its budget by Suffolk West PCT – which had suddenly transferred it to Addenbrooke's Hospital in Cambridge instead.[39]

Bemused onlookers struggled to make sense of it all. As early as March 2005, the West Suffolk Hospitals NHS Trust was reported as stating that the overspend forecast for the year was £6.8 million compared to £2.5 million overspend the previous year – even though it made savings of £5.5 million in the current year. Likewise, the Suffolk West PCT used the same language. It started the year with a £4.4 million deficit, was now predicting a £7.7 million year-end overspend – but was claiming to have saved £7.4 million in the intervening period.[40]

The logic was not quite clear. The projections anyway turned out to be misleading. By the time it launched its consultation in August 2005, the PCT was referring to a debt of over £20 million. Then, at the end of October 2005, the PCT announced that the debt was greater than it thought, to the tune of a further £6.6 million. This was because of the changing expectations of the strategic health authority.[41] In effect, the proposals in the consultation document no longer reflected the savings that would have to be made.

By the end of March 2006, the Suffolk PCTs had apparently been thrust into even further financial turmoil by central government itself. They were now threatened with a 'fine' for their overspending. A 10 per cent penalty would be imposed as interest on the money notionally borrowed to cover the deficit. The overall Suffolk fine to be imposed was reported to be some £5 million.[42]

In addition, a financial adjustment ('purchaser parity adjustment scheme') formula operated by central government was being removed earlier

38 Will Clarke, 'Second hospital is "too efficient".' *East Anglian Daily Times*, 12 August 2006.

39 'Job cut fears.' *EADT 24*, available via www.eadt.co.uk, 7 July 2006.

40 Mark Health, 'Health trusts still left £30 million debt.' *East Anglian Daily Times*, 14 March 2005.

41 'Health trust still needing to make £6.6 million cutbacks.' *East Anglian Daily Times*, 1 September 2005.

42 Rebecca Sheppard, 'Trusts face £5m penalty.' *East Anglian Daily Times*, 7 March 2006.

than anticipated. This would result in a further expected deficit for the PCTs across Suffolk for the year 2006–7. The total funding to be lost would be £11.5 million, of which Suffolk West would lose £4.73 million.[43] The Chairman of the PCT conceded that the loss had come as a 'surprise', and that the expected end-of-year deficit for 2005–6 would now be some £13.3 million.[44]

Yet even the Norfolk, Suffolk and Cambridgeshire Strategic Health Authority, which was meant to have a performance and financial oversight, seemed to be in the dark. In February 2005, the SHA's director of finance commented on an increased allocation of money to the PCTs. This was 'good news'. He stated, quite extraordinarily in the light of turmoil to come a mere few months later, that:

> the new allocation means the NHS can plan with more confidence over the next three years.[45]

By May 2006, it was announced that the strategic health authority was presiding over a forecast overspend of £100.4 million, the second highest debt of any strategic health authority. Only Bedfordshire and Hertfordshire were in a worse position.[46] Ironically, it was with these two counties that the Norfolk, Suffolk and Cambridgeshire Strategic Health Authority was shortly due to merge.

Notwithstanding the financial problems and the cuts to services being perpetrated across the county, upbeat responses from the local NHS continued. Suffolk West PCT was referred in February 2006 to the Audit Commission for a predicted deficit of nearly £14 million. A 'public interest' report was issued about the PCT. Such referrals and reports are normally regarded as serious. Nonetheless, the Chairman of the PCT was reported as almost nonchalant about it, saying it was nothing new and came as no surprise.[47]

Yet when, later in the year, the Audit Commission published a report about financial failure in the NHS – including, specifically, Suffolk West PCT and 24 other PCTs and acute NHS Trusts – it stated clearly that 'the

43 Craig Robinson, 'Health trusts suffer further £11.5m blow.' *East Anglian Daily Times*, 11 March 2006.

44 Dave Gooderham, 'Health shock as £5m funding is axed.' *East Anglian Daily Times*, 23 March 2006.

45 Rebecca Sheppard, 'MPs attack "less" Suffolk PCT cash.' *East Anglian Daily Times*, 10 February 2005.

46 Craig Robinson, 'Area's health debts over £100m.' *East Anglian Daily Times*, 8 June 2006.

47 'NHS Trust reported for cash crisis.' *Suffolk Free Press*, 16 February 2006.

origins of financial failure in the organisations we reviewed typically lay in ineffective management and weak or inadequate board leadership'.[48]

There was more to come. As the original consultation document had stated, all services would be reviewed and further substantial variations in service might be required.[49] Thus, in May 2006, it became known that the PCT had employed financial consultants, reputedly at a cost of nearly £100,000, to look at how further savings and potential cuts to services could be made.[50]

48 *Learning the lessons from financial failure in the NHS.* London: Audit Commission, 2006, Summary and p.13.

49 *Modernising Health Care in West Suffolk: consultation, 1 August – 31 October 2005.* Bury St Edmunds: Suffolk West PCT, 2005, p.10.

50 Will Grahame-Clark, 'Consultant move by PCT "unacceptable".' *East Anglian Daily Times,* 30 May 2006.

4

Declaring the Health Harvest and Concealing Ruined Crops

It is clear that governments are faced with the considerable problem of how to get elected and stay elected on the basis of promises about the health service – and then to deliver on those promises. The problem is exacerbated in proportion to the extravagance of the promises.

How then to live up to extravagant promises? One obvious way is to match their extravagance with equally ambitious claims about achievement. To have a chance of doing this, central government would have to choose and limit the terrain. Given the breadth of demands made on the NHS, detailed promises and claims made on all fronts would clearly invite perceived failure. However, if it could draw the journalists, its own MPs and the general public into accepting the limited ground of its choosing, then central government might win the NHS propaganda war. It could point to inviting but selective harvests; if other crops went to ruin, well, they could be concealed or ignored.

Setting up the targets and blanking out the rest

Specific targets and performance indicators were chosen against which NHS organisations could be measured and judged. From the point of view of dictating the terms of the debate, this was a masterstroke for a number of reasons.

First, even chronic doubters about the usefulness of targets are tempted to accept that a degree of 'objective' testing of the NHS is no bad thing. After all, which of us would complain if we no longer have to wait for hours on end at the local accident and emergency department? Or if we get to see a cancer specialist in a matter of a few weeks, rather than many months?

As the King's Fund has pointed out, there may be serious questions about how the extra money poured into the NHS has been used – but there have been real achievements in reduced waiting times, better cancer services and treatment of coronary heart disease.[1]

Even so, caution is required. Flattened out in one place, problems in the NHS – just like molehills – tend to reappear elsewhere. Thus, the nurse in charge of an acute medical ward wrote in April 2006 about the four-hour time limit imposed on trolley waits in accident and emergency:

> Three hours and that trolley has to go to the assessment unit, whether there are beds there or not. Failure to do so results in purple-faced people ringing each other and firing off emails saying the word nobody must utter: 'breach'. Hence people not on trolleys in A and E any more, but waiting on trolleys in the assessment unit, who are in turn trying to discharge patients to the wards, who in turn are trying to discharge patients.[2]

Margaret Cook, doctor and former wife of Cabinet Minister Robin Cook, had found herself submerged in meetings about 'staff partnerships, participative management, leadership drives and business plans'. She bemoaned the lack of insight into patient needs of NHS managers and the difference between official targets and the provision of good care.[3]

Obsession with targets and finance can lead NHS Trusts very far astray. In July 2006, the Healthcare Commission reported how one Buckinghamshire Hospitals NHS Trust had failed to follow advice on infection control at Stoke Mandeville Hospital. Instead the Trust Board prioritised other objectives, including Accident and Emergency department government-set targets, the control of finance and the reconfiguration of services. The result was two very serious outbreaks of the infection *Clostridium difficile* and the deaths of nearly 40 patients, as well as the infection of hundreds of others.

1 'True scale of NHS deficits masked, says King's Fund.' Press release. London: King's Fund, 7 June 2006.

2 Karen Moffat (a pseudonym), 'Nurses can't walk away.' *Guardian*, 28 April 2006.

3 Margaret Cook, 'A plague on NHS managers.' *Daily Mail*, 25 April 2006.

The Commission found that the Trust's executive team was perceived by staff to be close knit and to manage oppressively. It had 'appeared unwilling or unable to hear adverse messages. Staff were frightened to speak openly'. After the first outbreak, the Trust refused to compromise on its priorities. Even after the second had broken out, it still did not act on its infection control advice, until the story was leaked to the national media.[4]

Certainly it was an extreme case in terms of the consequences. But the pressures put upon the NHS Trust, finance and target-wise, were government-inspired. And, at the time of writing this book, shortly after the publication of the Health Commission's report, recruitment freezes, the shedding of NHS posts and the reduction in bed capacity of acute hospitals are all continuing apace. They are being driven by central government's demands via its regional conduits, the strategic health authorities. Which means the pressures, in terms of targets and finance, are if anything greater than ever. Likewise, the fact that the Trust only acted in response, apparently, to publicity is a particularly worrying – and almost sinister – aspect of what occurred.

NHS Trusts are under the direct control of strategic health authorities and the Department of Health. They do indeed jump this way and that at the whim of their political masters. In short, to vilify the Trust Board in such circumstances – and vilification there must be from the point of view of the patients and families affected – is only half the picture.[5] (In July 2006, the Health and Safety Executive and Association of Police Officers were considering what steps should be taken against the Trust.)

Thus, even the Healthcare Commission, in a somewhat restrained manner, stated that potential conflict between the government's targets and infection control affected all acute NHS trusts. Furthermore, this was nothing new. This conflict had been observed six years before by the National Audit Office.[6] In sum, if vilification must follow, it should arguably be aimed not just at local Trusts but also at least partly at the heart of central government. What happened is arguably the consequence, if not the intention, of its high pressure policy on targets and financial performance.

4 *Investigation into outbreaks of Clostridium difficile at Stoke Mandeville Hospital, Buckinghamshire.* London: Healthcare Commission, 2006.

5 John Carvel, 'Hospital's focus on waiting time targets led to 41 superbug deaths.' *Guardian*, 25 July 2006.

6 *Investigation into outbreaks of Clostridium difficile at Stoke Mandeville Hospital, Buckinghamshire.* London: Healthcare Commission, 2006.

In addition, the gathering of performance statistics and the reporting of them upward to central government can be very costly. For instance, in the case of local authorities it has been calculated that this 'performance regime' costs a typical council some £1.8 million each year. Unsurprisingly, local councils consider this to be disproportionate expenditure of scarce resources.[7]

Second, statistics can be massaged by NHS trusts in order to reach targets and indicators.[8] Central government might for political reasons not be inclined to be too fussy about such manipulation. Targets make good news if they are achieved. Even if they are seen not to be, nevertheless they sow the seeds of blame locally. Local NHS trusts and their managers are then cast into the role of whipping boys. Just as they were when the Department of Health admitted in 2006 that some 20 per cent of NHS ambulance trusts in England had misreported response times in order to give the appearance of complying with targets. The Department was suitably censorious and sanctimonious in its response.[9]

But all this was no surprise. In 2003, the House of Commons Public Administration Committee had reported on targets. From the Consumers' Association it had learnt of 'a range of near-corrupt practices' in ambulance services. These included the reaching of patients in less than one minute and, in one case, in less than zero seconds. It noted also that the National Audit Office had in 2001 found adjustments of waiting list figures by a number of NHS Trusts.[10]

Third, central government can cherry-pick which targets it chooses to hold up as reliable indicators, and on which it can base claims for wider NHS performance generally.

Fourth, and crucially, those services not included in, or directly related to, the targets start to slip from sight. For instance, in Bristol, waiting time targets for new outpatient appointments meant that follow-up appointments were neglected. This resulted in a number of patients losing their vision because of deteriorating glaucoma.[10] When the pressure is on, these other services get neglected. They no longer matter. More drastically, if services are

7 Patrick Wintour, 'Kelly to reduce number of Whitehall targets for councils.' *Guardian*, 3 July 2006.

8 National Audit Office (2001) *Inpatient and Outpatient Waiting in the NHS.* HC 221. London: HMSO. And: National Audit Office (2001) *Inappropriate Adjustments to NHS Waiting Lists.* HC 452. London: HMSO.

9 Nigel Hawkes, 'Ambulance trusts "fiddled statistics to meet targets".' *The Times*, 15 August 2006.

10 House of Commons Public Administration Committee (2003) *On target? Government by measurement.* HC 61-I. London: Stationery Office, paras 59–60.

simply too awkward, expensive and politically unglamorous, the NHS may even attempt to get rid of them altogether. It may simply cease to provide. Sometimes it attempts to pass on responsibility – for example, to local social services authorities (i.e. local councils) or indeed to people's informal carers at home.

Crucially, it should of course not be about whether performance targets are met, regardless of the damage done elsewhere. Good management is not about hitting targets for their own sake, but about 'achieving objectives without destroying the rest of the business on the way'.[11]

The way in which central government would covertly attempt to blank out the loss of crucial health services, by blindly referring to selected targets as an answer to everything, was illustrated explicitly by Tony Blair at Prime Minister's question time. Instead of answering a specific question put by Tim Yeo, MP, about health service cutbacks in Suffolk, his knee-jerk response was simply to refer to waiting times and targets, and not answer the question:

> I point out...that health funding has increased more than 30 per cent... The number of people there waiting more than six months for inpatient treatment has fallen [Hon. Members: 'Oh']. That is part of this Government's record.[12]

Of course if Tony Blair could stonewall, so could his ministers. For instance, in January 2006, Tim Yeo, MP for South Suffolk, made an impassioned speech about the loss of local services in Sudbury. In particular, he raised the issue of community hospital based rehabilitation for people with more complex needs:

> The truth is that if the trust wanted to improve services in Sudbury, it would revert to the previous evidence-based successful model of care, which included some inpatient beds...alongside improved services in the community. Ramming through bed closures by alleging that none of the patients who had used them in the past will in future ever need to be treated anywhere other than at home is absurd. Some patients will be inappropriately left at home to suffer or even die without proper community support. Others, as the trust admits, will have to be accommodated within West Suffolk Hospital, aggravating the problems of

11 Anthony Hilton, 'Soviet-style approach is no cure for the NHS.' *Evening Standard*, 25 April 2006.

12 Tony Blair, Prime Minister. *Hansard*, House of Commons Debates, 24 May 2006, column 1474.

> bed blocking and causing longer waiting lists, in direct contradiction of government policy.[13]

Liam Byrne, Under-Secretary for Health, purported to answer. At first, he avoided the question. Instead, by rote, he referred at length to overall NHS expenditure and waiting times. He then proceeded to show that both he, and his civil servants who must have briefed him, did not – or did not want to – understand the issue. His answer equated all rehabilitation with intermediate care in people's own homes. This was notwithstanding that his own departmental guidance warned against this equation.[14] He referred also to community matrons – even though they are primarily concerned with the ongoing management of people at home to avoid hospital admission, rather than concerned with rehabilitation. And he referred also to assistive technology in people's own homes, which has often little directly to do with rehabilitation and sometimes is even counter-productive.[15]

Visible targets and disappearing services across Suffolk

And so the pattern played out locally.

It seemed to be all about meeting throughput targets, not looking at patient outcomes. For instance, toward the end of 2005, the West Suffolk Hospitals NHS Trust closed 55 beds. A few months later, it justified the closures, and was reported as stating that rehabilitation had improved. However, a subsequent Freedom of Information Act request made by the Walnuttree Hospital Action Committee established that the presentation on which this claim was based appeared to relate to patient throughput, not patient outcomes. From the Trust's point of view its aim was apparently simply to reduce the number of hospital stays exceeding 28 days.[16]

The NHS Trust continued to attain targets relating to outpatient appointments, MRSA (methicillin-resistant *Staphylococcus aureus*) cases, accident and emergency waits. Of course in itself this was a most welcome and creditable achievement. But there was barely a word about rehabilitation outcomes of patients with more complex needs – at a time when both acute rehabilitation beds, and all the community hospital rehabilitation beds, were in the process of being culled.

13 Tim Yeo, MP. *Hansard*, House of Commons Debates, 24 January 2006, column 1404.

14 Health Service Circular 2001/01. *Intermediate Care.* London: Department of Health, para 10.

15 Liam Byrne, *Hansard*. House of Commons Debates, 24 January 2006, column 1409.

16 'Health chiefs say loss of beds has improved patient care.' *East Anglian Daily Times*, 26 January 2006.

By January 2006, the West Suffolk Hospitals NHS Trust reported that it had matched outpatient waiting targets for the first appointment following a GP referral. Yet, at the same time, it had an estimated £20 million debt and had already been forced to cut jobs and beds.[17] In May 2006, it was continuing to make good progress against targets concerning waiting times and MRSA infections, despite its continuing deficit.[18] But within a few days of this good news, it was announcing a further 30 bed closures and cuts in posts. It was also paying out £100,000 to financial consultants to advise it on how to make still further cuts and savings.[19]

Meanwhile, in formulating its proposals to save money and cut services, Suffolk West PCT appeared to target precisely those unglamorous services – basically its already neglected community services.

This was a fairly extraordinary thing to do. The government wished for more community services. Of the PCT's annual spending of over £250 million, the community services budget comprised a paltry £15.7 million, some 6.2 per cent of the entire budget. And the community services were not even the cause of the recurrent overspending.[20] Logic would be overruled by the sudden demands for short-term savings together with priorities imposed by central government.

In particular, the PCT aimed at community services affecting older people with more complex rehabilitation needs, recuperative and palliative care services, rehabilitation for younger adults, people with learning disabilities and people with mental health problems. Taking the policy cue from central government, not only did such people not count against targets in the modern NHS, but also maybe they could be shunted off elsewhere. Services could be closed, or somehow re-branded as a social care responsibility.

It would seem as if people's health-care needs could cease to exist, almost at the click of a PCT's fingers. In the West, the Suffolk West PCT's board was told in June 2005 that community hospital beds were 'part of an old fashioned model of care that often caters more for the social aspects of

17 Benedict O'Connor, 'Hospital waiting lists get shorter.' *East Anglian Daily Times*, 27 January 2006.

18 'Patient waiting times and instances of MRSA are both on the decrease.' *Sudbury Mercury*, 11 May 2006.

19 Laurence Cawley, 'NHS trust pays out £100,000 for advice.' *East Anglian Daily Times*, 25 May 2006.

20 *Modernising Health Care in West Suffolk: consultation, 1 August – 31 October 2005*. Bury St Edmunds: Suffolk West, 2005, p.5.

care occasionally required by older people'. Therefore people did not need to be there.[21]

This was despite the fact that hospital consultants and general practitioners referred people with medical needs there. And only a month previously, the PCT itself had been saying how important community hospital beds were and had been proposing to build a new hospital containing 32 such beds.[22] And a mere six months later, a government White Paper would heap praise on community hospital beds.[23]

Likewise in the East, the PCTs spoke of returning to their core services, and community hospitals and their beds would not feature because they were providing social care only.[24] Notably, neither West nor East PCTs could cite credible evidence for these claims. Even allowing for the desperation of the local NHS, the vanishing trick being perpetrated on people's needs was all too much for local residents. Referring to the many elderly patients in Walnuttree who would have worked from leaving school until retirement:

> They will remember the promise made by Clement Attlee (Labour Prime Minister) on July 5th 1948: 'You will be cared for from the cradle to the grave'... We must, now, demand that the care of the elderly and infirm should not be allowed to be dismissed by accountants whose sole aim is to balance mythical budgets.[25]

In summary, targets and performance indicators, for all their uses, appear to have had some serious and unwanted side effects. They constitute one method of papering over the cracks, of declaring false harvests and of creating a mirage of a comprehensive, universal health service. It is a classic case of a type of misleading metonymy, substituting the part of something for the whole.

21 *Proposed Local Delivery Plan and Financial Recovery Plan.* Bury St Edmunds: Suffolk West PCT, 2005, Appendix 3, para 15.

22 *Outline Business Case for the Development of Sudbury Health and Social Care Centre.* Bury St Edmunds: Suffolk West PCT, March 2005.

23 Secretary of State for Health (2006) *Our Health, Our Care, Our Say.* Cm 6737. London: HMSO, para 6.40.

24 Sarah Chambers, 'Packed meeting warned of cuts to care.' *East Anglian Daily Times,* 17 September 2005.

25 Andy Janes. Letter. *Suffolk Free Press,* 18 November 2006.

Concealing the ruined health crops

Running parallel with an attempt to declare selective, and sometimes false, health service harvests is the imperative for central government to conceal the ruined crops. These are the disintegrating health services that do not form part of the official harvest.

The need for central government of the moment to gloss over the inevitable gaps, failings and limitations of the health service is nothing new. However, during 2005 and 2006 the pressure to do so was perhaps greater on the New Labour government than it had been on any government for many years. It had injected large amounts of money into health services. Claims about how the health service was being transformed were at their highest pitch. Problems would have to be denied, minimised or blamed on somebody else. Everything had to be for the best.

In essence, central government adopted a threefold strategy. First, flat denial that anything was amiss. Second, if anything was amiss, it was financial and would not affect patient care. Third, if things really were amiss in respect of patient care, then somebody else was to blame. This was an unsophisticated strategy but one that government would come to push very hard. It would have to. This was because unwelcome stories about cancelled operations, wards closing, community hospital closures and NHS staff redundancies were commonplace as 2005 wore on. Things got worse in 2006. Despite central government's best endeavours, reality kept on breaking in. Even a government renowned for its ability to manipulate news was always going to struggle. It looked like a bonfire of NHS services.

Spoliation of the health landscape

Towards the last few months of 2005, the stories started picking up: bed and hospital closures, reduction in posts and huge deficits. The following gives a flavour.

Early on in July 2005, the *Sunday Telegraph* picked up on plans to close 55 beds at West Suffolk Hospital in Bury St Edmunds, 32 beds at Hartismere Hospital in Eye, 32 (in fact, 68) beds at Walnuttree Hospital in Sudbury, 26 geriatric beds and a children's ward at the Royal Bolton Hospital, 25 urology beds at Queen Elizabeth Hospital in Woolwich, 19 beds at Milford-on-Sea Hospital, and 38 beds at Evesham Community Hospital.[26]

26 Karyn Miller, 'Cash-strapped hospitals plan to close another thousand beds.' *Sunday Telegraph*, 31 July 2005.

The *Birmingham Post* reported that the Royal Wolverhampton Hospitals NHS Trust was facing a deficit of £12.8 million, and Good Hope Hospital a deficit of £4.5 million. The Sandwell and West Birmingham NHS Trust had projected a £5.1 million deficit and imposed a recruitment freeze on nursing staff. The University Hospitals Coventry and Warwickshire NHS Trust was to close a ward at Walsgrave Hospital as part of savings of £7.8 million. Likewise, the Shrewsbury and Telford Hospital NHS Trust had a £10.1 million overspend to tackle.[27]

It wasn't just local papers and broadsheets that were reporting the cuts, thus inviting dismissal by central government on grounds respectively of local exaggeration or a touch of middle-class angst. The tabloids weighed in also. Ahead of Christmas 1995, the *Sun* reported 'fears over NHS meltdown'. Its report included the 220 jobs being lost at West Suffolk Hospital in Bury St Edmunds, 300 in Lincolnshire, 1200 in Nottingham, 600 in Leeds, 500 in Southampton, 100 in Lewisham, 100 in Bradford on Avon, 100 in Westbury and 50 in Barnsley.[28] In fact, in November 2005, the West Suffolk Hospitals NHS Trust board agreed to cut a further 40 jobs, on top of the 220 already being lost, bringing the total to 260.[29]

The *Sunday Mirror*, too, knew a good headline: 'CASH CRISIS? LET'S SACK NURSES'. This referred to the threat to 40 jobs at Barnsley District Hospital, as well as the making redundant of 15 doctors at Oxfordshire Mental Health Trust.[30]

The story about surgery being delayed to save money came in December 2005, when Harrow Primary Care Trust instructed its hospitals to do the minimum required to meet national targets. It would treat the six-month maximum wait as a minimum.[31] Within three months, a memo had been sent by an NHS finance manager to PCTs in London, warning them not to overachieve. It went on to say that PCTs should not necessarily pay NHS trusts where patients had received treatment that could have been delayed without breaching the maximum waiting times.[32]

27 Jonathan Walker. *Birmingham Post*, 28 October 2005.

28 Adele Waters, 'Fears over NHS meltdown.' *Sun*, 12 December 2005.

29 Benedict O'Connor, 'Hospital says "yes" to extra 40 job losses.' *East Anglian Daily Times*, 30 November 2005.

30 David Hudson, 'Cash crisis? Let's sack nurses.' *Sunday Mirror*, 16 October 2005.

31 Nigel Hawkes, 'Surgery delayed to save money.' *The Times*, 3 December 2005.

32 Jeremy Laurance, 'London health trusts get cash warning over treating patients.' *Independent*, 9 March 2006.

At the same time, every NHS trust in London reportedly had to hand over 3 per cent of its budget to set up a special fund to deal with the £182 million overspend in London.[33] In May 2006, Leeds Teaching Hospitals NHS Trust announced that, ordered to make savings of £84 million over three years, it would be cutting 430 posts and closing 40 beds.[34] The East Sussex Hospitals NHS Trust announced a reduction of some 250 posts, aiming to ease its £5 million deficit.[35] The Worcestershire Acute Hospitals NHS Trust planned to shed 720 jobs over a period of 12 months in order to make inroads into accumulated deficits of £31.5 million.[36]

The Royal College of Nursing had begun to collate reports of cuts and the effects they were having on patients. For instance, children with cancer and leukaemia were no longer being treated by a community nurse, for whom funding had been withdrawn. Instead, they were having to make long journeys for treatment, with the result that they could not continue normal life in the community. Avon and Wiltshire Mental Health Trust had cut beds, thus affecting frail and vulnerable people. And ward closures in Skegness meant 40-mile journeys to Lincoln for patients.[37]

The government would claim that the job losses did not involve essential jobs, but the projected 10,000 student nurses who would not be offered jobs did not seem reassuring.[38] Even one of the new flagship services launched by central government, the NHS Direct phone line, was facing the loss of 1000 posts and the closure of 12 of its call centres. At the same time, Nottingham University Hospitals Trust planned to reduce posts by up to 1200 to avoid its deficit reaching £60 million.[39] Similarly, the new nurse-led NHS 'walk-in centres' were reported to be in jeopardy, coming under review as PCTs sought to make savings – now that the ring-fenced money provided by central government had run out.[40]

In 2006, the Royal Free Hospital in Hampstead, having already closed 70 beds in the summer, was now threatening more closures. This was against a backdrop of deficits in major London hospitals including St George's

33 Rebecca Smith, 'Trusts to cut £250m in London.' *Evening Standard,* 7 March 2006.

34 Vicki Robinson, '430 NHS jobs to be axed.' *Yorkshire Evening Post,* 12 May 2006.

35 Rebecca Smith, 'Debt forces NHS Trust to axe 250 posts.' *Evening Standard,* 25 April 2006.

36 John Carvel, 'More hospital job losses deepen mood of crisis in NHS.' *Guardian,* 7 April 2006.

37 John Carvel, 'NHS cuts hit cancer care for children.' *Guardian,* 24 April 2006.

38 Rebecca Smith, 'NHS cuts mean no jobs for 10,000 student nurses.' *Evening Standard,* 25 April 2006.

39 Paul Waugh, 'It's change or die, says Blair as health line axes jobs.' *Evening Standard,* 16 May 2006.

40 'Walk-in centres in danger of closure as ring-fenced funding to PCTs is scrapped.' *Nursing Times,* 23 May 2006.

Hospital (£22 million), North Middlesex Hospital (£4 million), and the Royal National Orthopaedic Hospital (£5 million).[41]

The rot had spread to Scotland as well, when Ayr was brought to a standstill. Thousands were protesting against the closure of an accident and emergency unit. A petition of 55,000 signatures had already been gathered.[42] Come April 2006, and the former Secretary of State for Health, John Reid, would be among the protestors in Lanarkshire, handing in a 45,000 signature petition against the downgrading of Monklands Hospital in Airdrie.[43]

In March and April 2006, it was more staff cuts that were hitting the headlines as well. On 17 March 2006, *The Times* headline announced North Staffordshire University Hospital planned to shed 1000 jobs in order to reduce debts of £15 million. The trigger had been a visit from a financial 'hit squad' sent in by Patricia Hewitt.[44]

In April 2006, the *Nursing Times* listed the job cuts that had been announced (if not yet implemented) as follows: County Durham and Darlington Acute Hospitals NHS Trust (700), Royal Cornwall Hospitals NHS Trust (300), Queen Mary Sidcup NHS Trust (190), Royal Free Hampstead NHS Trust (480), Plymouth Hospitals NHS Trust (200), Royal Wolverhampton Hospitals NHS Trust (300), Mayday Healthcare NHS Trust (100), Brighton and Sussex University Hospitals NHS Trust (300), Shrewsbury and Telford Hospital NHS Trust (291), NHS Direct (1250), Surrey and Sussex Healthcare NHS Trust (400), Medway NHS Trust (160), and the Royal United Hospital Bath NHS Trust (300).[45]

The Trafford NHS Trust announced the closure of two inpatient wards because of staff shortages and the resulting safety fears.[46] In North Staffordshire, the NHS Trust had reduced its deficit down from £34 million, but still remained £18 million overspent. And in March 2006, the *Guardian* carried details of some 26 PCTs that were in collective deficit of £264 million and 41 NHS trusts with a deficit of £467 million.[47]

41 Ellen Widdup, 'Wards shut to save NHS cash.' *Evening Standard*, 31 January 2006.

42 'Thousands protest over A&E axe plan.' *Scotsman*, 25 February 2006.

43 'Reid hands in hospital petition.' *News.bbc.co.uk*, 28 April 2006.

44 Sam Lister, 'Hospital's £15m shortfall to bring 1000 job losses.' *The Times*, 17 March 2006.

45 Richard Staines, 'Counting the costs.' *Nursing Times*, 11 April 2006.

46 'Depth of NHS cash crisis is revealed by cuts.' *East Anglian Daily Times*, 9 March 2006.

47 Hugh Muir, 'Old buildings, inefficient systems, delayed operations and £18m losses.' *Guardian*, 8 March 2006.

Alternatively, specific incidents would be indicative of the pernicious effect of just how desperately NHS bodies were trying to respond to the uncompromising demands of the Secretary of State. For instance, when a duty doctor for West Cornwall Hospital in Penzance called in sick, it was decided not to pay for a locum. Instead ambulance crews were instructed to send seriously ill patients 35 miles away to Treliske, Truro.[48]

Dissolution of the hospitals: turning out the vulnerable, the old and the young

Vulnerable groups of people would suffer, as rehabilitation, care of the elderly, and mental health wards were reported from every quarter to be closing. But the cuts went much wider, embracing all manner of local health services. As 2006 progressed, the likes of accident and emergency services, minor injuries units and maternity services were increasingly reported as being threatened and closed. Far from a measured improvement to local health services, the changes were clearly being driven by pressing financial deficits and hasty, knee-jerk decision-making. Rhyme, reason and measured change were absent. The following examples are but examples, fairly randomly collected – the tip of an iceberg.

Elderly care and rehabilitation beds typically seemed to feature in cuts, particularly – but not just – in the many rural areas reeling from the unprecedented scale of the assault on community hospitals. For instance, in Redbridge, London, such beds were to be reduced from 160 to 118.[49] Likewise, in Altrincham, Manchester, the Trafford Healthcare Trust attempted in June 2006 to close two rehabilitation wards without consultation.[50] Mental health, including dementia, wards were in the firing line, such as at Charterhouse Hospital in Trowbridge.[51]

Even the services that were meant to be about care closer to people's homes – supposedly government policy – would suffer, as well as other services. Up in Cambridge, for example, Addenbrooke's Hospital was reported as having to treat fewer people, Brookfields Hospital would lose its wards and have part of the site sold. Even, the hospice at home service – a crucial part of 'care closer to home', a flagship government policy – would

48 Sandra Laville, 'Trust refuses patients after doctor goes sick.' *Guardian*, 3 April 2006.

49 Dominic Yeatman, 'NHS may cut more beds.' *This is Local London*, 27 July 2006.

50 Caroline Jack, 'Axed wards win reprieve.' *Manchester Metro News*, 23 June 2006.

51 'Axe falls on more hospitals.' *Western Daily Press*, 7 April 2006.

also have its funding cut. Likewise, mental health services at Fulbourn Hospital would suffer permanent ward closures. The two Cambridge PCTs had a forecast debt of £45.9 million.[52] Suffolk West PCT, too, would support hospice at home in principle, but not fund it – despite the fact that it was closing all community hospital beds – including those that performed a palliative care function (as at Walnnuttree Hospital in Sudbury).[53]

But it was not just services specifically for vulnerable groups of people that were in the firing line. It was others affecting the population more generally, whatever people's age or health status.

Minor injuries units would be targeted, as in East Yorkshire, where the unit in Bridlington would be closed from 9pm to 9am – despite many tourists in summer and poor conditions along the coast road in winter. The North East Yorkshire NHS Trust was attempting to save £6.9 million.[54] Cockermouth Hospital, too, lost its minor injuries unit in August 2006, despite the Cumbria-wide petition of 70,000 signatures against community hospital closures or cuts.[55]

A step up from minor injuries units, accident and emergency (A&E) services, too, would be threatened. Emergency services in Cornwall were under review by the Royal Cornwall Hospitals Acute Care NHS Trust, as a £31 million projected debt loomed.[56] Also in Cornwall, minor injuries unit services were due for reduction or closure at Newquay, Bodmin, Launceston, Liskeard and Saltash. However, a 5500 name petition appeared to have prevailed in preventing closure of the unit at Stratton.[57]

The same pattern was playing out from the far flung south west of the country to north London – where Chase Farm Hospital A&E services in Enfield were being earmarked for closure.[58] Up the road in west Hertfordshire, it was being proposed that all A&E services be centralised in Watford. This would mean their removal from St Albans, Mount Vernon and Hemel Hempstead. The West Hertfordshire NHS Hospitals Trust faced a £28.3 million deficit.[59]

52 'Home hospice service and wards face axe.' *Cambridge Evening News*, 27 June 2006.

53 Dave Gooderham, 'No cash for 24-hour home care scheme.' *East Anglian Daily Times*, 10 June 2006.

54 Alex Wood, 'Anger as trust cuts hospital centre's hours.' *Yorkshire Post*, 16 August 2006.

55 'Hospital injuries unit to close.' *News & Star*, 21 August 2006.

56 'Hospital plan to cut £31m deficit.' *News.bbc.co.uk*, 10 August 2006.

57 'Injuries unit to close at night.' *News.bbc.co.uk*, 27 February 2006.

58 Tommy Norton, 'Rally of support for Chase Farm.' *Enfield Independent*, 10 August 2006.

59 Louisa Barnett, 'NHS Trust moves to cut Herts services.' *This is Local London*, 20 June 2006.

However, Watford General Hospital was itself set to lose 50 beds, in the face of a £13 million deficit.[60] Even the A&E Unit nearest Wembley Stadium in London became threatened, as the North West London Hospitals Trust struggled with a £25 million deficit. London Health Emergency campaigners referred to this as 'dangerous nonsense'.[61]

Mothers, babies and children were not sacrosanct. In the New Forest, three birthing centres (maternity units) were being targeted for closure by the Southampton University Hospitals NHS Trust.[62] Baby care services were reported under threat of centralisation in Greater Manchester, with residents fearing that seriously ill babies would have to be flown by helicopter as far as Oldham.[63] Enfield PCT would look to close the majority of its eighteen baby clinics. Five would close immediately; over time the total would reduce to four. Health visitors would also make fewer visits to new mothers and babies.[64]

At Trafford General Hospital, it was planned to close a children's ward within the next two years.[65] Nearby, Salford City Council felt moved to threaten a judicial review against the local NHS plans to reorganise maternity services. It would mean Bury, Trafford and Rochdale hospitals losing children's inpatient services, maternity and neo-natal wards – and the Hope Hospital in Salford losing its maternity unit.[66] In Heywood, Lancashire, the Fairfield Hospital found its special care baby unit under threat, together with acute surgery and accident and emergency services.[67]

The fact that the country has serious sexual health problems did not save family planning clinics from the firing line. Facing a monthly overspend of £2 million, the East Lincolnshire PCT would consider closing all such clinics.[68] Similarly, Haringey Teaching PCT, trying to save £160,000, planned to close three of its family planning clinics.[69]

60 Louisa Barnett, '£13m debt forces Watford ward closures.' *This is Local London*, 28 May 2006.

61 'A&E downgrade plans under attack.' *News.bbc.co.uk*, 12 July 2006.

62 Matt Smith, *This is Hampshire.net*, 4 August 2006.

63 Caroline Jack, 'Axed wards win reprieve.' *Manchester Metro News*, 23 June 2006.

64 Kate Southern, 'Clinics close in shake-up.' *Enfield Independent*, 2 August 2006.

65 Paul Taylor, 'Children's hospital ward set to close.' *Manchester Metro News*, 5 May 2006.

66 'Threat to baby units shake up.' *Manchester Evening News*, 11 January 2006.

67 'Baby unit protest march again.' *Heywood Advertiser*, 30 November 2005.

68 'Contraception clinics may close.' *News.bbc.co.uk*, 3 May 2006.

69 Kay Murray, 'Family planning clinic closure plan defended.' *Muswell Hill & Crouch End Times*, 1 June 2006.

A last example. West Suffolk Hospital NHS Trust's reaction to concerns about the steeply increasing incidence of obesity and diabetes was to withdraw the dietetic and nutrition clinic from Sudbury, a town with significant pockets of mortality and deprivation. The Trust was trying to save money against a £12 million deficit.[70] This closure was despite the fact that the number of new cases of diabetes in West Suffolk had risen by 50 per cent in three years. Furthermore, by 2010, it was expected that 1.25 million adults and nearly 170,000 children in the East of England would be obese. A public health consultant for the area stated that 'obesity and being overweight is [sic] a very complex issue and often people need help and support to be able to tackle it'.[71] And yet, despite such detrimental cutbacks, the people of Suffolk – and across the country – had been continually lectured by local NHS executives and chairmen that the changes to their health service were all about modernisation and improvement.

Laying waste to the Suffolk health services

And so the stories kept on coming. Down in Suffolk, it might have been easy to dismiss these reports from around the country as selective, unrepresentative, political scaremongering.

Unfortunately, if anything, it appeared that Suffolk was in the vanguard and ahead of the game in terms of the speed and scale of the cutbacks. By August the proposals by the Suffolk PCTs had been formulated and put out for consultation. In the West, beds had been eroding at the West Suffolk Hospitals NHS Trust anyway and were now to do so at an increasing rate, along with hundreds of posts. All community hospital beds were threatened with closure, as well as consultant outpatient services in Sudbury. Some community mental health services were to be closed down too, together with learning disability support and respite services.

In the East, community hospitals at Eye and Felixstowe were to be closed, as well as a range of day hospitals including services for people with learning disabilities and with mental health problems. Beds were to be lost in Ipswich where, by April 2006, Ipswich Hospital NHS Trust had agreed to the cutting of 105 posts also.[72] Some months earlier, general practitioners in

70 Paul Holland, 'Anger as clinic shuts.' *Suffolk Free Press*, 8 June 2006.

71 Lorraine Price, 'Doctors warn of massive rise in diabetes.' *East Anglian Daily Times*, 24 August 2006. And: Craig Robinson, 'Obesity fears: shock rise in number of overweight forecast for region.' *East Anglian Daily Times*, 26 August 2006.

72 Craig Robinson, 'Health reform given the green light.' *East Anglian Daily Times*, 29 April 2006.

East Suffolk had been told by the PCTs that they might not be paid to run services during the month of March 2006 – in which case, they would only treat patients with life-threatening emergencies – and otherwise shut up shop for a month.[73] In the event, this drastic step was averted by the East Suffolk East PCTs in consultation with the strategic health authority – doubtless to avoid the disastrous publicity that would have ensued.[74]

In late July 2006, it was announced by the Norfolk and Waveney NHS Mental Health Trust that up to 230 posts would be lost over the next few years – including 40 redundancies being implemented immediately.[75]

A spot of turbulence

Undaunted by all of this, central government would set about trying to convince the public that all was well and to prove beyond doubt that it was the master of publicity and of the Press, if not necessarily of the health service. Its threefold strategy unfolded as follows.

First, it would simply deny anything much was wrong. For instance, during much of 2005, Sir Nigel Crisp (NHS chief executive) and the Department of Health tended to refer to mild turbulence. By September 2005, dire predictions about the overspend were made by a pressure group called Health Emergency, predictions that would turn out largely to be true. At the time, Sir Nigel dismissed them as completely misleading and the worst type of scaremongering.[76] In fact, the turbulence was not only to undermine seriously local services across the country but also to claim Sir Nigel's job some months later.

Throughout 2005 and early 2006, central government would continue to insist that the NHS problems were caused by only a few NHS trusts that were attracting a disproportionate amount of Press attention. This remained a preferred theme of the Department of Health and elements of the Press, both of whom seemed to be in denial about the scale of what was happening. For instance, as late as May 2006, some newspaper columnists would continue to swallow the line, equating protests about the NHS with the shrieking of doctors and nurses, their 'mouths stuffed with silver'.[77] This was

73 Craig Robinson, 'Surgery crisis over funding.' *East Anglian Daily Times*, 20 December 2005.

74 John Howard, 'Surgery closure averted.' *East Anglian Daily Times*, 20 January 2006.

75 'Health trust cuts 230 jobs.' *East Anglian Daily Times*, 29 July 2006.

76 John Carvel, '£1.6bn deficit to force cuts in NHS.' *Guardian*, 7 September 2005.

77 Polly Toynbee, 'This may be the beginning of the end for Labour itself.' *Guardian*, 9 May 2006.

a no doubt unwitting, but insensitive dismissal of all those fearful local residents involved in widespread petitions, letters and protest marches across England. They feared for good reason. Their local health services were about to disappear.

The Royal College of Nursing had in February 2006 reported on the results of a survey that showed 38 per cent of NHS trusts had closed wards and 27 per cent having delayed treatments.[78] Health service experts such as Professor John Appleby were indicating that it was not just a 'few rotten apples in the barrel' but more like 40 per cent of NHS trusts with underlying financial problems.[79]

This was an unsurprising conclusion, since the National Audit Office and Audit Commission had identified that even for the financial year 2003–4, 18 per cent of NHS bodies had failed to achieve in-year financial balance, 24 per cent of NHS trusts did not break even, and 14 per cent of PCTs did not stay within their revenue resource limits.[80] The Healthcare Commission had then reported in July 2005 that a third of NHS hospital trusts failed to balance their books in the financial year 2004–5 – and crucially that patient care could suffer. The Commission, not noted for over-statement, considered this to be a 'very serious issue'.[81]

Besides which, and most importantly, it became abundantly clear that measuring the health of the NHS in terms of financial deficits alone would be inadequate. For instance, nearly all NHS mental health trusts managed to avoid deficits in 2005–6, but in most cases this was achieved only by implementing recruitment freezes and service reductions. These included both temporary and permanent closures of wards or other service units.[82] In the same vein, a Unison survey had suggested that up to 70 per cent of NHS trusts in England were reducing services, 90 per cent had recruitment freezes and 60 per cent were both implementing redundancies and making cuts in training.[83]

In other words, it seemed as if central government was not so much concerned about patient care – as about finance and those NHS Trusts and

78 John Carvel, 'Overspending crisis hitting patient reforms, hospitals are warned.' *Guardian*, 27 February 2006.

79 'The NHS Blame Game.' *Panorama*, BBC1, 26 January 2006.

80 *Financial Management in the NHS.* London: National Audit Office and Audit Commission, 2005, p.2.

81 James Meikle, 'Budget crisis may hit patient care.' *Guardian*, 27 July 2005.

82 *Under pressure: the finances of mental health trusts in 2006.* London: Sainsbury Centre for Mental Health, 2006, pp.5, 15.

83 Celia Hall, 'Job cuts, ward closures…and more to come.' *Daily Telegraph*, 9 March 2006.

PCTs that had not yet succeeded in making sufficiently timely and drastic cuts to services.

Even so, the local Suffolk PCTs needed no second asking to maintain that all was well. Given the imperative of slashing services, they argued that patient care would not be adversely affected. The widespread closures and cutbacks would constitute modernisation and improvement. It was all about changing for the better. Throughout the dogged, bitter and contentious conflict to come, the PCTs continued to maintain that local communities, including clinicians, simply misunderstood. Local communities had fallen victim to a 'misconception' about what was happening.[84]

Patient care will not be affected: the harvest is safe

To the extent that there might after all be a problem, government would argue that it was financial only, and that patient care would not be affected.

By late 2005, it was clear that a significant number of NHS trusts were in serious financial trouble, notwithstanding the extra resources received. The government riposted that it would respond by forcing local NHS trusts into 'surplus'.[85]

It was not going to be a question of saving on fringe spending. Some individual trusts were now boasting individual deficits of £10 million and more. Health care regions (strategic health authorities) could boast tens of millions of overspending, deficit or debt – whichever was the most apt word to describe what was happening in an NHS financial system, the precise workings of which few people seemed to understand.

Unless central government seriously believed that NHS trusts were simply dissipating resources in a reckless and frivolous fashion, the slashing of these large deficits without affecting patient care would obviously be a contradiction in terms. This did not deter the Secretary of State for Health. 'Turnaround teams', popularly labelled financial hit teams, were duly sent into some NHS trusts by Christmas 2005. The shifting of priorities from patient care to finance seemed evident. These teams comprised accountants, generally with commercial backgrounds, who rapidly looked at projected figures but were not qualified to consider the implications for patient care.

84 Carole Taylor-Brown (2006) *Decisions on Changing for the Better: next steps, 25th January 2006, combined boards.* Ipswich: Suffolk East PCTs.

85 John Carvel, 'Hewitt names worst trusts to rein in health service's big spenders.' *Guardian*, 26 January 2006.

It was as if the Department of Health, having heaped multiple and sometimes incoherent demands on the NHS, had waited for things to go wrong before sending in the private sector – in the form of legions of management consultants at great public expense – 'to pick over the corpse'.[86] But even then, the government had not been prepared to reveal the true scale of this exercise. Its claim that only 50 trusts were involved was shown up to be less than accurate. The Freedom of Information Act was used to obtain figures revealing that the turnaround teams had in fact been sent to 29 PCTs, 33 hospital trusts, and 20 out of the 28 strategic health authorities.[87]

The government also deployed one desperate last measure at the end of the financial year for 2005–6. In late February 2006, it stated on a Thursday that, by the following Monday, all strategic health authorities had to sign off a plan, contributed to by all PCTs, to save some £400–£500 million by the end of March.[88] The 'High Noon' ultimatum, at least as it was reported in the newspapers, appeared absurd for two reasons.

The notice given was derisory, given that a mere five weeks of the financial year remained. In addition, the implications were that central government really did believe that NHS trusts were after all reckless, dissipated spenders. It had declared that these savings would have to come from discretionary spending, so leaving patient care unaffected. This knee-jerk, desperate ultimatum appeared more Canute-like than ever, when juxtaposed with a report published by Reform shortly before in December 2005. This had predicted an inexorable rise of the NHS 'debt' to some £7 billion by 2010.[89]

A variation on the theme of government denial was that, if patient care was by chance affected, this would only be because the NHS was performing so well. In other words, any patient care affected would only be the extra, or surplus, so to speak. A levelling off was no bad thing. But this explanation, nationally or locally, could simply not account for the brutal cutbacks in services, with elderly people perhaps most affected. Such closures were nothing to do with hospital consultants exceeding their targets a little too enthusiastically or efficiently.

86 'Dump the debt.' *Private Eye*, 23 June – 6 July 2006, p.12.

87 Sam Lister, 'Hospitals shut wards as cash crisis bites.' *The Times*, 19 January 2006.

88 John Carvel, 'NHS chiefs get "high noon" deadline to cut huge deficit.' *Guardian*, 25 February 2006.

89 N. Bosanquet *et al.* (2005) *The NHS in 2010: reform or bust.* London: Reform.

Flattening out the financial bumps

The implications of regarding trusts as business units, and no more, were perhaps inadvertently given away by the Chief Executive of Norfolk, Suffolk and Cambridgeshire SHA. Commenting on the overspending in Suffolk, he simply stated that saving £20 million was fairly straightforward. Since each £1 million of expenditure equated to about 40 staff, you simply needed to shed 800 jobs.[90] Not a word about the effect on local services and patient care.

Both central government and local NHS bodies would refer also to the statutory duty not to overspend under s.10 of the NHS and Community Care Act 1990 and under the Government Resources and Accounts Act 2000. However, the fact that overspending had previously been tolerated made this pronounced reference to the duty seem disingenuous. For example, the PCTs in Suffolk had been set up with an inherited overspend that was then tolerated for some three to four years.

Suffolk West PCT would refer to this financial duty in its consultation document.[91] Nevertheless, perhaps in a sign of the times, it would fail to refer to its other competing duty to provide local health services under the NHS Act 1977. So, too, in the East of Suffolk. It seemed to be only after the general election of May 2005 that the PCTs began really to scaremonger about the overspending of £2500 per hour every day.[92]

Just like central government, so too the Suffolk West PCT began to talk increasingly of local health in terms of finance. In December 2005, the Department of Health sent in financial hit teams to three NHS organisations in Suffolk (as well as in other parts of the country): West Suffolk Hospital NHS Trust, Suffolk West PCT, and the Suffolk East PCTs.[93]

Consequently, Christmas cheer from the Chairman of the Suffolk West PCT stemmed not from patient care issues but from the approval given to the PCT by the turnaround team. Composed of accountants, the team could not, and did not, directly consider patient care, but only whether the books would begin to balance over the next year or so. Nevertheless, the Chairman was 'delighted to have received this vindication of the competence and effectiveness of our management team'. The PCT received the highest

90 Benedict O'Connor, 'Debts of £20m are "not that bad".' *East Anglian Daily Times*, 25 June 2005.

91 *Modernising Health Care in West Suffolk: consultation, 1 August – 31 October 2005*. Bury St Edmunds: Suffolk West PCT, 2005, p.3.

92 *Changing for the Better: next steps*. Ipswich: Suffolk East PCTs, 2005.

93 Will Grahame-Clark, 'Check on health finances.' *East Anglian Daily Times*, 10 December 2005.

possible ranking. The three members of the team, all from a private consultancy firm, had commercial backgrounds and had spent a week with the PCT.[94]

Spurred on by this approval from the accountants, the Chairman referred in April 2006 to the significant savings his PCT was making, and said that this was a tremendous achievement and a tribute to staff who had continued to provide good-quality services.[95]

The Chief Executive would likewise repeat that it was a tremendous achievement and that it called for public recognition, although it seemed the PCT would remain with a £13.3 million deficit at the financial year's end. This was part of a deficit of some £90 million across the whole area of the Norfolk, Suffolk and Cambridgeshire Strategic Health Authority.[96]

A little later, it seemed that the end of year deficit had actually turned out at £11.6 million. The PCT heaped further plaudits on itself. Clearly, the Chief Executive had made financial inroads and this was a significant achievement. To the newspapers, the PCT mentioned reduction in management costs, prescribing costs, out-of-county placements of patients, and commissioning with NHS trusts.[97] Nonetheless, it did not mention at what cost all this was being achieved, and all the cuts to services still in the pipeline – both those it had already approved and those it had yet to approve. This was left to the Walnuttree Hospital Action Committee. It pointed out, for instance, that the Chief Executive had stated:

> that the PCT had made £9.6 million savings and continued to provide high quality health services. What he did not add is that staff morale is low, staff confidence in senior management and the Trust board has been severely compromised and patient services have suffered. For example, a sweeping recruitment freeze is in place... [and] has led to outpatient physiotherapy waiting times to reach nearly 12 months for some patients. This can lead to unnecessary pain, suffering and sometimes permanent disability that could have been avoided – for people of both working age and older.[98]

94 Dave Gooderham, 'Top score for health trust.' *East Anglian Daily Times*, 24 December 2005.

95 Colin Muge, 'We've all worked hard to cut PCT's debts.' Letter. *East Anglian Daily Times*, 15 April 2006.

96 Danielle Nuttall, 'Region's NHS still in debt.' *East Anglian Daily Times*, 24 April 2006.

97 Lawrence Cawley, 'Cheaper drugs help reduce trust debts.' *East Anglian Daily Times*, 23 May 2006.

98 Walnuttree Hospital Action Committee, 'Savings do affect health service quality.' Letter. *East Anglian Daily Times*, 27 April 2006.

In addition, the PCT did not mention that, as had been reported by its own Director of Finance, the savings had been achieved only by putting staff under huge pressure and by running the highest vacancy level (6.7 per cent) across Norfolk, Suffolk and Cambridgeshire.[99]

Overall, despite a growing wave of protests from around the country, not least from Suffolk, central government attempted to hold firm. By April 2006, the Prime Minister had stepped in to what was now a gaping breach, and referred to the holding of nerve and confidence about reform and change. For Tony Blair, 'turnaround' could be done and would be done. The old way of working was dead and not in the interests of patients. It would nonetheless be a 'challenging' year ahead, he added.[100]

For residents in Suffolk and many other parts of the country, reference to a 'challenging year' ahead was an ominous and unwelcome reference to the crisis already affecting their health services.

Scapegoats and blame: flushing out the health reactionaries

To the extent then that central government spin could not keep the lid on events, another strategy had to be found. This was the language of blame. By definition, it seemed, central government must be right. Anybody not toeing the line could only be a reactionary.

An obvious ploy with a long pedigree is to accuse others of the very thing that you wish to do yourself. Thus, the 2005 manifesto talked of 'defeating those who would dismantle the NHS'.[101] Yet within three months, the notorious Nigel Crisp letter of 28 July would suggest just such a breaking up.[102] This letter demanded that primary care trusts prepare to shed all service provision, and instead farm it out – together with the staff – to the independent sector.

Local NHS managers would come to be blamed by Patricia Hewitt, Secretary of State for Health. At times, they would be treated almost as local renegades, when in fact they were of course effectively appointed through, and answerable to, central government. Nonetheless, this would not stop the Health Secretary emphasising that 'where managers are letting patients down, that will not be tolerated'. She was referring not to patient care,

99 Alison Taylor (2006) *Finance Report: PCT medium term financial strategy, 26th April 2006.* Bury St Edmunds: Suffolk West PCT, para 2.7.

100 Nigel Hawkes, 'You've run out of time, ministers tell failing NHS trusts.' *The Times,* 13 April 2006.

101 *Labour Party Manifesto: Britain forward not back.* London: Labour Party, 2005, p.57.

102 Sir Nigel Crisp, *Commissioning a Patient-led NHS.* Letter, 28 July 2005. London: Department of Health.

however, but to financial deficits.[103] This was a particularly important distinction because some of the NHS organisations suffering from serious financial failings had a good record on patient care. For instance, Suffolk West PCT could boast achievements on waiting times, and its GPs scored highly against quality assurance checks. Without its financial deficit, it might have scored two or three 'stars', rather than the one it had been awarded.[104]

Sir Nigel Crisp, Chief Executive of the NHS, had already tried to deflect blame away from himself down to local managers. He would state that overspending was not acceptable and that poor management eroded public confidence in the NHS.[105]

At a meeting with captains of industry in May 2006, the Chairman of Cable and Wireless suggested that the Prime Minister should get rid of anybody on an NHS trust board who was 'sympathetic to the whingers among the staff' who opposed change. One third of NHS managers, who were probably opposed to change, should also be fired. Tony Blair replied that he thought this was 'absolutely right'.[106] The blunt local implications of this approach were captured accurately by the *East Anglian Daily Times*, following an interview with Patricia Hewitt:

SORT IT OUT – OR ELSE.[107]

Strategic health authorities, too, had both to ward off blame and apportion it. The Norfolk, Suffolk and Cambridgeshire SHA had previously all but approved Sudbury's new community hospital but had now withdrawn its support. It 'instilled' in local PCT chief executives the 'need to balance their books'. The riot act had been read. However, when the SHA's new Chief Executive was asked if he had wondered 'what on earth had been happening' before he took up his post, he replied 'yes'. This was implicit condemnation of his predecessors at the SHA, as well as of the local PCTs. Also, he made clear, the SHA would not be held responsible for drastic measures

103 John Carvel, 'Hewitt names worst trusts to rein in health service's big spenders.' *Guardian*, 26 January 2006.

104 Colin Muge, 'Our work is laudable in very many respects.' Letter. *East Anglian Daily Times*, 25 October 2005.

105 John Carvel, 'NHS chief criticises trusts for running up £250m deficit.' *Guardian*, 17 September 2005.

106 John Carvel, 'Blundering ministers are making NHS patients suffer say consultants' leader.' *Guardian*, 7 June 2006.

107 *East Anglian Daily Times*, 30 September 2005.

implemented by local PCTs. This was because it was not the SHA's responsibility to manage PCTs' debts, but to ensure they did so themselves.[108]

Strategic health authorities, NHS trusts and PCTs were and are in effect regional and local branches of the 'head office' occupied by the Secretary of State. Blaming them excessively could easily backfire and be turned into criticism of head office. So other reactionaries or incompetents have to be found. If it were not local managers then it would be recalcitrant professional groups that were obstructing central government from giving us the health service we all wanted and needed. Patricia Hewitt duly blamed 'clinical resistance' for the delay in NHS reforms.[109]

Local PCTs would faithfully follow suit in the blame game. Suffolk West PCT did, in unguarded moments, point the finger at central government and the SHA – for example, at a public meeting held in Sudbury in June 2005. It would also concede to MPs that it was under the 'financial cosh' of the SHA.[110] However, the PCT could scarcely bite publicly the hand of the very government that paid its salaries (or other remuneration in case of the PCT non-executives). So it soon moved on to softer targets.

Clinicians and other experts would be dismissed as incompetents. When general practitioners in Sudbury publicly criticised the PCT's own plans, the Chief Executive told them that they had misunderstood, and had not read the proposals properly.[111] When an independent expert (who had previously carried out the very work for the PCT that underpinned its intermediate care strategy) produced a critical report, she was dismissed out of hand. The PCT stated that because she was an expert on community hospitals, her report could not be considered to be truly independent. Her particular criticisms were not responded to.[112]

By Christmas 2005, the PCT had branched out and had begun to make what were perceived as personal attacks on prominent members of the local community. It blamed them for the fact that the local community was so fearful about the closure of their much-loved local services, and for deliberately misleading people.[113]

108 Benedict O'Connor, 'Major cutbacks in bid to save £7.4 m.' *East Anglian Daily Times*, 25 June 2005.

109 Melissa Kite, 'It's the doctors' fault the NHS is in financial trouble, says Hewitt.' *Daily Telegraph*, 12 March 2006.

110 Benedict O'Connor, 'Sparks fly as MPs meet with health bosses.' *East Anglian Daily Times*, 12 July 2005.

111 'Town GPs express "serious worries" for patients.' *Suffolk Free Press*, 8 September 2006.

112 Dave Gooderham, 'Health cuts plan "flawed".' *East Anglian Daily Times*, 31 October 2006.

113 Mike Stonard, 'Read the document before you respond.' Letter. *East Anglian Daily Times*, 12 December 2005.

The PCT had already complained that campaigners, politicians, union representatives (and even the church) were repeatedly exaggerating and distorting facts, thus hindering mature and informed public debate.[114]

When, in desperation, patients in Sudbury attempted to launch a judicial review case, the PCT referred to this in a memo to staff as 'deeply regrettable', and that it would result in a reduction of frontline patient services. A press release stated that the PCT was very 'disappointed' and that the judicial review case would put the proposed future health services in West Suffolk at 'great risk'. It was not a 'sensible route to take'.[115] Whatever the intention, these comments were interpreted locally as blaming and threatening. The MP, Tim Yeo, labelled the Chief Executive's comments as deplorable threats.[116]

By implication, it was almost at times as if NHS management, local, regional and national, was blaming patients. For instance, the strategic health authority, which had already linked overspending in Suffolk to personal debt, emphasised that it had to be paid back.[117] But, of course, the analogy was totally inapt. The debt had effectively been incurred by civil servants appointed by central government and unaccountable to their local communities. Yet it was local people having to pay it back in terms of their health and welfare. The total injustice of this occurring in a national health service was obvious. As Unison stated about Suffolk:

> Our workers can't understand why they and the patients are having to pay the price for mistakes that may have been made by the managers.[118]

A Sudbury town councillor, Nick Irwin, likewise articulated the same, compelling point:

> This situation is not Sudbury's fault, so why should we pay the price and be left with virtually no health facilities at all?[119]

114 Mike Stonard, 'Health debate hindered by inaccuracies.' Letter. *East Anglian Daily Times*, 27 August 2005.

115 'New Health Plans Delayed to Judicial Review.' Press release, 24 May 2006. Bury St Edmunds: Suffolk West PCT.

116 Paul Holland, 'Health chiefs' threat to delay town plans.' *Suffolk Free Press*, 25 May 2006.

117 'Politics Show: Health.' *BBC Look East*, 18 September 2005.

118 Patrick Lowman, 'Resign over debts crisis – bosses are urged.' *East Anglian Daily Times*, 24 June 2005.

119 'Residents urged to fight proposals.' *East Anglian Daily Times*, 25 June 2005.

5

Uprooting the Traditional Health Fields

On one level, central government was attempting unsuccessfully to make the current system look as though it was working. On another, it was revealing an altogether more radical and rushed agenda.

Following the 2005 general election, it was clear that it had in mind not just tampering, but a deeper uprooting of the NHS. This would entail very substantial changes. Even without the financial crisis, these changes promised to introduce considerable instability. The changes appeared radical and inconsistent with what the electorate had expected. A leading health policy expert, Professor Chris Ham, who had until recently run the Department of Health's strategy unit, commented. He referred portentously in December 2005 to the unleashing by central government of a wave of 'creative destruction' that would result in the closure of district general hospitals.[1]

The changes included throwing the NHS open to the private sector, organising it along the lines of local, semi-independent business units, and introducing a system of funding called 'payment by results'. Coupled with the financial instability already affecting the NHS, these changes promised to be extremely unsettling. Worryingly, the reassuring noises from central government that it was all for the best appeared not to be based on convincing evidence.

1 Sam Lister, 'Health reforms "will bring hospital closures".' *The Times*, 19 December 2005.

Taking us all to market: letting loose independent enterprise

The government had talked previously in policy documents about the wider involvement of the independent sector in the delivery of health services. Its May 2005 general election manifesto commitment was to use independent providers, private and voluntary, 'where they add capacity or promote innovation'.[2] Such a general and innocuous phrase could scarcely be linked by the average voter to what followed. New Labour was acting with no political mandate, but this was no deterrent.

Speed and covertness seemed to be key. In the middle of the summer holidays and Parliamentary recess, on 28 July 2005, central government betrayed both its impatience and the true extent of its aims. It wrote a letter to NHS primary care trusts, the so-called 'Nigel Crisp' letter.[3] Its timing suggested an awareness of the controversy it might spark. So it proved.

The import of the letter was that NHS primary care trusts should by and large neither be providing services directly nor employing staff. At an extreme this would mean that hundreds of thousands of staff, including nurses and therapists, would no longer be NHS employees but would transfer to the independent sector. The tone of the letter appeared radically to depart from the manifesto commitment. There was no mention of spare capacity or innovation being the trigger for going out to contract with the independent sector. In short, central government seemed logically to equate the private sector with service delivery in either all or at least most circumstances.

Furthermore, the speed demanded would brook little pause for thought. Strategic health authorities would have to put forward plans by October 2005, with changes to PCT service provision to be complete by December 2008. This hardly seemed consistent with the definitive statement made in 2002, that:

> above all, any capacity used in the private sector must augment, not subtract from, the number of precious skilled clinical staff already working in the NHS.[4]

New Labour had indeed betrayed its hand and a great deal more. In 1997, its manifesto had stated that it would 'end the Conservatives' internal market in

2 *Labour Party Manifesto: Britain forward not back.* London: Labour Party, 2005, p.57.

3 Sir Nigel Crisp, *Commissioning a patient-led NHS.* Letter. 28 July 2005. London: Department of Health.

4 Secretary of State for Health (2002) *Delivering the NHS Plan: next steps on investment, next steps on reform.* Cm 5503. London: HMSO, para 6.1.

healthcare'.[5] What it had not explained was that it would go one better by throwing the NHS wide open not just to an internal, but to an external, market.

The outcry was predictable, for example, from the Royal College of Nursing (which threatened a judicial review challenge, subsequently dropped) and other relevant unions. Outrage in such quarters did not appear to bother central government. It seemed almost as if it would gauge the value of its proposals in direct proportion to the degree of opposition they attracted – from what it considered to be entrenched and reactionary interests.

Following alarm raised in its own backyard, in the form of its own backbench MPs, central government signalled an apparent retreat later in the year from the 28 July letter. The retreat was more tactical and temporary than strategic. By early 2006, central government had learned the lesson that greater stealth was required. The evidence as to whether the Nigel Crisp letter had been abandoned was ambiguous. Certainly, the White Paper issued in January 2006 still envisaged that PCTs would shed services, with other organisations, including voluntary or private sector, taking them over. The proviso about using the independent sector only to add capacity or innovation to NHS provision, was absent. Now it was a question of quality, with PCTs having to justify continued in-house provision.[6] Follow-up guidance similarly stated that there was now no requirement or timetable for PCTs to divest themselves of provision, but that they would have to consider the lost opportunities if they did not get the private sector involved.[7] This suggested pressure behind the scenes would continue for PCTs to invite the private sector to run health services.

The House of Commons Health Committee had been scathing. Referring to the Nigel Crisp letter, it pointed out that it represented a major change in policy direction and should properly have been the 'subject of full and open debate'. Instead, central government's 'numerous announcements and subsequent retractions mean that it is still unclear what its policy is on the divestment of PCTs' provider services'. All this amounted to a 'clumsy and cavalier approach to NHS staff'. Furthermore, the Committee referred to 'important concerns' about the consequences of independent sector

5 *New Labour Because Britain Deserves Better.* London: Labour Party, 1997, p.16.

6 Secretary of State for Health (2006) *Our Health, Our Care, Our Say.* Cm 6737. London: HMSO, para 7.83.

7 *Our health, our say, our community: investing in the future of community hospitals and services.* London: Department of Health, 2006.

provision, such as 'fragmentation of community services', which would make the provision of joined-up care even more problematic.[8]

Nonetheless, the local warning signs were evident. Suffolk West PCT in May 2006 were reported to have taken on United Health as financial consultants to audit their services and make recommendations for further savings and maybe cuts to services.[9] Reputedly at a cost of some £90,000–100,000 (the PCT did not say), this gave rise to some concerns. United Health were large-scale providers of health care, and were currently trying to get into the market to run services for the NHS. United Health Europe are one of those private companies waiting in the wings to bid to run substantial parts of NHS primary care, including general practitioner services. Its president, Simon Stevens, is the former health policy adviser to Prime Minister Tony Blair.[10]

One issue was whether the financial consultancy was the thin end of a wedge which could see the PCT shedding its services and forcing its staff to work for a private provider. In particular it was feared that the staff recruitment freeze currently in place, together with the apparent running down and shedding of services for people with more complex needs (by closing community hospital beds), could be a prelude to just such a move.[11]

Fanning out across the private sector

The move toward privatisation of the health services was not confined to community health services. By 2005, privately operated diagnostic and treatment centres were increasingly being used by the NHS.

By mid-2006, the House of Commons Health Committee reported that these centres had made no direct contribution to increased capacity, that any good practice to be found within them could be found also within the NHS, that they were poorly integrated into the NHS, and that the centres could have a significant and destabilising impact on the finances of NHS hospitals. On the question of value for money, the Committee could not reach a fully informed view, since the Department of Health refused to disclose detailed figures on grounds of commercial confidentiality.

8 House of Commons Health Committee (2005) *Changes to Primary Care Trusts.* HC 646. London: HMSO, p.4.

9 Will Grahame-Clark, 'Consultant move by PCT "unacceptable".' *East Anglian Daily Times,* 30 May 2006.

10 Allyson Pollock, 'The politics column.' *New Statesman,* 1 May 2006.

11 Peter Clifford, 'PCT questions are in need of answers.' Letter. *East Anglian Daily Times,* 6 June 2006.

The Committee's report further hinted at the reluctance of central government to explain, fully and transparently, the rationale and justification for promotion of these centres:

> The Department of Health and Secretary of State have, over the course of our inquiry, given answers which have shifted in both fact and emphasis as time has gone by, and the statement of the current position by the Secretary of State leaves several important questions unanswered.[12]

There is additional concern that independent treatment centres are sometimes being contracted to carry out operations but not to deliver the necessary post-operative rehabilitation. This then leaves NHS rehabilitation services to pick up the pieces, something they may not always have the resources to do. Patients might then fall through the net.[13]

The Private Finance Initiative (PFI), too, was now well advanced. Private companies built hospitals and sometimes ran certain services within them. Serious concerns were being raised that this initiative might not represent value for money. This was for a number of reasons, one concerning the amount of money paid back to the private companies by the NHS. Another was that the NHS might find itself 'locked' into paying for buildings and services that in, for example, 30 years time were not clinically required.[14] In addition, equivalent private sector involvement in primary care premises came in the form of LIFT (Local Improvement Finance Trust) projects. The higher costs of LIFT projects, and implications for NHS spending and for patients – as the House of Commons Public Accounts Committee pointed out – needed to be carefully weighed up by PCTs before entering into them.[15]

It might not just be the longer term that was a problem. In May 2006, the House of Commons Public Accounts Committee published a report into the Norfolk and Norwich University Hospital PFI scheme. Only five years into the contract, the private companies had trebled their rate of return from

12 House of Commons Health Committee (2006) *Independent sector treatment centres.* HC 934-I. London: Stationery Office, Summary.

13 Joanna Clarke-Jones, 'Minor ops cause major problem for therapists.' *Therapy Weekly*, 22 June 2006.

14 For more detail: Allyson Pollock (2005) *NHS plc: the privatisation of our health care.* London: Verso, p.72.

15 House of Commons Committee of Public Accounts (2006) *NHS local improvement finance trusts.* HC 562. London: Stationery Office.

16 per cent to 60 per cent by means of a refinancing arrangement affecting the loans they had taken out to build the hospital.[16]

The Committee's report indicated that the NHS came off very badly. Part of the reason for this was instructions from the Department of Health and the Treasury.[17] By March 2006, some 39 PFI schemes had been approved and completed to the value of £6.2 billion, on which large repayments by the NHS were due.[18]

The increasing scale of PFI, and the financial burden it was generating, meant that by 2006 it was perceived to be increasingly responsible for the size of the NHS debt, together with related bed closures and service cutbacks. For instance, it was reported that the capital charge paid to the Treasury in 2005 for use of land and buildings by a major NHS Trust (Barts and the London) was £8.62 million per year. But, under PFI, this would rise in future to £67 million. Similarly, some £9 million of the £19 million deficit of the Queen Elizabeth Hospital in Greenwich was reported as stemming from PFI – even though the hospital had become increasingly efficient over the last five years.[19]

Taking the hint from central government, local NHS bodies would grasp at any private straw if they could. For instance, desperate to make short-term gains even at the risk of long-term disadvantage, West Suffolk Hospitals NHS Trust decided to lease out for seven years the running of its car parks for a one-off payment of £3.8 million.[20] The car parks made an annual profit of £660,000, and the deal was defended on the basis that an upfront payment of £3.8 million was worth more than £4.6 million over seven years.[21]

It is beyond the scope of this book to discuss private sector involvement in detail. But there are cogent arguments that a marketised NHS private sector involvement will not only bring about the demise of the NHS as we know it, including its three key principles, but is anyway not a cost-effective means of delivering the nation's health. This is because of, for instance:

16 House of Commons Committee of Public Accounts (2006) *The Refinancing of the Norfolk and Norwich PFI Hospital.* HC 694. London: HMSO.

17 George Monbiot, 'The man who treats public services as a pension fund for fat cats.' *Guardian,* 9 May 2006.

18 Jeremy Laurance, 'How did things go so wrong for the NHS?' *Independent,* 9 March 2006.

19 Alysson Pollock, 'The exorbitant cost of PFI is now being cruelly exposed.' *Guardian,* 26 January 2006.

20 Liz Hearnshaw, 'Hospital bids to lease car parks.' *East Anglian Daily Times,* 1 December 2005.

21 Dave Gooderham, 'Anger at "cheap" deal on hospital car parks.' *East Anglian Daily Times,* 31 March 2006.

1. higher transaction and administration costs attendant on the numerous contracts required
2. fragmentation of services and risk pools
3. loss of mechanisms for fair distribution and monitoring of fair allocation of resources
4. loss of central and local accountability, and
5. an increase in the likelihood of fraud and embezzlement.[22]

By 2006, it was estimated that market-related costs – including invoicing, marketing, advertising, drawing up of contracts, legal disputes with providers and rival hospitals, and the widespread use of management consultants – accounted, at a conservative estimate, for between 6 and 14 per cent of the NHS budget.[23]

Other privatisation plans included the possible contracting out wholesale of pathology (blood testing etc.) services in England, of NHS supplies (a contract worth up to £4 billion annually) to a Texas-based company under investigation in the United States for financial impropriety, and of the management and commissioning functions of PCTs.[24]

On 29 June 2006, the Department of Health was caught out placing a £64 billion advertisement in the European Union official journal – apparently for multi-national companies to manage PCT commissioning functions and services, lock, stock and barrel. At 3.45pm that day, a government minister defended the advertisement. At 6.05pm he changed his mind and withdrew it. A former New Labour health minister, Frank Dobson, described it as privatisation of the health service and as putting multinational policies in the 'driving seat' of the NHS.[25] The advertisement was reissued some weeks later in a watered down form.

The leasing out of car parks is an example of peripheral privatisation. And leased out or not, some patients are charged very substantial sums to attend hospital and park their cars. For instance, charges in England vary from 30

22 *Briefing note for the House of Commons Health Committee on proposed changes to the functions of NHS primary care trusts, 10th November 2005.* Edinburgh: The Centre for International Public Health Policy, School of Health in Social Science, University of Edinburgh.

23 Alysson Pollock, 'The politics column.' *New Statesman,* 1 May 2006.

24 'Private firms "may do NHS tests".' *News.bbc.co.uk,* 2 August 2006. And: Nigel Hawkes, 'Firm handed £4bn NHS contract was investigated for overcharging.' *The Times,* 31 July 2006.

25 John Carvel, '£64bn NHS privatisation plan revealed.' *Guardian,* 30 June 2006.

pence to £4 per hour, and a 24-hour stay can cost up to £30. Patients attending regularly clearly suffer, although some hospitals do offer them concessions. Even then, such concessions may not be advertised clearly or may be difficult to obtain.[26] A further trend emerging in 2006 was the 'outsourcing' of the work of medical secretaries. For instance, Southampton General Hospital announced it would contract out such work to South Africa – with information emailed to and fro. Dozens of medical secretaries would be made redundant.[27]

Local fields into prairie lands: NHS reorganisation

By late 2005, central government decided to throw in yet one more combustible ingredient. This was the reorganisation and reduction of the number of NHS primary care trusts and of strategic health authorities. This was despite, in January 2006, the House of Commons Health Select Committee having reported itself unhappy with this reorganisation, because of 'well-founded concerns that patient care will suffer'.[28]

Apart from the ill-advisedness of too much simultaneous change, there were other criticisms. The reorganisation might in many places effectively restore the equivalent of the very health authorities that central government had disbanded only five years before. There was concern not just about the costs of this bureaucratic and circular change, but also the redundancy costs involved. The previous creation of the PCTs was estimated to have cost £63 million. The costs associated now with the demise of many of them (from 302 down to some 130–150) would be considerable.[29]

The reorganisation plans appeared to involve centralising, rather than localising, effective control of the NHS – despite central government's claims precisely to be giving trusts, staff and patients more local control. And not only were PCTs to be reduced in number and increased in size, but so too were strategic health authorities. Yet, almost in contradiction, this pulling back could lead to disorganised fragmentation of services at local level by private sector providers – a point picked up by the House of Commons

26 House of Commons Health Committee, *NHS charges.* HC 815-I. London: Stationery Office, paras 76–83.

27 'Hospital's typing pool in Africa.' *The Times,* 15 August 2006, p.21.

28 House of Commons Health Committee (2006) *Changes to Primary Care Trusts.* HC 646. London: HMSO, p.4.

29 Robert Watts, 'Primary care trusts face deep cuts in NHS efficiency drive.' *Sunday Telegraph,* 9 October 2005.

Health Committee.[30] A reversion to local, self-interested, profit-driven strip farming, so to speak.

Destabilising the machinery and blighting the crops

By late 2005, the same theme was being played out with police forces, as well as fire and ambulance services. Regionalisation and centralisation was being proposed across the East of England.[31]

For instance, MPs and local police authorities would express themselves opposed to mergers that would create huge regional forces and reduce local accountability, responsiveness and sensitivity. Although there was meant to be consultation, central government ruled out certain options in advance, thus tying the Suffolk Police Authority's hands.[32] Into 2006, it became clear that the Home Secretary remained determined to rule out certain options. In the case of Suffolk, he rejected out of hand, first, the option of Suffolk remaining a 'stand-alone' force and, second, the merger option favoured in the region (an Essex, Suffolk and Norfolk force).[33] In fact, a change of Home Secretary during 2006 saw these plans for police force amalgamations shelved or put on hold.

It should be noted that such centralisation of the NHS runs directly counter to what central government has repeatedly stated and trumpeted in the *NHS Plan* of 2000:

> Local hospitals cannot be run from Whitehall. There will be a new relationship between the Department of Health and the NHS to enshrine the trust that patients have in frontline staff. The principles of subsidiarity will apply. A new system of earned autonomy will devolve power from the centre.[34]

Although stripping out more local layers of senior management might save administrative costs, it was by no means clear how this could contribute to decentralised planning. For example, the town of Sudbury felt neglected by the Suffolk West PCT based in Bury St Edmunds; how much more would it

30 House of Commons Health Committee (2006) *Changes to Primary Care Trusts.* HC 646. London: HMSO, p.4.

31 Rebecca Sheppard, 'Merger worry: Suffolk at risk.' *East Anglian Daily Times,* 19 October 2005.

32 Craig Robinson, 'MPs criticise proposals to merge police forces.' *East Anglian Daily Times,* 21 December 2005.

33 Craig Robinson, 'Police to fight merger.' *East Anglian Daily Times,* 4 April 2006.

34 Secretary of State for Health (2000) *The NHS Plan: a plan for investment, a plan for reform.* Cm 4818-1. London: HMSO, p.11.

be neglected by a Suffolk-wide PCT based in Ipswich, which would still be taking orders direct from government? The House of Commons Health Committee expressed itself outraged at the whole exercise:

> Despite the government's repeated assurances, it is clear from our evidence that the consultation has been a 'top down' process: change has been imposed on local NHS organisations by central government for financial reasons and as a result solutions that would best meet local needs are being overruled because they do not meet the required savings.[35]

In Suffolk, it was decided by the Norfolk, Suffolk and Cambridgeshire strategic health authority that five PCTs should be rolled up into one. This was a direct return to the old Suffolk Health Authority (although this decision was later modified by the Secretary of State). The Norfolk, Suffolk and Cambridgeshire SHA itself – already covering a sizeable part of the country – was to be swallowed up and become part of an even larger organisation covering those three counties, together with Essex, Bedfordshire and Hertfordshire. This was confirmed by April 2006.[36]

As early as September 2005, the three Suffolk East PCTs had already in effect been merged in advance. Two of the chief executives were made redundant with 'golden handshakes' of £350,000. Revealed two days after the plans had been made known to sell off the Felixstowe and Bartlet Hospitals for £6 million, the payments were heavily criticised.[37] Payoffs were not the preserve of Suffolk. For instance, a termination payment to a chief executive in East Sussex amounted to £231,000. The NHS Trust there had a deficit of £1.9 million.[38]

In addition to the costs attendant on such constant reorganisation are those associated with the inevitable planning blight, and effect on service delivery. This was conceded by the Suffolk PCTs in 2005, although they stated this in restrained manner, referring to the ill-timing of the reorganisation, its short timescales, its unfortunate combining with financial recovery plans and the difficulty of involving the public.[39]

35 House of Commons Health Committee (2006) *Changes to Primary Care Trusts.* HC 646. London: HMSO, p.3.

36 Rebecca Sheppard, 'New health authority to cover region.' *East Anglian Daily Times,* 13 April 2006.

37 Craig Robinson, '"Outrageous": fury as hard-up Suffolk health trusts pay out £350,000 to two redundant managers.' *East Anglian Daily Times,* 26 September 2005.

38 'MP attacks trust chief's payoff.' *News.bbc.co.uk,* 26 July 2006.

39 *Suffolk Primary Care Trusts Reconfiguration Options.* Ipswich: Suffolk West PCT, Waveney PCT, Suffolk East PCTs, 2005, para 6.1.

The House of Commons Health Committee felt no such restraint:

> there were well-founded concerns that patient care will suffer because of the proposed reforms.[40]

Locally, at least the Chairman of the Suffolk West PCT's Professional Executive Committee had the courage to speak out. He suggested that the reorganisation could be a 'vast mistake'.[41]

The inevitable uncertainty incidental to such reorganisations was also illustrated when on 11 April 2006, the Suffolk West PCT board voted through serious cuts to services but did leave some outpatient services in place in Sudbury. At a public meeting the next day, the PCT's Chief Executive conceded that that the new Suffolk-wide PCT, to be operational in October 2006, would not be bound by what the current PCT had decided.[42] Sure enough, in June 2006, the PCT conceded that organisational change had caught up with it and intermediate care implementation should be suspended. In future the new PCT would have to review its plans for intermediate care as a matter of priority.[43] So there were no guarantees, then.

This effectively devalued the nine-month consultation process and final decision. It was in spite of an SHA spokeswoman having some months earlier stated that 'any responsibilities for decisions made by the current PCTs will transfer to successor organisations'. However, even this statement of course stopped short of saying that those successors would actually implement previously made decisions. On this very theme of blight, once more the House of Commons Health Committee did not hold back:[44]

> After the immediate disruption of reorganisation, it is thought to take a further 18 months for the benefits to emerge – a total of three years from the initial reforms. Thus, just as the benefits of PCTs (established in 2002) are about to be realised, the government has decided to restructure them. The cycle of perpetual change is ill-judged and not conducive to the successful provision and improvement of health services.[45]

40 House of Commons Health Committee (2006) *Changes to Primary Care Trusts.* HC 646. London: HMSO, p.4.

41 'Merger "could save region's NHS £11m".' *East Anglian Daily Times,* 29 September 2005.

42 'It's a question of trust, says health chief.' *Suffolk Free Press,* 13 April 2006.

43 Jonathan Williams, untitled letter. Bury St Edmunds: Suffolk West PCT, 23 June 2006.

44 '"No-one answerable" for hospital closure.' *Suffolk Free Press,* 19 January 2006.

45 House of Commons Health Committee (2006) *Changes to Primary Care Trusts.* HC 646. London: HMSO, p.4.

Payment by piecework: results and tariffs

The government was attempting to set in motion, from April 2006, a new funding mechanism for the NHS. It would be known as 'payment by results'. Basically, this would more closely link NHS funding services actually provided rather than simply allocating block finance to NHS services. Payment would be against basic tariff costs for different types of treatment, calculated by the Department of Health. While attractive on its face, the widespread and swift application envisaged by central government could bring serious problems in its wake. Some of these seemed to be as follows.

First, it could result in local services being closed if they were seen not to be cost-effective – begging the question of just where local people would then go to find the services they needed.

Second, it presupposed that there would be in place sophisticated enough tariffs that were adjusted for profitable and unprofitable treatments – to avoid a perverse incentive not to provide services for 'non-profitable' patients.[46]

Third, such payment by results would underpin a system of 'contestability' between the NHS and the independent sector. The main driver behind payment by results seems to have been the need to have a market oriented pricing system, in order to make the privatisation of NHS clinical services possible.[47] In other words, by measuring patients as business and financial units, the system would become the basis for wholesale contracting out of the health service to the independent sector. In turn, people who did not get 'better' reliably and predictably within too crude a 'care pathway' could be at most risk of being unprofitable. That is, the most vulnerable in our society, for example older people with multiple needs, and other people with physical disabilities, learning disabilities and mental health problems.

There has been concern that oversimple 'care pathways' can sometimes mean no more than 'conveyor belts', based on uniform, predictable patients. Business models and competition have their drawbacks:

> It is the business model that makes NHS 'bed managers' behave, against their will, like bailiffs acting for a ruthless landlord, eager to evict one set of patients to make room for another (the existing patients have used up their quota of care, the next patients bring new cash). Lack of bed capacity, and pressure for the earliest possible discharge, see patients

46 Alison Talbot-Smith and Alysson Pollock (2006) *The New NHS: a guide.* Abingdon: Routledge, p.9.

47 Alysson Pollock, 'The exorbitant cost of PFI is now being cruelly exposed.' *Guardian*, 26 January 2006.

> moved from ward to ward, or marooned in remote parts of the hospital. There is even a label – 'medical outliers' – for these orphans of the system, while those who can't be evicted soon enough to make room for new patients are known as 'delayed discharges', or 'bed blockers' – second-class citizens cluttering up the wards. As hospitals compete for trade, they trade away care and humanity.[48]

Indeed, the Department of Health's code of conduct on payment by results refers particularly to the ability of providers to offer a restricted range of services – as long as this is consistent with their contracts from commissioners.[49] Since NHS commissioners might be only too keen to shed responsibilities for vulnerable groups of patients, this would appear in itself to be no barrier to the 'cream skimming' of patients and services. Payment by results could mean 'over-diagnosis and over-treatment for some, and neglect and under-treatment of others'.[50]

A King's Fund report identified just such risks in relation to primary care and general practice based commissioning of services. For instance:

> open lists for general practice teams may reallocate the current, already scarce, workforce away from more challenging populations... It may also serve to decrease profitability of practices in other geographical areas, leading to instability and greater incentives to 'cherry pick' less needy patients.[51]

It observed also that public health, geographical planning and commissioning on the basis of local population need (of both health and social care) could suffer in a system of contestability. Commissioners might only be prevented from targeting disproportionate numbers of 'healthy patients' by heavy regulation; and inter-professional and inter-organisational collaboration is likely to suffer.[51] The ability or will of central government to regulate and control such market forces is questionable.[52]

The great danger appears to be that payment by results will essentially be about volume of activity and speed of delivery, playing surrogate for high-quality health care based on properly measured patient outcomes. Not

48 Allyson Pollock (2005) *NHS plc: the privatisation of our health care.* London: Verso, p.88.

49 *Code of Conduct for Payment by Results.* London: Department of Health, 2006.

50 Allyson Pollock (2005) *NHS plc: the privatisation of our health care.* London: Verso, p.231.

51 Richard Lewis and Jennifer Dixon (2005) *The Future of Primary Care: meeting the challenges of the new market.* London: King's Fund.

52 Allyson Pollock (2005) *NHS plc: the privatisation of our health care.* London: Verso, p.261.

only might complex conditions or needs be shunned, but there will be an incentive to operate at 'below tariff', in order to generate a profit. This would create a perverse incentive to reduce the quality of care.[53]

Fourth, by the time of the 2005 New Labour election manifesto, there was reference to use of the independent sector to add capacity and innovation – but also to 'drive contestability'.[54] In 2006, plurality and contestability were key objectives, 'enabling funds to go to any provider (whether NHS or Independent Sector) who can treat patients at tariff and at NHS standards, enabling providers to compete on an equal basis to provide services'.[55]

Fifth, the code of conduct issued by the Department of Health itself pointed out not just some of the pitfalls that need to be avoided, but as well its own flimsiness. It conceded unreassuringly that it was not enforceable directly. It would only be enforced indirectly through contractual, regulatory and performance management mechanisms.[55]

The potential instability of the system of payment by results, in relation to more specialist or complex needs, began to surface already in April 2006. For instance, the chairs and chief executives of four children's hospitals – Great Ormond Street, Alder Hey, Birmingham and Sheffield – stated that the new system would result in a £22 million shortfall in funding. This would mean a reduction of vital children's treatments.[56]

Levelling the fields: business contestability and financial balance

A suspicion arose that the financial crisis to which Patricia Hewitt constantly alluded from late 2005 onwards was not just a question of concern over the public finances and pressure from the Treasury. It was also the fact that local balancing of the NHS books was crucial to facilitate a system of contestability and competition.

The overspending had not arisen overnight. It had been known about for many years. Thus, in Gloucestershire, there had been a £5 million historical debt inherited by the Cotswold and Vale PCT. Given an ultimatum by central government to wipe out the debt almost immediately, the PCT

53 Rory O'Connor and Vera Neumann (2006) 'Payment by results or payment by outcome? The history of measuring medicine.' *Journal of the Royal Society of Medicine 99*: 226–231.

54 *Britain Forward Not Back.* London: Labour Party, 2005, p.63.

55 *Code of Conduct for Payment by Results.* London: Department of Health, 2006.

56 Patrick Wintour, 'Children's hospitals warn ministers of £22m funding.' *Guardian,* 18 April 2006.

responded by threatening and then deciding to close its cottage hospitals at Tetbury, Fairford, Bourton-on-the-Water, Moreton-in-March and Cirencester.[57] The King's Fund press release summed it up:

> many trusts have had underlying deficits for a number of years, which their boards, auditors, strategic health authorities and by implication the Department of Health, must have been aware of for some time. Many of the deficits were dealt with by short-term fixes by trusts, encouraged to prioritise hitting targets above achieving financial balance.[58]

And so it was in Suffolk, too, where the Suffolk West Primary Care Trust, on its creation in 2002, apparently inherited a pattern of service provision that cost nearly £11 million more than it was funded to provide. (Although Audit Commission figures for the PCT at its inception refer to a pure deficit of some £1.5 million only.[59]) This represented 6.5 per cent of the PCT's funding. By 2005, it had reduced the annual overspend to 4.5 per cent.[60] Central government, post-election in 2005, nevertheless demanded that the books be balanced within the next 12 months or so.

In other words, it began to look as though government might at least in part have engineered a crisis for ulterior motives. Notably, it had not complained of the overspending before the general election when, under its own instruction, NHS trusts were throwing money at government targets with gay abandon. It had also become apparent by April 2006 that central government itself was directly responsible for up to as much as £300 million of the debt, owing to a miscalculation over the pay of general practitioners.[61]

It was further baffling, because the Health Secretary would both overplay and underplay the significance of the underspend. On the one hand it was a crisis brought about by poorly managed, free-wheeling local NHS trusts and primary care trusts who were threatening the entire NHS. On the other, it remained less than one per cent of the NHS budget and so was not unduly serious. Which was it?

57 Geoffrey Clifton-Brown, MP for Cotswold. *Hansard*, Westminster Hall, 2 November 2005, column 269WH.

58 *NHS Must Avoid Short-term Fixes to Cure Financial Ills, Warns King's Fund.* Press release, 26 April 2006. London: King's Fund.

59 *Learning the lessons from financial failure in the NHS.* London: Audit Commission, 2006, p.13.

60 Dr Andrew Hassan. Letter. *The Green Sheet*, 7 July 2005.

61 'Scoring points reaps rewards.' *Guardian*, 19 April 2006.

Perhaps an indication of central government's true motives was its consistent blaming of local NHS trusts and PCTs. The implication was that although it was a 'national' health service, and although most local trusts' spending is dictated by rules and targets set by central government, nevertheless, the overspending was due to the failure of local NHS trusts to break even as autonomous business units. Furthermore, this would mean local patients suffering. This was the type of language that would appear to betray central government's wish to see health services delivered in fragmented fashion by a range of private and independent providers – as opposed to a coherent national health service.

6

Cultivation of Local Health Services

Central government has made great play of keeping the NHS local. This aim is to be found littered across any number of policy documents. There are many commonsense advantages. These include convenient access, less travel for patients and their relatives, environmental issues, car parking difficulties, the exhaustion of patients having to travel for regular day treatments, cheaper treatment costs and so on.

For instance, one key policy, known as 'intermediate care', is to avoid people being admitted to, or staying unnecessarily long in, acute hospitals. It aims to get people back home or at least near their homes, or to avoid admission in the first place. Care closer to home is the watchword; have local services, both inpatient and outpatient.

Were there any doubt about this, central government even published a major policy document going by that name: *Keeping the NHS Local.* It would be an 'exciting time for smaller hospitals in particular'.[1] The government's White Paper of early 2006 made the same point, explaining the value of community hospitals, which not only delivered care closer to home, but provide better care and were cost-effective.[2] It sounded fine, but local communities had no idea just what sort of excitement central government had in mind for them – as PCTs attempted, all over the country, to shut down or diminish their community hospitals. And it would not just be rural areas

1 *Keeping the NHS Local: a new direction of travel.* London: Department of Health, 2003, p.4.

2 Secretary of State for Health (2006) *Our Health, Our Care, Our Say.* Cm 6737. London: HMSO, para 6.40.

affected. Towns and cities, too, would see whole swathes of local services threatened with cutback and closure.

In rural areas, the issue of local health services takes on added importance in terms of both health and social care. The reasons, all too obvious, nevertheless continue to be ignored by central government, largely – some people suggest – because most rural areas in England do not return New Labour candidates. The issues include longstanding under-investment in rural services, poor public transport, geographical isolation, rural poverty, ageing communities and the continued closure of local services.[3]

Even central government recognises some of the problem at least in principle. Urban dwellers tend to move on retirement – resulting, for instance, in a net shift of 780,000 people into rural areas between 1991 and 2001.[4] The Commission for Rural Communities revealed that people living in rural areas of East Anglia had dramatically less choice of and access to a range of key services, such as health and education – compared to those living in urban areas.[5]

The great thing about some of New Labour's policy documents is that much of what they say is hard to disagree with. We all want our services local and convenient. The policies keep on saying the right thing. However, a harsh rule seems to operate. The more sensible the policy in principle, all too often the greater the departure in practice. Unfortunately for its residents, Suffolk would provide a glaring illustration.

Rural massacre of the community hospitals

The New Labour 2005 election manifesto stated that:

> we will over the next five years develop a new generation of modern NHS community hospitals.[6]

It said nothing about closing down or severely reducing the capacity of nearly 30 per cent of existing community hospitals, without replacement community hospitals in sight, built or even planned – thus leaving local communities bereft of vital local health services.

3 J. Glasby, 'Out in the field.' *Community Care*, 15–21 September 2005.

4 Secretary of State for Health (2005) *Independence, Well-being and Choice: our vision for the future of social care for adults in England.* Cm 6499. London: HMSO, para 2.12.

5 Danielle Nuttall, 'Rural residents "hit by lack of services".' *East Anglian Daily Times*, 12 December 2005.

6 *Labour Party Manifesto: Britain forward not back.* London: Labour Party, 2005, p.63.

Yet within months of the election this was precisely what was being proposed with the approval of strategic health authorities (and thus of central government) all over the country. In some cases, the instructions appeared to be coming directly from those SHAs. Central government could not claim ignorance. Both the professional and the national Press had rumbled the story. By December 2005, the *Nursing Times* reported it as 'terrifying' that at least 80 out of 320 such hospitals in England were losing beds and services – as well as facing closure.[7] By January 2006, the *Daily Telegraph* could refer without exaggeration not only to the 'massacre' of community hospitals, but also to central government's refusal:

> to offer any public comment or justification for the irreversible extinction of dozens of hospitals, hiding resolutely behind civil servants who are themselves anonymous.[8]

Follow my White Paper: the Secretary of State rides out

The new year had been rung in gloomily. However, during January 2006, the local communities for a moment believed that rescue was in sight.

Richard II had ridden out 625 years earlier to confront and inspire the peasants. Now, in the same vein, Patricia Hewitt's White Paper stated that community hospitals were after all important, and should include those very services and facilities that local communities were fighting for. These included inpatient beds for the elderly and vulnerable in the community, as well as consultant outpatient clinics. It stated that, compared to acute district general hospitals, they provided better rehabilitation and recuperation for older people and did this more cost-effectively.[9]

National newspapers, naively as it transpired, took the White Paper and its Secretary of State author at face value. Even local people, 'the peasants', did. The next day, the *Daily Mail* announced on its front page:

> REPRIEVE FOR THE COTTAGE HOSPITAL.[10]

The national press appeared to have demonstrated its potential gullibility in the face of New Labour's claims. Notably, it was a regional newspaper, the

7 'Community hospitals in crisis.' *Nursing Times*, 6 December 2005, p.2.

8 Boris Johnson, 'Forget the "porno sirs": the real scandal is going on in the NHS.' *Daily Telegraph*, 19 January 2006.

9 Secretary of State for Health (2006) *Our Health, Our Care, Our Say*. Cm 6737. London: HMSO, para 6.40.

10 James Chapman, 'Reprieve for the cottage hospital.' *Daily Mail*, 31 January 2006.

East Anglian Daily Times, that cut to the chase. On the very same day that the national press was fooled, its editorial made quite clear that Suffolk hospitals would not be saved. This had followed an interview with Liam Byrne, the junior health minister.[11] The PCTs were not for turning; nor was the Secretary of State minded to turn them. It was as if a new round of promises had been made and broken in the same day. The peasants would after all be betrayed, much as they were all those centuries ago when they were rounded up and killed following the monarch's assurances. The national press subsequently picked it up of course:

> 'Reprieve for the cottage hospitals.' The newspaper headlines fluttered merrily like bunting at a village fete. All's well with middle England – those ivy-clad war memorial hospitals and wisteria-decked community hospitals are safe thanks to health secretary Patricia Hewitt and her white paper on healthcare outside hospitals...but many of those that were under threat on 29th January were still due for closure on 30th January...[12]

The MP for South Suffolk, Tim Yeo, had foreseen the doubtful reliability of the Secretary of State's apparent policies and statements. Even prior to the White Paper, Patricia Hewitt had referred to the importance of community hospitals, at the Labour conference at Brighton. She had stated that 'what people want are good local hospitals'.[13] Given that his own community hospital was facing closure, he had thought 'her words were unbelievable – we just hope they were not words by the seaside'.[14]

It seemed too late. Many local primary care trusts had the bit between the teeth. They were determined to get rid of their community hospitals. The White Paper seemed to make no difference. The NHS continued in its headlong rush to close down local hospitals and associated services and to sell off valuable capital assets in the search for short-term savings. This was to stave off the wrath of Patricia Hewitt's financial hit squads of accountants, brought in from private consultancy firms to 'turnaround' the NHS trusts in financial trouble.

11 Graham Dines, 'Our hospitals seem doomed.' *East Anglian Daily Times*, 31 January 2006.

12 Mark Gould, 'No closure on campaigns to save cottage hospitals.' *Health Service Journal*, 23 February 2006.

13 'Yeo takes Hewitt to task over local hospital closures.' *Sudbury Mercury*, 14 October 2005.

14 Dave Gooderham, 'MP takes health boss to task over hypocrisy.' *East Anglian Daily Times*, 12 October 2005.

The Secretary of State did go through the motions of saying she would support her own White Paper, announcing that another set of 'hit squads' would meet the heads of strategic health authorities to ensure that community hospitals were not improperly closed.[15] But the SHAs seemed to lack the will. In West Suffolk, weeks after the PCT had taken the decision to close its community hospital beds and begun to make arrangements to do so, it was discovered that the SHA had not yet tested or approved its proposals. The PCT had purported to proceed regardless.

When the SHA finally did conclude its appraisal, it fully approved the PCT's proposals. The manner in which it did so, effectively by filling in a series of boxes – seemingly by rote – appeared highly unsatisfactory. The SHA appeared simply to have taken the PCT's word for everything, and not genuinely to have listened to, or taken seriously, any other voices. However, the content of the completed boxes bore little relation to what the local community saw was happening in reality – or to what the White Paper apparently demanded concerning the involvement of the local community.

Much of what the SHA concluded was at the very least contentious; certainly the evidence for its conclusions was not obvious. Some of it was plain wrong. For instance, the SHA referred to an analysis of local responses to the consultation by CLEAR – a consultancy that had analysed the responses in the east of Suffolk. However, CLEAR had had nothing to do with the west of Suffolk. In all, it seemed to be a whitewash.[16]

It was a contest between logic, long-term planning, local services and patient care on the one hand – and short-term financial savings driven by panic and fear on the other. It was of course no contest at all. Within a month, the BBC reported that despite government statements, local community hospitals remained under serious threat.[17] In March 2006, *Public Finance* carried an article, entitled 'Community scare', confirming this.[18] The article seemed in part to be prompted by the long list of threatened hospitals which at that time was roughly as follows:[19]

15 Jo Revill, 'Hit squads aim to save community hospitals.' *Observer*, 19 February 2006.

16 Dr Norman Pinder. *Suffolk West Community Hospitals proposals: assessment for White Paper compliance.* Agenda item 17c. Cambridge: Norfolk, Suffolk and Cambridgeshire Strategic Health Authority, 28 June 2006.

17 Jane Dreaper, 'Community hospital battles continue.' *News.bbc.co.uk*, 17 February 2006.

18 Tash Shifrin, 'Community scare.' *Public Finance*, 17 March 2006.

19 List kindly supplied by Helen Tucker.

Avon, Gloucestershire and Wiltshire SHA

- Bradford-on-Avon Hospital
- Westbury Hospital
- Melksham Community Hospital
- Trowbridge Community Hospital
- Devizes Community Hospital
- Warminster Hospital
- Malmesbury Community Hospital
- Tetbury Hospital
- Cossham Hospital
- Moreton-in-Marsh Hospital
- Moore Cottage Hospital, Bourton-on-the-Water
- Fairford Hospital
- Thornbury Hospital

Cumbria and Lancashire SHA

- Alston Cottage Hospital
- Cockermouth Hospital
- Millom Hospital
- Brampton War Memorial Community Hospital
- Keswick Community Hospital
- Maryport Hospital
- Penrith Hospital
- Workington Community Hospital
- Pendle Community Hospital, Nelson

Hampshire and Isle of Wight SHA

- Emsworth Hospital
- Fordingbridge Hospital
- Romsey Hospital
- Milford War Memorial Hospital
- Havant War Memorial Hospital
- Alton Community Hospital

- Andover War Memorial Hospital
- Fenwick Hospital
- Hythe Hospital

Norfolk, Suffolk and Cambridgeshire SHA

- Hartismere Hospital
- Aldeburgh and District Community Hospital
- Felixstowe General Hospital
- Bartlet Hospital
- Newmarket Hospital
- Walnuttree Hospital, Sudbury
- St Leonards Hospital, Sudbury
- Doddington Hospital

Surrey and Sussex SHA

- Weybridge Community Hospital
- Cranleigh Community Village Hospital
- Farnham Community Hospital
- Dorking Hospital
- Emberbrook Care Centre, Thames Ditton

North and East Yorkshire and Northern Lincolnshire SHA

- Hornsea Cottage Hospital
- Withernsea Community Hospital
- Alfred Bean Hospital
- Bridlington Hospital
- Whitby Hospital

Trent SHA

- Skegness Hospital
- Newholme Hospital
- Cavendish Hospital, Buxton

Shropshire and Staffordshire SHA

- Ludlow Community Hospital
- Bridgnorth Hospital
- Whitchurch Hospital

South West Peninsula SHA

- Moretonhampstead Hospital
- Okehampton Community Hospital

Thames Valley SHA

- Townlands Hospital, Henley
- Bicester Community Hospital

Kent and Medway SHA

- Sittingbourne Memorial Hospital
- Edenbridge and District War Memorial Hospital

Dorset and Somerset SHA

- Clevedon Hospital
- South Petherton Hospital

West Midlands South SHA

- Evesham Community Hospital

The government's own White Paper stated that community hospitals should not be closed (or run down) to make short-term savings – unless they were not clinically viable or local people did not want to use them.[20] Accordingly and predictably, ever ready to circumvent a new rule, PCTs teemed out of the woodwork and argued that their local hospitals were not clinically viable – although they could scarcely argue that people did not want to use them.

Central government lent a hand in this when the acting Chief Executive of the NHS disingenuously – or ignorantly – stated that it was amazing how hospitals 'in the worst possible workhouse conditions' suddenly became the

20 Secretary of State for Health (2006) *Our Health, Our Care, Our Say*. Cm 6737. London: HMSO, para 6.42.

'best loved in the community' when threatened with closure.[21] He did not apparently pause to think that the reason why they were loved might have been because they provided valued and effective services. Nor that, in most instances, people were not being offered any, or at least comparable, alternatives. And so the Department of Health just denied it all, referring to the 'bright future' of community hospital services.[22] The government mantra seemed now to be that all community hospitals were old and that all old hospitals were not clinically viable.

This was derisory. Not only of course had many community hospitals long been loved for the high standard of local care they provided, but the PCTs were anyway being indiscriminate. They were targeting modern community hospitals as well. For instance, Potters Bar community hospital, barely 10 years old, was to lose 15 out of 45 beds.[23]

Withington Community Hospital had only been officially opened in September 2006 at a cost of £19.5 million. A year later, the South Manchester PCT was concerned about its viability because of under-use of the surgical facility at the hospital. This situation apparently posed a financial risk to the PCT of some £600,000 per annum. However, the reason for this state of affairs was in the form of an apparently absurd, vicious circle. This was that the PCT itself would not fund the hospital to perform more operations and so reduce the waiting lists. It was thus a catch-22 situation.[24]

Down in Wiltshire, the mayor pointed at the plaque on the hospital in Westbury showing its opening year, '1989'. A stroke rehabilitation unit was added five years ago: 'if it was good enough to invest in then, what's wrong with it now?'[25] A bemused patient (and journalist), who had just had a cataract operation in the Westbury hospital, noted:

> I was so struck by the friendly atmosphere and the speed and efficiency with which the operation was completed... Westbury seemed an absolute model of everything the NHS should be. I was then told that, thanks to a shock decision, the hospital was being closed down – starting the following week with the removal of its 12 elderly in-patients. Unsurprisingly, news of the closure provoked uproar. A

21 Graham Dines, 'Sort it out yourselves.' *East Anglian Daily Times*, 13 April 2006.

22 Dave Gooderham, 'Hospital protestors join in March.' *East Anglian Daily Times*, 21 March 2006.

23 James Clappison, MP, Hertsmere *Hansard*, House of Commons Debates, 5 July 2006, column 827.

24 Emma Scott, 'Hospital is a financial risk to NHS.' *South Manchester Reporter*, 20 April 2006.

25 Cassandra Jardine, 'The government wants community hospitals to be a template for health care in the 21st century. So why are 80 of them still under threat?' *Daily Telegraph*, 16 February 2006.

> thousand people met to protest. Friends of the hospital have in recent years raised £1 million to improve its services.[26]

Likewise, Newmarket Hospital in West Suffolk was a modern building, but still stood to lose its beds. And the whole dispute in Sudbury, Suffolk, concerning the loss of community hospital beds and outpatient services, was about a planned new community hospital, not the old workhouse buildings.

In any case, as 2006 wore on so did the paradox. Community hospitals, old or new, continued to be threatened and closed – essentially by a government and NHS claiming to be committed to community hospitals. All Hallows Hospital at Ditchingham in Norfolk was informed in July about a severe cut in funding that would put the charitable hospital's future at risk – despite its provision of terminal, rehabilitative, respite and post-acute care.[27]

In Yorkshire, the chief executive had, it was claimed, 'halved, literally overnight' the beds at Castleberg and Ripon community hospitals, reducing them to a figure below the level of historical demand. In Surrey, it was reported that the general hospital was losing its status rapidly, and the three community hospitals were being 'starved of revenue'. Patients were being sent home, on arguably unsafe discharges. Doddington community hospital in Cambridgeshire had just lost two inpatient bed units. Three wards were threatened in the Brookfields hospital, also in Cambridgeshire. Down in Kent, services were threatened at the Sevenoaks, Edenbridge and Tonbridge Hospitals. Buckland Hospital in Dover stood to have its basic services stripped away. Westbury and Bradford on Avon had already lost services in Wiltshire; Warminster, Melksham and Trowbridge continued to be threatened. Grantham community hospital, it was announced in June 2006, would lose all acute surgery, the consultant-led A&E department, and critical care.[28]

And the Suffolk PCTs – well they gave the impression of barely glancing up from their efforts to close or cut back community hospital services across the county.

26 Christopher Booker, 'Hospitals must go, to pay for the managers to close them.' *Sunday Telegraph*, 12 March 2006.

27 'Hospital faces survival fight.' *East Anglian Daily Times*, 17 July 2006, p.14.

28 *Hansard*, House of Commons Debates, 5 July 2006, columns 817–832.

Over the hills, down the dales and all round the houses: chasing the disappearing health services

By 2006 the government had firmly committed itself to what it called a new generation of community hospitals, a policy spelt out in its White Paper of 2006.

In July, the government issued a further policy document, referring again to the new generation of community hospitals in which it would be investing. To take the document at face value was to be seduced into believing in a seventh heaven, underpinned by community hospitals responsive to the needs of local communities. It was full of the familiar feelgood jargon and aspiration about choice, diversity, suiting everybody's needs, facilitating rehabilitation by adjusting the way in which NHS tariff payments work, making people feel they are in control of their own health and care, hubs, patient journeys and pathways, community ventures (run as a commercial enterprise but on a not for profit basis). And so on.[29]

However, quite apart from the widespread attack on existing community hospitals, other indications suggested that the policy was not all that it might have seemed. As the chairperson of Community Hospitals Acting Nationally Together (CHANT) remarked:

> The NHS Plan in 2000, the 2003 policy document, *Keeping the NHS local*, and the recent white paper all promised to save community facilities. None have stopped the relentless closure of community beds and services.[30]

Further suspicions arose, in Parliament and elsewhere. At the same time as investment in community hospitals was being announced, the Department of Health had been talking of the possible downgrading or closure of district general hospitals. MPs were amongst those onlookers raising the following question:

> Does the Secretary of State envisage that at the end of this process – at the end of her vision – there will be more community hospitals than the Government inherited? Can she also clarify whether she will be counting in her total figure former district general hospitals such as Frenchay hospital, which will be reduced to a community hospital? Will we find that the Secretary of State comes back to the House to tell

29 *Our health, our care, our community: investing in the future of community hospitals and services.* London: Department of Health, 2006.

30 'Community hospital closures on hold after funding boost.' *Nursing Times*, 11 July 2006, p.5.

> us that she has opened Frenchay community hospital, while overlooking the fact that she has closed a district general hospital?[31]

In other words, it seemed as if district general hospitals might be rebadged as community hospitals – with possibly a net loss, rather than an increase, of local services.

In West Suffolk, for instance, there was particular concern about the district general hospital in Bury St Edmunds being closed down or at least diminished. This was in response to the acting NHS Chief Executive, Sir Ian Carruthers, referring to possible closures – particularly in areas of high deficit such as East Anglia.[32]

Two months later, the BBC was reporting that at least ten major hospitals in England faced closure or downgrading – with more set to be affected. Even the NHS Confederation admitted that acute care could end up centralised and in too few hospitals.[33] The downgrading, 'rebadging' or closure of district general hospitals and the closure of local community hospitals could mean that both specialist services (increasingly regionalised) and basic services would be further away. In effect, the complete opposite of what government policy was saying about having enhanced local health services.

This could lead to situations where people are seriously penalised in terms of travel, time, fatigue and money. It could increasingly mean that long trips are no longer the exception. For instance, an 87-year-old cancer patient living in Wales was facing 500 miles of travel each week for treatment in Cheltenham. In another case, a husband took his wife to Cheltenham to receive cancer treatment – a total of 7,000 miles, 210 hours of travel and £750 in petrol costs.[34]

The context is not just rural. For instance, in Leeds the potential removal of renal services from Leeds General Infirmary would mean longer journeys – many on public transport – for very sick patients.[35] It was feared that even helicopters for sick babies might be required if maternity services were centralised in Greater Manchester.[36]

31 Steve Webb, MP, Northavon. *Hansard*, House of Commons Debates, 5 July 2006, column 821.

32 Dave Gooderham, 'Hospital's closure is unlikely: consultant.' *East Anglian Daily Times*, 26 June 2006.

33 Nick Triggle, 'Doubts over future hospitals.' *News.bbc.co.uk*, 18 August 2006.

34 Steven Morris, 'Cancer patient, 87, forced to travel five hundred miles a week.' *Guardian*, 4 April 2006.

35 Debbie Leigh, 'Patients in pledge to challenge cutbacks.' *Leeds Evening Post*, 3 February 2006.

36 Caroline Jack, 'Axed wards win reprieve.' *Manchester Metro News*, 23 June 2006.

It wasn't just specialist services. Throughout 2006 many local people would point to the real and obvious risk of avoidable deaths occurring if local A&E departments are withdrawn. By July 2006, it wasn't just local people. The British Association for Emergency Medicine referred to the increasing rate of closure. The result was that some patients were being 'left miles from essential services' and would be put at risk. In addition, the logic was highly questionable because hospitals had invested in A&E departments in order to meet government-set waiting times. One NHS manager effectively agreed with the Association's view that the motive was to save money. The manager referred to a 'slash and burn policy going on just so the government can keep its promise' – for the NHS to break even by March 2007. He concluded that these cutbacks were not in the best interests of either patients or the health service generally.[37]

Likewise, in Grampian, a unanimous vote by NHS Grampian meant that four rural hospitals would lose their maternity services. For some mothers, this would mean journeys of up to 60 miles to Aberdeen Maternity Hospital, unless they chose to have their babies at home. Access problems would be exacerbated by people on benefits not having easy access to transport, not to mention snow.[38] Even in tamer Suffolk, an hour's long, bumpy bus trip round the villages – from Sudbury to Bury St Edmunds (or longer for some people, who might require two buses) – followed by an uphill walk at the other end – could prove daunting and difficult for frail, older people.[39] Even for those with cars, parking at the hospital in Bury was all but impossible (it had been proposed that consultant outpatient clinics be withdrawn from Sudbury, to the district general hospital at Bury).

Beyond the bricks and mortar of local hospitals

Central government and local PCTs would tend to accuse local action groups of being sentimentally wedded to buildings and not concentrating on services. In fact, the reverse was the case. For the NHS, if it was a slightly older community hospital building – or even if it wasn't – it must be bad. It was the NHS that had got hung up on buildings and lost sight of what it should have been evaluating, empirically, in each individual case – namely the effectiveness of services against local population need. The Suffolk West

37 Nick Triggle, 'NHS cash crisis hitting A&E units.' *News.bbc.co.uk*, 9 July 2006.

38 Frank Urquhart, 'Fears over maternity unit closures across Grampian.' *The Scotsman*, 2 August 2006.

39 Nicki Harvey, 'Yeo calls on health chiefs to try the bus.' *Suffolk Free Press*, 14 July 2006.

PCT would refer to misconceptions and claim that the discussion seemed to be about the hospital building rather than the services.[40]

Yet, it was the other way around. The local community were not bothered about losing the old hospital building; they were concerned that local people should have appropriate services, some of which would quite rightly be in their own homes, but some of which would need to be in the community hospital.[41] In order to understand the issues, you have to look beyond the building – as a local nurse and historian implied in the title of her book, *Beyond the bricks of Walnuttree Hospital Sudbury.*[42]

This all begged the question as to just how and why these community hospitals had operated hitherto, if they were so clinically flawed. But, in any case, even where buildings were not up to the job any more, a measured approach to change could have been proposed. This would first of all have ensured that alternative, modern community hospitals – together with community intermediate care services – were available, before closures took place. It would have been a gradual change. The unseemly, destructive rush of so many PCTs was quite the opposite and amounted in some people's view to sheer recklessness. As ever, it fell to local residents, at a public meeting, to state the obvious:

> old fashioned care is better than no care at all.[43]

Similarly, replacing a ferry before a new bridge is built seemed absurd, especially as it was not clear whether the bridge could span the distance:

> Would it not be ludicrous if a local authority proposed replacing a ferry across a river or between an island and the mainland with a bridge, and then scrapped the ferry before building the bridge? Yet that is precisely what Suffolk West PCT is proposing by taking away our current healthcare provision before introducing an untried new model in a time of diminishing resources, and in an area with a growing population and poor transport links.[44]

40 Barbara Eeles, 'Have your say on future of health care.' *Suffolk Free Press,* 18 August 2005.

41 Walnuttree Hospital Action Committee, 'The state of our health services in Sudbury.' Notice. *Suffolk Free Press,* 8 June 2005.

42 Phyllis Felton (2006) *Beyond the bricks of Walnuttree Hospital Sudbury.* Sudbury: private publication. Available from Tourist Information, Sudbury.

43 D. Green, 'Health bosses challenged on hospital axe.' *East Anglian Daily Times,* 7 October 2005.

44 R. Anthony Platt, 'PCT's community care plan wasn't convincing.' Letter. *East Anglian Daily Times,* 5 May 2006.

Community hospitals have fulfilled a tremendously important role, particularly, but not only, in more rural areas. As Boris Johnson, MP, pointed out, community hospitals were relied upon by local people, provided recuperation and relieved the pressure on general hospitals. Why, then, close them?[45]

In Sudbury, Suffolk, Dr Donnelly, a prominent local GP and Chairman of the League of Friends of Walnuttree Hospital, was in no doubt about the value of community hospitals and their beds (in 2004, 25 of the 68 beds were GP referral beds):

> If someone is not extremely ill, but not well enough to be left at home, we can admit them to Walnuttree, where they are under our care and where we can keep an eye on them. These beds are not for the acutely ill and are used in cases of respite, recovery and investigatory work.

Without them people would have unnecessarily to be referred to the acute hospital.[46]

Attacking community hospitals in Suffolk: the PCTs lead the field

Notwithstanding the views of local clinicians, Suffolk would epitomise the events occurring more widely across the country. The PCTs not only hit the ground running a mere month or two after the general election; but the extremeness of their proposals would also set the tone. It was as if they were determined to lead the field.

In the East, the Hartismere and Bartlet hospitals were targeted for rapid closure. In the West of Suffolk, the PCT abandoned without ceremony the carefully laid plans for a new Sudbury community hospital. This was even though it would have been completely in line with the forthcoming White Paper, containing inpatient beds for rehabilitation and recuperation. It also proposed to close down rapidly the two existing community hospitals in Sudbury, and that consultant outpatient clinics should retreat to Bury St Edmunds, leaving sometimes long and difficult journeys for patients. The rehabilitation beds at Newmarket Hospital would all be shut.

In fairness to Suffolk West PCT, the abandonment of assurances, promises, undertakings – whatever you choose to call them – was not peculiar to it. Such about-turns had come to characterise NHS decision-

45 Boris Johnson, 'Hewitt and her appointees are bad news for our hospitals and health.' *Daily Telegraph*, 13 October 2005.

46 Patrick Lowman, 'Doctors in fight to save hospital.' *East Anglian Daily Times*, 16 November 2004.

making on a much a wider scale. Abandoned assurances about the future of community hospitals are commonplace at local level. As one MP complained:

> Is the Secretary of State aware that at a public meeting last September in my constituency, which I chaired, her local NHS officials told that Red House Hospital – that is Harpenden Memorial Hospital – was safe, but that eight months later they announced it was to close all beds to save £1 million a year?[47]

All this was of course counter to the notion of having local services. It went further. A Parliamentary Command Paper had spoken of fast access to local emergency care.[48] Yet Suffolk West PCT had also scrapped the plans for a local minor injuries unit, which had been planned for the now abandoned new community hospital.

The Suffolk West PCT seemed to be acting without rhyme, reason or logic. To all appearances, it had torn up and disowned its own carefully laid and evidenced plans, swallowing without murmur the financial imperative to make short-term savings. According to the PCT itself, the community hospitals in West Suffolk were not the cause of the recurrent overspend.[49] Thus, at most, the savings achieved by closing the Sudbury hospitals would seem to represent no more than an extremely short-term sticking plaster – at the cost of losing a range of local services serving a population in excess of 50,000. As for published government policy, election manifestos and evidence-based practice, they appeared to fall by the wayside.

National rebellion over community hospitals

By Christmas 2005, a national organisation had been created, called Community Hospitals Acting Nationally Together (CHANT). At short notice, it campaigned vigorously to save the community hospitals threatened across England. The supreme irony of this campaign was that CHANT was arguing three main planks of government policy, all of which were epitomised by community hospitals: care closer to home, local services and patient choice. Yet CHANT was campaigning, ultimately, against central

47 Peter Lilley, MP, Hitchin and Harpenden. *Hansard*, House of Commons Debates, 5 July 2006, column 824.

48 Secretary of State for Health (2002) *Delivering the NHS Plan: next steps on investment, next steps on reform.* Cm 5503. London: HMSO, para 5.9.

49 *Modernising Health Care in West Suffolk: consultation, 1 August – 31 October 2005.* Bury St Edmunds: Suffolk West PCT, 2005, p.5.

government, which was allowing, and even encouraging, widespread closures that flatly contradicted its own policy.

Nonetheless, central government was in no mood to listen to local voices, reason, its own White Paper or CHANT. This was despite the fact that on 28 March 2006 there was a record of 44 individual petitions (concerning just one issue) submitted to the House of Commons about community hospital reductions and closures.[50] There followed a rally of hundreds of people in London on 28 March 2006, organised on behalf of all the community hospitals in England facing cuts and closures.

By that date 300,000 signatures had been collected across the country protesting against the cuts to community hospitals. The Joint League of Friends of North Cumbria alone presented a petition to Downing Street of 69,381 signatures relating to the nine community hospitals under threat in the Cumbria and Lancashire SHA.[51]

Central government could not help but betray signs of the contradictions by which it was riven, and which were sowing such local discord. On the one hand, responding to pressure from CHANT and others, Lord Warner, a health minister, issued a press release on 28 March referring to the bright future of community hospitals. He reiterated that community hospitals should not be lost to short-term budgetary pressures, and – almost surreally – said that it was a 'myth' that community hospitals needed to be closed to save money.[52] Yet, a mere two weeks later, Sir Ian Carruthers, NHS Chief Executive, was dismissive of the fuss about community hospitals.[53]

The absurdity of this full-scale assault on community hospitals was best summed up perhaps by New Forest MP, Julian Lewis. He pointed out that closure of such hospitals would mean it 'will cost more money to provide a worse service'. The supply of services in rural areas 'is likely to be grossly inefficient and inadequate...which is why the network of small hospitals evolved in the first place'. Furthermore, their closure would cause more bed blocking in general hospitals, and the financial crisis would not be significantly diminished by closing such hospitals since they 'cost only a tiny

50 Graham Stuart, MP, and Others. *Hansard*, House of Commons Debates, 28 March 2006, columns 819–823.

51 'One thousand campaigners from across the country attended a rally in Westminster yesterday to protest against closures and cutbacks to community hospitals.' News release, 29 March 2006. London: CHANT (Graham Stuart, MP, Chair, House of Commons).

52 Lord Warner. Press release, 28 March 2006. London: Department of Health.

53 Graham Dines, 'Sort it out yourselves.' *East Anglian Daily Times*, 13 April 2006.

fraction of the sums and deficits involved'. Referring to the reorganisation of PCTs:

> Finally it is worth noting that the PCT responsibilities for such matters such as these are due to change in the next few months. It is outrageous that a body with such an atrocious financial record with a serious question mark over its future, should seek to bring about the headlong destruction of inpatient facilities for no viable financial savings and in the name of a half-baked philosophy of care in the home which will undoubtedly be discredited sooner rather than later.[54]

Another voice raised in concern was that of Linda Nazarko, a consultant nurse and visiting lecturer:

> It is cold and dark. We are expecting very cold weather. There is a shortage of flu vaccine and an epidemic is predicted. People are falling ill and the hospitals are crammed to capacity... Acute hospitals are closing beds, freezing posts, cutting back on agency staff and even making staff redundant in order to save money. Yet many people considered medically fit may not be well enough to go home. Community hospitals can help ease these pressures... They offer sub-acute care so that acute hospitals can discharge quicker, and provide ongoing rehabilitation following illness or injury and high-quality palliative care... However, now it seems that PCTs may close up to 100 community hospitals to save money.[55]

Ripping the heart and history out of local communities

Another reason why community hospitals are so loved and also provide a high standard of care is that often they have sprung from, and been supported by, local people. They tend also to have stable, dedicated workforces drawn from the local community. That is why it is so difficult for government ministers and local primary care trusts to convince the local communities that it is all for the best simply to shut them down without more ado.

For instance, in Felixstowe both the Bartlet and Cottage Hospitals had been 'gifted in perpetuity' to the people of Felixstowe by Dr Bartlet and Mr Croydon respectively. At a local meeting, the latter's granddaughter had substantiated the latter's wishes. How, then, could the PCT contemplate selling

54 Quoted in *Challenge, Community Hospitals Association Newsletter*, Issue 45, 2005, p.4.

55 L. Nazarko, 'It is the worst possible time for cuts in the NHS.' *Nursing Times*, 3 January 2006, p.13.

the properties, thereby 'contravening the two gentlemen's wishes'?[56] Mr Croydon had given the Croydon Cottage Hospital in 1909 to the people of Felixstowe. It then consisted of ten beds, to serve a population of some 1840 people. In 2005, with a population of 33,000, the hospital was to be closed.[57]

Adding insult to injury, it transpired that Dr Bartlet had originally left £250,000 for the building of a convalescent and rehabilitation unit in Felixstowe. It cost only £100,000 to build. So, in 1923, the Court of Chancery set up the Bartlet Trust Fund containing £150,000. With interest, this would have been worth millions of pounds by 2006. But by then, the NHS could not say what had happened to the fund. It had simply vanished from sight, swallowed up without trace.[58]

In Sudbury in Suffolk, after the war, the town with a population of some 9000 was served by two hospitals, Walnuttree and St Leonards. The latter was built mainly with money transferred by the Charities Commission from an old leper home dating back to the reign of Edward II. However, local people had paid for the running of the hospital through voluntary subscriptions of a few pence a week, together with fundraising through fetes, regattas and gala days. In 1948, the town effectively gifted the hospital to the state. The implications, by 2005, had at last become clear:

> The local people who turned out to see the Princess Helen Louise open the new wing of St Leonards Hospital in Sudbury, Suffolk, in 1938 would not have recognised the term 'stakeholder', but they would have seemed to have fitted perfectly Tony Blair's vision of a breed of socially responsible citizens helping to run the country's public services... It has taken the Blair government, for all its blather about 'stakeholding' and for all the billions it has ploughed into the NHS, to rob the town of a hospital for the first time in 140 years... Plans for a brand new hospital...have been scaled down to a 'glorified GP surgery'.[59]

By contrast, during the postwar period, a wide range of services and other facilities had been available in Sudbury. For example, at Walnuttree Hospital, these included at one time up to 220 beds (in 1946) reducing to 140 beds (in 1959), accommodation for nurses (Stour House, sold in 1990), a nurse

56 B. Adams, 'How can hospitals sale benefit townsfolk?' *East Anglian Daily Times*, 19 January 2006.

57 Gill Ib, 'Our vanishing hospitals.' Letter. *Spectator*, 24 September 2005.

58 'Bartlet: thousands missing.' *East Anglian Daily Times*, 8 August 2006, p.16.

59 Ross Clark, 'Fear in the community.' *Spectator*, 17 September 2005.

training school (closed in 1970), acute wards, long-stay beds (for both 'chronic' and 'able-bodied' people), a range of outpatient clinics, day hospital and so on. Meanwhile over at St Leonards, there were during the 1960s some 20 general beds (including those for children), 13 maternity beds, a casualty unit run by GPs, an operating theatre, an X-ray department, various outpatients clinics, and a home for nurses (sold, now Hill Lodge Hotel).[60]

This gives a flavour. And it was not just sentimentality for the past. The hard facts were that in 2005, with a vastly increased population (50,000 covering Sudbury and the surrounding area), the Suffolk West PCT's proposals were to close both hospitals, close all beds (although only 68 were now remaining), and transfer all the consultant outpatient clinics away from Sudbury.[61] Is it any wonder that statements about modernisation and improvement – from an NHS body in severe financial deficit and disarray – should have fallen on so many unbelieving local ears?

60 Thanks for this information are due to Phyllis Felton, author in 2006 of *Beyond the Bricks of the Walnuttree Hospital* (Private publication. Available from Sudbury Tourist Information, Town Hall, Market Hill, Sudbury, Suffolk CO10 1TL), and Barry Wall, local historian and author of *Sudbury: history and guide.* Stroud: Tempus, 2004.

61 *Modernising Health Care in West Suffolk: consultation, 1 August – 31 October 2005.* Bury St Edmunds: Suffolk West PCT, 2005.

7

Choosing the Method of Cultivation: Patient Choice

The term 'patient choice' was becoming more and more prevalent in New Labour's discourse. By 2005 and 2006, it had risen to a crescendo. It appeared closely allied to the idea of comparison and 'contestability' between health-care providers – not just NHS providers but also the independent sector. In other words, it was going to be about opening up the NHS to market forces and competition.

Taken at its barest, this notion of choice represented a departure from the core principles of the NHS. The Beveridge report on *Social Insurance and Allied Services* of 1942, Aneurin Bevan's White Paper on the NHS of 1944, and the NHS Acts of 1946 and 1977 did not talk about choice – but need (see Chapter 2).

Of course, if need remains the main focus but, in addition, we are given extra choices, we are unlikely to complain – although questions could be raised about whether any extra expenditure involved would be justifiable and whether people would wish to pay more tax in this connection. The Audit Commission has raised such issues in relation to local council social services.[1] However, this does not appear to be what central government had in mind.

First, this idea of patient choice and consumerism tends to be linked with the more able among us, generally or at any particular time. That is, those of us with the physical and mental capacity to choose, as well as with

1 *Choosing well: analysing the costs and benefits of choice in local public services.* London: Audit Commission, 2006, Summary.

the time and inclination. Indeed, the extension of choice, typically taken up by the better informed and educated, might tend to increase inequality.[2]

Second, there was considerable irony that New Labour appeared to be forcing patient choice on people, when the evidence was unclear as to whether people wanted that choice. In other words, what many, indeed most, people wanted appeared to be good local health services.[3]

Third, it was uncertain whether, in this brave new world, it would be consumers or central government (aided by the independent sector) who would be choosing what was good and viable by way of health care. To all appearances it was going to be the latter who would decide which hospitals and other health services remained or went to the wall. This would be according to what targets, clinical and financial, had been set and met. Local people's choice would seem not to count. This would be not least because there would be no mechanisms for democratic local control.[4]

Taking the above points, the disparity between New Labour's idea of choice and that of patients seemed only too apparent. By early 2005, New Labour in its general election manifesto had boasted that its 'one principle' was 'putting patients centre stage. And extending patient power and choice is crucial to achieving this.'[5] But, as it entered its third period of power, the government lost little time in exposing its own manifesto and itself to complete ridicule. By the end of the year, hospitals and wards closed, and demonstrations, anger and petitions spread across the country. Forcing local communities into truly bitter fights with the local NHS – fights born mainly of fear and anger – was a truly perverse way of delivering patient choice.

Meeting, marching and petitioning

Already by September 2005, some 5000 marchers presented a 20,000 signature petition protesting against the closure of a 26-bed ward in Stamford Hospital and the possible total closure of the hospital. The Peterborough and Stamford NHS Foundation Trust was some £8 million in debt.[6]

2 David Lipsey, 'Too much choice.' *Prospect*, December 2005, p.26.

3 Secretary of State for Health (2006) *Our Health, Our Care, Our Say: a new direction for community services.* Cm 6737. London: HMSO, p.15.

4 Allyson Pollock (2005) *NHS plc: the privatisation of our health care.* London: Verso, p.83.

5 *Labour Party Manifesto: Britain forward not back.* London: Labour Party, 2005, p.63.

6 'Marchers fight hospital closure.' *News.bbc.co.uk*, 10 September 2005.

In November, problems were surfacing up the East coast. The Queen Elizabeth hospital at Kings Lynn faced cutbacks; in Skegness residents were protesting about closure of a ward in the local cottage hospital; and in East Yorkshire protests were being made about the threat to the minor injuries unit at Hornsea community hospital.[7] The *East Riding Mail* ran a 'Hands off our hospital' campaign, collecting more than 15,000 signatures.[8]

In November, too, hundreds of protestors marched through Oxford to campaign against cuts being implemented across the county to save £34 million.[9] By December, hundreds of protestors were on the streets of Cambridge to oppose £3 million worth of cuts to mental health services.[10] In the same month, the leader of Shropshire County Council vowed to oppose the sudden proposed closure and sale of community hospitals. This was especially as a recent report – from the local PCT no less – had stated that 'community hospitals are both a valued and valuable asset within a large, rural county'.[11]

Into 2006 and these marches – together with petitions – would proliferate up and down the country. In Ludlow, Shropshire, more than 4,000 people marched on a freezing January day at the beginning of 2006. By July, a second march was being held in protest about threatened cuts to services at Ludlow Hospital.[12] In Wellington (Wrekin), 1000 people took to the streets to protest about the mooted removal of A&E services from the Princess Royal Hospital. As the local MP explained, they were fighting not for money, not for wealth but for life.[13]

In northwest Wales, too, 1000 people marched through Llandudno to oppose proposed closure of a ward for mentally infirm elderly people, a coronary care unit and a breast cancer unit.[14] Five thousand uniformed workers, union members and residents protested in the centre of Stoke-on-Trent in April 2006. Attempting to reduce debts of £15 million, the University Hospital of North Staffordshire NHS Trust had planned 1000 job losses. The posts involved were expected to include 15 consultants, 370

7 'Yorkshire and Lincolnshire: your good health?' *News.bbc.co.uk*, 11 November 2005.

8 Graham Stuart, MP. *Hansard*, Westminster Hall, 2 November 2005, column 257WH.

9 'Marchers rally against health cuts and privatisations.' *Socialist Worker*, 26 November 2005.

10 '300 protestors march to fight big health cuts.' *Cambridge Evening News*, 19 December 2005.

11 'County Council to lead campaign against NHS closures.' Press release, 22nd November 2005. Shropshire County Council.

12 Sally Jones, 'New protest at NHS cuts.' *Shropshire Star*, 10 July 2006.

13 'Hospital protest hits the streets.' *Shropshire Star*, 11 March 2006.

14 'Protest march a success.' *Thebestof.co.uk/llandudno*, 24 July 2006.

nurses and 200 nursing assistants. Of these losses, 75 per cent were expected to be compulsory.[15]

Anticipating the worst for St Richard's Hospital in Chichester, 4000 people brought the centre of the town to a halt – mindful of the huge deficit (of some £80–100 million) hanging over the strategic health authority. Sir Patrick Moore, astronomer, highlighted just how intuitive and visceral, literally, such health issues are: 'If we lose it with it's A&E, the people are going to die.'[16] And threats to Stroud Maternity Hospital and Weavers Croft mental health unit brought 3000 people to the streets of Stroud.[17]

In Worthing, some 6000 people marched and converged on Worthing Pavilion for a public meeting about the threat to Worthing and Southlands Hospitals, including accident and emergency services. There were banners waving, fancy dress outfits, and hordes of people of all ages, colours, shapes and sizes. Nine hundred people packed into the Pavilion; a video link relayed the meeting to a large crowd outside. Des Lynam, television presenter, would comment that he had never seen Worthing people 'so cross'. As the local newspaper summed up: 'if the NHS suits think it's all over, they've got another think coming'.[18]

If the Worthing protests were colourful, the people of North Cumbria surely took the biscuit. They staged a remarkable two-day protest – on the roads, streets and waterways – spanning all nine of the towns facing closures and bed cuts: Wigton, Brampton, Alston, Penrith, Keswick, Cockermouth, Maryport, Workington and Millom. A different form of transport was used to pass rings on from town to town, illustrating at the same time the geography and environment of the area – and in effect the potential impact on delivery of health care.

The means included a vintage tractor from Wigton to Brampton, a gyro-copter (planned but not used because of the weather), a bright red VW beetle to Alston, 50 bikers riding Harley-Davidsons and a quad bike over the moors through hail and rain to Penrith – then a carriage drawn by four horses to Keswick. This marked the end of the first day. At the crack of dawn the next day, a lone canoe set off from Derwentwater to Cockermouth. A group of 20 runners then took up the rings on a nine-mile run to Maryport Hospital. From there a group of cyclists went on to Workington. The final

15 'Rally to fight hospital jobs cuts.' *News.bbc.co.uk*, 29 April 2006.

16 'Thousands in NHS cutbacks rally.' *News.bbc.co.uk*, 23 July 2006.

17 'Town rallies against health cuts.' *News.bbc.co.uk*, 10 June 2006.

18 'Thousands join hospital march.' *Worthing Herald*, 3 August 2006.

stage saw classic cars deliver the rings to Millom Cottage Hospital.[19] All this on the back of a petition of some 70,000 names collected by the Friends of North Cumbria.

Gloucestershire was similarly embattled, facing cuts and closures involving the Dilke Hospital, Colliers Court, Lydney Hospital, Stroud Maternity Hospital, Fairford Hospital, Tetbury Hospital, Delancey Hospital, Winchcombe Hospital, Berkeley Hospital, Sandpits Clinic – not to mention ongoing bed reductions at Gloucestershire Royal Hospital and Cheltenham General Hospital. Unsurprisingly, not only did a petition run to many thousands of signatures but 600 protestors from the Forest of Dean chartered a train to take them to Downing Street.[20] Neighbouring Oxfordshire too was under serious assault. From Banbury alone came a petition of 15,000 names. It declared:

> of all the Trusts in England, it is Oxfordshire which receives the lowest funding for treatment per patient. ...the blatant discrimination in the funding system for the NHS is not fair, cannot be justified, and means that in Oxfordshire NHS jobs are under threat, community care is under threat, mental health care is under threat and operations and beds are under threat.[21]

Sometimes people conjured up petitions single-handedly and from nowhere. When mental health day hospitals were threatened in Tooting and Roehampton, a patient and her brother-in-law, who cared for her, swiftly collected 1000 signatures and set about forming a pressure group.[22] The threat to just one mental health ward at Loughborough Hospital elicited a petition of 6000 names; its closure was confirmed anyway. The chief executive of the PCT explained that he wished to shed such services, redirecting them to the independent sector and social services.[23]

Equally, petitions could go to the other end of the scale, and involve tens of thousands of views – not that the sheer weight of opposition tends to make any difference to the response from NHS decision-makers. For instance, the closure of an accident and emergency unit in Monklands,

19 Pamela McGowan, 'Hospital cuts protesters take to the roads and waterways.' *News & Star*, 3 April 2006.

20 'Health campaigners charter train.' *News.bbc.co.uk*, 18 July 2006.

21 Tony Baldry, MP, Banbury. *Hansard*, House of Commons Debates, 22 June 2006, column 1572.

22 Carron Taylor, 'We pose as carer – and expose NHS "closures".' *This is Local London*, 30 June 2005.

23 'Ward to close despite opposition.' *News.bbc.co.uk*, 18 July 2006.

Scotland, attracted 50,000 signatures. The decision was still to close it.[24] In Stockton, North Tees, 20,000 people unsuccessfully opposed the removal of specialist maternity services – despite the fact that the North Tees centre had been opened as a specialist centre only four years earlier, and had millions of pounds invested in it.[25] Even before the march in Llandudno to oppose proposals to cut three key services at the hospital, 17,000 people had signed the petition.[26]

People do not give up. Eighteen months after Crawley Hospital lost its accident and emergency services, the town's Labour MP was part of a delegation that presented a petition of 30,000 names to Patricia Hewitt, Secretary of State for Health.[27]

A strategic health authority debt of £102 million led the local population in Hastings to fear for its accident and emergency, children's, maternity and cardiology services at the Conquest Hospital. This was before even consultation had begun; still, 19,000 signatures had already been collected.[28]

Nor was the campaigning confined to rural areas; the large towns and cities followed too. For example, in the Manchester area, the group Health in Trafford, led by a former a hospital nurse, took judicial review proceedings against the local NHS Trust to resist closure of rehabilitation wards.[29]

The great unrest in Suffolk

Suffolk saw particularly marked agitation as one community after another realised the uncompromising nature of the threats now being levelled against them.

In August 2005, several hundred people attended a public meeting at the Jubilee Hall in Aldeburgh, protesting against the loss of a minor injuries unit and beds. Local people agreed to form an action group and start a letter-writing campaign.[30]

24 Kathleen Nutt, 'Closure of hospital accident unit is a sham, says Reid.' *Sunday Times*, Scotland, 6 August 2006.

25 'Hospital shake-up plans approved.' *News.bbc.co.uk*, 22 February 2006.

26 'Protest march a success.' *thebestof.co.uk/llandudno*, 24 July 2006.

27 'A&E campaign goes to Westminster.' *News.bbc.co.uk*, 31 January 2006.

28 Richard Gladstone, 'Trouble at the Conquest.' *Bexhill Today* (Bexhill-on-Sea Observer), 12 July 2006.

29 Caroline Jack, 'Axed wards win a reprieve.' *Manchester Metro News*, 23 June 2006.

30 Sarah Chambers, 'Action group to fight closure bid: hospital crisis meeting packed.' *East Anglian Daily Times*, 1 August 2005.

Come September and a petition had been launched to save the Violet Hill day hospital in Stowmarket, which provided therapy, medication and other support for people with mental health problems. It was regarded as vital by those using it and their carers. The petition was lauched by a former RAF pilot with obsessive compulsive disorder, who had used the centre for years, and his wife.[31]

In September 2005, too, 15,000 people had signed a petition opposing the plans to close the Bartlet Hospital in Felixstowe and to sell it off for conversion into luxury flats.[32] Back in Aldeburgh, over 400 people attended a public meeting at the parish church, to register their disquiet at the proposed cuts to their hospital – which would mean long journeys (50-mile round trips) to Ipswich Hospital for relatives. Furthermore, they felt that care in people's homes was doubtful because of the shortage of professional carers and the great difficulty in recruiting them.[33]

On 18 September 2005, the Gislingham Silver Band led a march of several hundred people through Eye to protest against the closure of the Hartismere Hospital. Marchers ranged from young children to 91-year-old former patients of the hospital. Over 2000 letters had already been sent to the Suffolk East PCTs in protest.[34] In the same month, over 200 people attended a public protest meeting in Newmarket concerning the closure of all the beds at Newmarket Hospital. The depth of feeling was palpable, summed up by the local MP, Richard Spring:

> This is bureaucracy gone mad. Those who brought this about must know just how angry and dismayed people are, whether they are local residents or hospital staff.[35]

By October, another packed public meeting was held at Stradbroke Community Centre to challenge the PCTs about closure of Hartismere Hospital.[36] And, following up the public meeting of the previous month,

31 John Howard, 'Petition launched in bid to save hospital.' *East Anglian Daily Times*, 14 September 2005.

32 'Thousands sign hospital protest.' *East Anglian Daily Times*, 16 September 2005.

33 Sarah Chambers, 'Packed meeting warned of cuts.' *East Anglian Daily Times*, 17 September 2005.

34 David Lennard, 'Hospital supporters in march against closure.' *East Anglian Daily Times*, 19 September 2005.

35 Lisa Cleverdon, 'Public meeting vows to fight hospital cuts.' *East Anglian Daily Times*, 22 September 2005.

36 David Green, 'Will closures be bad for patients?' *East Anglian Daily Times*, 7 October 2005.

hundreds now marched through Newmarket to oppose the loss of all the beds at Newmarket Hospital.[37]

And so to Sudbury, where activity was as intense and advanced as anywhere. Already in November and December 2004, a successful campaign had been run to save the Walnuttree Hospital from closure. This had been threatened on the basis of a fire risk, the safety and cost implications of which had turned out to have been exaggerated by the West Suffolk NHS Hospitals Trust. A large public meeting of some 500 people had then been convened to show just how deep feelings ran. A 10,000 signature petition had followed. The success of this 2004 campaign was, however, to be shortlived.

In June 2005, another highly charged public meeting took place in response to the renewed threat to close both Sudbury's community hospitals. By November, a march through the town and a second public meeting had taken place. A second petition was delivered to Patricia Hewitt and Tony Blair. The wording was forceful, but the desperate tone of it was suggestive of the vast imbalance in power between local people and all-powerful Secretaries of State and Prime Ministers. The plight of local people in such situations is all too evident, caught as they are between anger and fear on the one hand – and on the other, a feeling of helplessness and even a pleading tone:

> To: Rt. Hon. Tony Blair, Prime Minister
> Rt. Hon. Patricia Hewitt, Secretary of State for Health
>
> 2 November 2005
>
> Saving Sudbury's Health Services
>
> We, the people of Sudbury in Suffolk and the surrounding area, petition and implore you to save our local health services.
>
> We are not Luddites. Like yourselves, we want NHS modernisation. Up to June 2005, we were going to get it. A new community hospital on modern lines had been approved by Suffolk West Primary Care Trust (PCT), the strategic health authority and central government. Then the project was withdrawn literally overnight.
>
> Instead, sudden destruction of Sudbury's health services at Walnuttree and St Leonards Hospitals is now proposed, with no adequate replacement services. This is a slash and burn approach. The new proposals

37 Will Grahame-Clark, 'Hundreds march to stop bed cuts.' *East Anglian Daily Times*, 31 October 2005.

> contain no options. The PCT is simply telling us what will happen. The consultation is a sham. There is no partnership or working with the local community. It is decision-making by diktat.
>
> The services and model of care proposed will not meet local needs. Patient care will suffer. There will be no choice. The proposals will result in greater disability and dependence amongst local people. There will be more acute hospital admissions, and more care home admissions. Local services will be lost, and care will move further away from people's homes. A group of dedicated, experienced and skilled staff will be lost to the NHS and many made redundant.
>
> All this is contrary to government policy and to clinical governance. The PCT's own clinicians are alarmed. The PCT is not modernising. It is imposing an old-fashioned model of care that threatens the health, welfare and lives of elderly, vulnerable and disabled people.
>
> Local people are angry, bewildered but most of all very frightened. Please will you exercise your powers to intervene before it is too late.
>
> People of Sudbury and the Surrounding Area

The Suffolk West PCT would, to the end, deny that there was substance to such views. Nevertheless, across the country, and across Suffolk, patients were clearly expressing their 'choice' in no uncertain terms. To local communities, it appeared that the Secretary of State for Health and her placemen at regional and local level simply didn't want to know.

Ploughing up choice: 'no' means 'yes'

During 2005 and 2006, the PCTs in Suffolk demonstrated graphically how the central government policy of 'patient choice' could end up achieving the exact opposite. It is the sort of demonstration that gives NHS consultation exercises a bad name in local communities. The PCTs may have protested that they had conducted legally acceptable consultations, in a 'proper and robust' fashion as the Suffolk West PCT put it.[38] But there is no gainsaying what local communities felt about the consultations: that they were a sham. It all seemed to depend on what side of the fence you stood.

For instance, in the East of Suffolk, the PCTs employed a marketing consultancy to analyse responses to the PCTs' consultation document. These were overwhelmingly opposed to the PCTs' proposals. Taking not just the

38 Dave Gooderham, 'Legal battle to save beds at hospital.' *East Anglian Daily Times*, 6 June 2006.

responses to the consultation document, but also other representations (including petitions), there were over 30,000 expressions of opinion. Of the formal responses to the consultation, some 90 per cent were opposed to the Suffolk East PCTs' proposals. For example, three separate questions asked people whether they agreed with the proposed developments in Eye, Felixstowe and Aldeburgh. The responses were, respectively, 80 per cent, 89 per cent and 86 per cent opposed – the majority of the rest of the responses constituting 'no opinion'.

But the consultancy gave the PCTs an apparent way out. It explained that the PCTs had drafted the consultation questions poorly. This had, it argued, led people to provide negative answers, which were therefore of limited value. Furthermore there was little way of knowing whether the responses received were representative. Therefore, it went on, the health community would be well advised not to place undue weight on the quantity of opposing views.[39]

How gratefully the Suffolk East PCTs appeared to snatch at this escape route. No wonder, since of the 31,302 responses, 29,541 were contained in petitions that called for the retention of services and hospitals. And of the other responses and letters, the overwhelming majority were also opposed. For good measure, the PCT would also add that the 'difficult and contentious consultation' had been influenced by misconception and anxiety in the local community. From the PCTs' point of view, the consultancy had given them a way out it seemed, and it had been money well spent. Quite how much money, the PCTs refused to disclose, citing commercial confidentiality.[40]

This was true sophistry and was staggering. In effect, it seemed that the consultancy was arguing that the PCTs had fallen into the pitfall of asking straightforward questions and of getting straightforward answers. It was as if such straightforwardness was dangerous and tantamount to heresy in the world of the modern NHS. For good measure, the consultancy would state also that, whether or not the expressions of opinion were representative, the exercise was anyway not a 'public vote'. In fairness, that is true and the Cabinet Office code of practice makes this point. Nonetheless, that does not mean that large-scale opposition should simply be dismissed. In sum, heads or tails, the PCTs would win.

39 *Changing for the Better: next steps, NHS consultation in East Suffolk, Independent Summary and Analysis Report.* London: Clear Communication Consultancy and Training, 2006, p.2.

40 Richard Smith, 'Health trusts set to close hospitals.' *East Anglian Daily Times*, 21 January 2006.

The Chief Executive of the Suffolk East PCTs sought further to downplay the opposition to the closure of the Hartismere and Bartlet hospitals by referring to it as 'strong localised opinion'.[41] This drew a heated response in the newspapers, referring to the 'tens of thousands of impassioned responses', the letters, lobbies, petitions, marches – all of which had amounted to what MPs had described as an unprecedented public response. The writer went on to refer to how exceptionally strong arguments had been used, only for people to feel brushed aside by the reference to a localised response:

> How insulting is that? Can anyone define this word 'localised', narrow and ignorant perhaps? Tell that to the knowledgeable people in the frontline of delivering services, GPs and other professionals who are being treated so disrespectfully... I have no words of comfort for those elderly and vulnerable people I work with daily.[42]

Likewise, it was pointed out that concern about local closures inevitably and quite naturally would be localised. Furthermore, if most responses came from people who had benefited from services, then 30,000 (out of a 360,000 population) is a great number.[43] Another correspondent thanked the *East Anglian Daily Times* for its help in trying to avert mental health closures, but felt it had been a 'waste of time' meeting with the PCTs. This was because, although they promised to 'look at all of our reasons', the writer felt that the PCTs 'knew what was going to happen anyway'.[44]

In the West, the PCT, too, sought in part to explain away the overwhelming opposition to its proposals by stating that its consultation was not a 'referendum or public vote'. In the report provided to the Board for its final decision on 11 April 2006, the extent and the nature of the opposition appeared to be underemphasised. For instance, aware of the existence of some 5500 letters that had been sent to Patricia Hewitt, the PCT failed to acknowledge their existence in the Board papers underpinning its final decision.

41 Carole Taylor-Brown, 'Working hard to offer best local health care.' Letter. *East Anglian Daily Times*, 27 January 2006.

42 Jennie Buckle, 'Stop wasting money, and give us health care.' Letter. *East Anglian Daily Times*, 6 February 2006.

43 M Newell, 'Closures will hit those already vulnerable.' Letter. *East Anglian Daily Times*, 7 February 2006.

44 Thelma Price, 'Meeting with PCTs was a waste of time.' Letter. *East Anglian Daily Times*, 11 February 2006.

Likewise, the opposition of the Patient and Public Involvement Forums (PPIFs) – meant to be representing patients – was not acknowledged. This was especially notable, because the PPIF was mentioned for its role in verifying the analysis of the consultation responses, but not in respect of its trenchant criticisms of the proposals themselves. It seemed as if the PCT was both being highly selective and verging on a disingenuous approach.

Two expert reports full of carefully collated evidence and submitted by the Walnuttree Hospital Action Committee – one produced by independent experts – also gained no mention. Furthermore, some of the key issues raised in the reports were not dealt with in the board papers.

Statistics, in the form of graphs, indicating the extent of the opposition were included in the Appendices to the PCT's Board papers. But nowhere in the main body of the papers was there a simple sentence spelling out and linking the overwhelming nature of that opposition, its degree, its provenance (for example, in terms of expert or representative bodies) and the evidence it cited.[45]

Chorus of disapproval: local councils and voluntary bodies raise their voices

The extent of opposition to the Suffolk PCTs from and on behalf of the public was quite astonishing. That it was in large part disregarded was even more so.

Furthermore, it came not just from tens of thousands of individuals across Suffolk, but also from representative bodies, including many councils and voluntary organisations. The response illustrated the fear and distress, but also expertise and insight, coming not only from individual patients and families, but from both local councils and voluntary organisations.

A joint statement by all the PPI Forums across Suffolk (November 2005) did not hold back. The proposals, it stated, were badly thought out, lacked a factual cost justification and were likely to cause unnecessary pain and suffering to people in need. It went on to suggest that it might all be a cynical exercise in change for change's sake with little thought as to how it would affect those in need and their carers.[46]

45 Michael Stonard (2006) *Modernising Health Care in West Suffolk: report for decision, 11th April 2006.* Bury St Edmunds: Suffolk West PCT.

46 Tim Holland Smith, Joint Statement by all Suffolk PPI Forums. Letter. November 2005.

This statement came from the Forums for Suffolk West PCT, West Suffolk Acute, Suffolk Mental Health, Ipswich Acute, Ipswich PCT, Suffolk Coastal PCT, Suffolk Central PCT, East Anglian Ambulance NHS Trust, and Waveney PCT. The public opposition from local communities across Suffolk had rained in from every direction during the consultation period. The leader of Suffolk County Council, Jeremy Pembroke, stated that the government:

> needs to be aware that, here in Suffolk, there is a widely-held perception that there could be a total collapse of local health services'.[47]

Indeed, a joint group of councillors from the county council and other councils across Suffolk went to London to meet with the health minister, Rosie Winterton.[48] And, following a county council meeting specially on the health services during December, the leader wrote formally to Patricia Hewitt, protesting against the nature of the cuts being imposed and indicating the 'strength of feeling running throughout the county'.[49] The Suffolk Association of Local Councils expressed itself to be really concerned, suggesting that at best the proposed closures were a short-term, knee-jerk reaction. At worst they would inflict substantial damage on the most frail and needy in society.[50]

In East Suffolk, the Stradbroke Parish Council opposed closure of Hartismere Hospital in Eye, being 'emphatic that current services should be extended and not reduced'.[51] Leiston-cum-Sizewell Town Council would send a letter to the Suffolk East PCTs about closures in Aldeburgh, expressing how 'horrified' it was and its strong disagreement.[52] Diss Town Council, Eye Town Council and South Norfolk District Council all registered with the PCTs their opposition to the closure of the Hartismere Hospital.[53]

Chilton Parish Council chairman Peter Clifford predicted the proposals would lead to 'a collapse in adequate health provision, particularly for the elderly'.[54] The Chairman of Suffolk Pensioners warned that:

47 Rebecca Sheppard, 'Health service collapse fear.' *East Anglian Daily Times*, 8 September 2005.

48 Jonathan Barnes, 'Health crisis: a plea to minister.' *East Anglian Daily Times*, 27 October 2005.

49 Jeremy Pembroke, 'Plea for hospital services to health secretary Hewitt.' Letter. *Suffolk Free Press*, 5 January 2006.

50 Jonathan Barnes, 'Health cuts branded.' *East Anglian Daily Times*, 27 August 2005.

51 'Council plea over health service cuts.' *East Anglian Daily Times*, 19 July 2005.

52 Sarah Chambers, 'Concern over bed cuts plan.' *East Anglian Daily Times*, 3 September 2005.

53 'More back NHS fight.' *East Anglian Daily Times*, 2 December 2005.

54 Peter Clifford, Chairman. *Response to Suffolk West Primary Care Trust's Consultation*. Letter/report, 11 December 2005. Sudbury: Chilton Parish Council.

> We are deeply concerned. Suppose your GP says you have to go to hospital but if you are blocked from a hospital bed and consultant care and bundled back into your own bed, you will perhaps not see a nurse or somebody until two days later. You could be dead by then. I think quite honestly that people have already died because of the cutbacks and let's be frank about it, you do not hear all the statistics about death.[55]

The Sudbury Society expressed its disquiet and concern about the closure of all NHS community hospital beds.[56]

Dispersal in the mist: playing down the protests and opposition

In its final report on the consultation exercise, the Suffolk West PCT failed to list all the organisations that had sent in responses. Nor did it explicitly acknowledge the extent of the opposition from clinicians, other health professionals and representative bodies, be they councils or voluntary organisations. By omission, this appeared to be a tactic designed to play down the opposition and its provenance.

The PCT would in other ways appear to undermine the status of the opposition. It would refer to 'strength of emotion' attached to the 'old' model of care. By implication therefore, evidence, reason and modernity lay on the side of the PCT – even though it stated that it had 'been very keen to engage with stakeholders including the public and to listen to their issues and concerns raised'. This suggested condescension for the following reasons.

The PCT had been inundated with evidence. Tremendous expertise lies with patients and their carers who actually experience care, both in hospital and the community. In addition, the PCT received expert evidence – both national and local – from a range of sources, including many of its own clinicians (general practitioners and rehabilitation therapists), as well as expert reports from the Walnuttree Hospital Action Committee. But in its final report to its Board, the PCT made minimal reference to this expert evidence that it had received. Instead, it seemed quietly to damn the opposition

55 Richard Smith, 'Lives at risk in NHS crisis.' *East Anglian Daily Times*, 1 August 2005.

56 Sudbury Society, 'Response by the Sudbury Society Executive Committee'. Letter. December 2005.

collectively and by implication, with those references to 'emotion', and 'strong public feeling'.[57]

Subtly, but most importantly, the PCT did not link the questions and objections raised with particular sources. For instance, it is one thing if doubt about 'care in the community' is raised quite validly by one respondent member of the public. It is quite another if it arises collectively from a group of experienced general practitioners. The PCT made no distinction. Its Board could have no idea by whom particular issues had been raised. The intention of the PCT to play down the authority of opposition cannot be proven; but the effect was achieved nonetheless.

The Suffolk East PCTs did better in one respect. The consultancy employed to analyse the public response did itemise various concerns raised by particular bodies. But it did so in a fragmented way, and there was still no clear overall statement in the relevant Board papers that most – or even all – of these bodies opposed the proposals. Again, this seemed to be a way of playing down the strength of opposition from councils, voluntary bodies, advocacy organisations, patient organisations etc.

Nevertheless, the list speaks for itself in terms of just how widespread was the opposition in the East. The councils listed included:

- Suffolk County Council
- Mid Suffolk District Council
- Suffolk Coastal District Council
- Suffolk Association of Councils
- Felixstowe Town Council
- Hadleigh Council
- Benhall and Sternfield Parish Council
- Eye Town Council
- Aldeburgh Town Council
- Stradbroke Parish Council
- Wickham Skeith Parish Council
- Syleham Town Council
- Old Felixstowe Parish Council
- Woolverstone Parish Council

57 Michael Stonard (2006) *Modernising Health Care in West Suffolk: report for decision, 11th April 2006.* Bury St Edmunds: Suffolk West PCT, p.14.

- Occold Parish Council
- Rickinghall Parish Council
- Friston Parish Council
- Bawdsey Parish Council.

Patient groups and advocacy groups included:

- Suffolk User Forum
- East Suffolk Advocacy Network
- Ipswich Hospital NHS Trust Carers User Group
- Suffolk Coastal Patient Participation Group
- Ipswich Hospital Older People's User Group
- Ipswich Acute PPI Forum and Central Suffolk CPPIH Forum
- Suffolk Rethink Group
- Maternity Services Liaison Committee
- Suffolk Acre
- Hospital Advisory Group.

The voluntary and campaign organisations included:

- Lioness Club of Felixstowe
- Brackenbury Women's Institute
- Eye Women's Institute
- Felixstowe Morning Women's Institute
- Respite
- Felixstowe and District Citizen's Advice Bureau
- Friends of Old Whitwell and Kesgrave Day Hospital
- Sue Ryder Care
- Suffolk Association of Voluntary Organisations
- Royal British Legion (Aldeburgh Branch)
- Save Felixstowe Hospitals Group
- Ipswich and District Council for Voluntary Service
- Heartbeat
- Aldeburgh Hospital Action Group
- League of Friend of Aldeburgh and District Community Hospital

- Suffolk Family Carers
- Hartismere Hospital League of Friends.

Even industry and business organisations expressed opposition, including:

- Hutchinson Ports in Felixstowe
- Felixstowe Port Users Association
- Hollies Enterprise and Hollies Trading
- Wickham Market Partnership.[58]

58 *Changing for the Better: next steps, NHS consultation in East Suffolk, Independent Summary and Analysis Report.* London: Clear Communication Consultancy and Training, 2006, pp.21–27.

8

Alienating and Spreading Fear in the Community

Central government talks of patient choice and local services. Local communities are meant to be involved in local NHS decision-making. The local NHS is meant in some way to be accountable.

Central government issued a specific policy document, entitled *Strengthening Accountability*. It referred to the duty to consult about change with the public under s.11 of the Health and Social Care Act 2001. It stated that real:

> patient and public involvement is not about ticking boxes, it is about NHS organisations developing constructive relationships, building strong partnerships and communicating effectively.

Further, it was about 'designing services with local populations, not for them'.[1] The 2006 White Paper likewise used strong language on this score. It stated that when services were being reconfigured locally, local people should be:

> engaged from the outset in identifying opportunities, challenges and options for change… It is important that the local community feels a real sense of involvement in and ownership of the decision.[2]

1 *Strengthening Accountability: involving patients and the public. Policy guidance, section 11 of the Health and Social Care Act 2001.* London: Department of Health, 2003, pp.2, 7.

2 Secretary of State for Health (2006) *Our Health, Our Care, Our Say: a new direction for community services.* Cm 6737. London: HMSO, para 6.59.

As ever it sounded all too good. All too often the process seemed to be complied with in principle rather than spirit. Local PCTs and NHS trusts take their cue in this respect from the Secretary of State for Health. For the best part of a year Patricia Hewitt batted away all representations made to her about Suffolk – in the form of many thousands of items of postal correspondence, petitions, council delegations and marches. When receiving vigorous protests from local MPs about proposed closures across West Suffolk, she would simply state that she did not want to express a view.[3] Otherwise, she would refer people back to their local PCT, saying that responsibility for local decision-making lay there, and not with her.

Of course, central government may run publicity stunts such as 'a national listening event' in Birmingham at the cost of some £500,000, but local residents are singularly unimpressed. For instance, one local Sudbury resident, who had received an invitation to it, was incensed – given that the continual large-scale protests to the NHS about Walnuttree Hospital had 'fallen on deaf ears'.[4] Actions speak louder than words. Early in 2005, a 2000 signature petition was delivered to the previous Health Secretary about closure of beds at a Cheltenham hospital. A matter of weeks later, it was found 50 miles away in a skip in Oxford.[5]

Similarly, having received over 5500 items of correspondence and a petition of 11,500 signatures from Sudbury over the community hospital closures, the Secretary of State remained unmoved. She even refused to pass down the letters or the petition to the Suffolk West PCT, so that they could be taken account of in the local consultation process. It was of note that, post-general election, any notion of democracy involving some 17,000 expressions of view did not concern the Secretary of State. Yet, pre-election, when a 10,000 signature petition had been delivered about Walnuttree Hospital in November 2004, it was a different story. Then, the previous Secretary of State for Health (John Reid) had written to the prospective local Labour candidate, Kevin Craig, saying:

> Kevin...you have ensured that the voices of local people have been heard at the highest levels of government.

3 Dave Gooderham, 'United in fury at health cuts.' *East Anglian Daily Times*, 20 July 2005.

4 Dave Gooderham, 'Health event attacked as waste of cash.' *East Anglian Daily Times*, 15 October 2005.

5 Ross Clark, 'Fear in the community.' *Spectator*, 17 September 2005.

Even more notably, the Chancellor of the Exchequer was quoted subsequently as congratulating Kevin Craig on his role in the successful hospital campaign.[6]

Even those PCTs who wish to take collaborative working seriously find it difficult to do so when they are ordered instantly to make rapid savings and cuts to services at the whim of central government. Of course it is at such times that it is all the more important that local communities are engaged, so as to explore all options for ameliorating matters and finding solutions. As pointed out by Helen Tucker, an expert on community hospitals:

> Primary care trusts across the country have, until recently, taken seriously their obligation to engage with patients and the public. However, there has been shocked reaction by the public to rapid changes in direction and the abandonment of their involvement. Public engagement needs to be sustained rather than abandoned at this time… Public trust and confidence needs to be gained to support major changes to services.[7]

The Department of Health and NHS bodies would ride roughshod over local communities throughout 2005 and 2006. Still, central government remained determined to maintain the fiction that local communities should be involved in changes to health and social care. Yet one more document duly followed a long line of ineffective predecessors in July 2006. Entitled *A stronger local voice*, it proposed amongst other things the abolition of the relatively toothless Patient and Public Involvement Forums – which themselves had only been formed a mere three years earlier when the stronger community health councils had been abolished. The document referred to a strengthening of local involvement in decision-making. But neither its content, nor the continuing highhandedness that appeared to be endemic to the Department of Health and the NHS generally, suggested that it would make any difference.[8]

Consulting with the peasants

Central government might claim it really does believe that local communities should be consulted about, and involved in, NHS decision-making. After all,

6 Tim Yeo, MP. *Hansard*, House of Commons Debates, 24 January 2006, column 1404.

7 Helen Tucker, 'Where is the trust: community hospitals under threat?' *Challenge 45*, December 2005, p.3.

8 *A stronger local voice.* London: Department of Health, 2006.

it did put in place the legal machinery of consultation, embodied in the Health and Social Care Act 2001.

Under this Act, when significant changes are being made to the way in which services are delivered, consultation is required both with the public and with a 'health scrutiny committee' (attached to the relevant local council). This duty of consultation is further strengthened by a Cabinet Office code of practice, which sets out the basic principles of fair consultation.[9]

Health scrutiny committees have the power to refer proposals for local health service change to the Secretary of State for Health for her consideration. She in turn can refer such proposals to an Independent Reconfiguration Panel. Such referrals are potentially a brake on the excesses of NHS Trusts and PCTs and, if nothing else, can buy local communities time to work out how to fight or otherwise avoid local closures. Nonetheless, it appears that the Secretary of State relatively seldom takes the part of the local community and refers to the Panel. It is not clear how effective the whole process really is. For instance, she basically rejected the Suffolk Scrutiny Committee's referral of the proposals of the Suffolk East PCTs, but did ask the PCTs to rethink their strategy concerning closure of Hartismere Hospital. The local community in Eye celebrated, but not for long. Within a few days, the PCT had issued a letter stating that it would close the hospital anyway.

Even under what might be wholly unfair pressure, some NHS bodies do seem to do better than others. For instance, after New Forest Primary Care Trust had announced the closure in 2005 of five local community hospitals, it did draw back following the submission of a 40,000 signature petition. It agreed to shelve the immediate proposals and re-consult with the local community.[10] A similar rethink took place at Wells-next-the-Sea in Norfolk, following strong local community protest about the closure of community hospital beds.[11]

Likewise in Shropshire, plans to close community hospitals altogether were dropped, although substantial change was still proposed, in the light of a county wide £55 million deficit.[12] Nonetheless, frequently, NHS bodies are

9 *Code of Practice on Consultation.* London: Regulatory Impact Unit, Cabinet Office, 2004.

10 Sarah Jones, 'Health care trust announces community hospitals have been saved.' *Southern Daily Echo*, 27 October 2005.

11 'We Won.' *www.savewellshospital.com.* 3 May 2006.

12 'Hospitals' closure plan dropped.' *News.bbc.co.uk*, 24 March 2006.

perceived to go through the formal hoops of consultation but not to adopt the true spirit of it – thus ignoring local views. For instance:

> Is the Secretary of State aware that her references to consultation and local decision making will be treated with anger and contempt by man people who have been embittered by an empty consultation procedure...? I chaired a meeting in Alverstoke in my constituency, at which 800 people unanimously demanded the retention of the hospital at Haslar, which has excellent facilities. Those are not stupid, uninformed people. In many cases, they are former patients who know that the facilities are outstandingly good.[13]

Unfortunately, legislation and government guidance are all too easily undermined, if the will and spirit is lacking. In this respect, it is difficult to conclude anything other than that, behind the scenes, local NHS Trusts and PCTs take their cue from central government.

Accusations that NHS consultations are frequently sham processes come from many quarters. These include government ministers, as well as local communities. After 50,000 expressions of view had opposed the closure of an A&E unit at Monklands, NHS Lanarkshire decided to close it anyway. John Reid, former Secretary of State for Health and current Home Secretary, agreed that the consultation had been a sham and that the closure would be grossly unfair.[14]

Other MPs, too, end up similarly exasperated. After removing funding from a local mental health service, highly respected by both patients and clinicians, the local MP commented that 'transparency, openness and consultation seem to be alien concepts to Hounslow PCT'.[15] The Worthing Herald captured most aptly the flavour of how consultations are perceived. After 6000 people had protested about the threat to two local hospitals. It reported the overwhelming feeling as being that it had already been decided. It was just:

> a gruesome fandango to show 'due process'. A terrible ticking of boxes for people who think they know what's best for you.[16]

13 Peter Viggers, MP, Gosport. *Hansard,* House of Commons Debates, 5 July 2006, column 827.

14 Kathleen Nutt, 'Closure of hospital accident unit is a sham, says Reid.' *Sunday Times,* Scotland, 6 August 2006.

15 'Dakers calls on Hounslow NHS to explain closure of respected counselling service.' *http://hounslowlibdems.org.uk,* 8 June 2006.

16 'Thousands join hospital march.' *Worthing Herald,* 3 August 2006.

Back in Scotland, following the decision to close Jedburgh and Coldstream Cottage Hospitals by NHS Borders, an MP (Christine Grahame) referred to the consultation as a 'whitewash', which had not listened to local views.[17]

Unsurprisingly, local communities and their representatives often perceive that decisions have been made, before proposals ever go out to consultation. To the extent that, as one councillor in Bognor Regis put it, 'it is too late when it gets to the consultation stage'. Especially when the NHS in the relevant area is overspent by £85 million.[18] Understandably then, suspicions are easily aroused at an early stage. The Oxford Radcliffe Hospitals Trust would deny it had any intention of closing Horton Hospital – even though it had just been included in a local district council plan for residential development.[19] Hundreds of people had already protested about the downgrading of the children's ward and the maternity unit.[20]

If they think they can get away with it, NHS Trusts and PCTs will indeed sometimes attempt to push through closures and cutbacks with no consultation. The West Suffolk Hospitals NHS Trust managed to withdraw the closure of 55 beds from a consultation actually half way through the process. They were shut by the time the consultation had finished. Similarly, it was reported that the Royal Cornwall Hospitals Trust had decided to shed 300 jobs, stop emergency surgery at the West Cornwall Hospital, concentrate all accident and emergency work in Truro, and had plans (which had been leaked) to shut St Michael's Hospital (with 70 beds) in Hayle. The Penwith Council chief executive promptly queried the legality of doing all this without consultation.[21]

Consulting on the hoof: taking shortcuts and sidewinds

The PCTs across Suffolk must have been subject to unremitting and ruthless pressure from central government. There would be no such conciliatory response to community protests, and no sitting down in a collaborative manner – despite repeated requests that they should do so. For instance, in the West:

17 'Borders hospital closures agreed.' *News.bbc.co.uk*, 14 June 2006.

18 'March over hospital cutback fears.' *News.bbc.co.uk*, 13 July 2006.

19 Julian Dancer, 'Developers eye up hospital site.' *This is Oxfordshire*, 3 August 2006.

20 'Protest against hospital cutbacks.' *News.bbc.co.uk*, 19 June 2006.

21 'Anger over "legality" of NHS cuts.' *News.bbc.co.uk*, 19 July 2006.

> For the last ten months, WHAC has repeatedly invited the PCT to pause, and to sit down with WHAC, local clinicians and other key parties. This is what the White Paper says PCTs should do. Our PCT has not done so. We have been expertly advised of various ways to proceed – in line with what the White Paper says about community hospitals. We believe that goodwill and compromise on both sides would go a long way. We would far rather put our energies and expertise into working with the PCT, than remain in a state of conflict. Once again, we urge the PCT as a matter of urgency to take up our invitation.[22]

In Suffolk, the PCTs would be regarded as attempting to take all manner of shortcuts with the consultation process. The PCTs would deny this, arguing that they had attempted to rectify some of the original, perceived faults, by publishing more information and extending the consultation period.

They had launched their 12-week consultation during the summer holidays, despite the Code of Practice's warning that longer consultation periods should be considered if a summer holiday period is involved. Likewise, the Code states that there should be active informal consultation with interested groups prior to the formal written consultation.[23]

Suffolk West PCT omitted this informal stage altogether, announcing its proposals in mid-June 2005, adopting a financial recovery plan on 29 June and the very same evening telling a public meeting in Sudbury what the PCT was going to propose. This was abandonment of the new community hospital, and closure of the two existing hospitals, with the timing and extent of replacement services unclear. This type of failure to engage with the public at an early stage, before consulting on formal options, is exactly what a government minister, Lord Warner, warned against.[24]

The Code also states that the consultation should as far as possible be open with no options ruled out. The PCTs in Suffolk paid little heed to this. They put forward the imperative of financial savings and basically only one way of achieving them – widespread closures, with ill-defined replacement services. Logically, this meant only one overall option and indeed nothing to consult about. Such an approach inevitably suggested to the public that the PCTs had already made up their minds on the main issues. In East Suffolk,

22 Walnuttree Hospital Action Committee, 'The State of our Health Services in Sudbury'. Notice. 8 June 2006.

23 *Code of Practice on Consultation.* London: Regulatory Impact Unit, Cabinet Office, 2004, paras 1.2,1.3.

24 Lord Warner, 'Consult before conclusions.' *Health Service Journal,* 3 November 2005, p.8.

this led Sir Michael Lord, MP, to describe the consultation process concerning Hartismere Hosptial as 'dictation' and 'farcical'. He explained to the Health Scrutiny Committee of Suffolk County Council that he had been a:

> member of Parliament for 22 years for my part of Suffolk. This is the worst case by far I have ever seen in my experience as an MP. Before the General Election, we had five options. Immediately after the General Election, those were reduced to two. In a matter of days, I had communication there is only one option now and that's the closure of Hartismere Hospital.[25]

The reasons for pre-consultation, and for putting forward a range of options at a formative stage of the process, are various. One at least is pragmatic. There is a greater chance of gaining the trust of the public. By contrast, as the Health Scrutiny Committee put it, concerning the East of Suffolk consultation exercise, this trust was never gained. This was because of the rush to consult during the summer holidays brought about by financial pressure from the strategic health authority, the lack of options on offer and no prior consultation. This led to a 'mood of distrust and concern amongst the general public'. The impression given was of haste and ill-thought-through proposals. In sum, the PCTs had failed to take the public with them.[26]

Suffolk West PCT would claim that the lack of detail in its consultation document showed that it had not made up its mind and that its ideas were not yet fully formed.[27] The problem with this argument was that the original consultation document did actually contain very considerable detail – on closures, but with no comparable detail on replacement services.[28] The PCT was forced to attempt to rectify this, when the Health Scrutiny Committee demanded further information. However, other factors in West Suffolk appeared to the public to undermine the spirit of the consultation process. One such arose in the form of pre-emptive decision-making, which by definition is anathema to true consultation.

For instance, before the end of the consultation process, 55 beds at West Suffolk Hospitals NHS Trust – which were being explicitly consulted on by the PCT – were closed anyway. The PCT explained this away, by saying that

25 Danielle Nuttall, 'The worst case in my 22 years as MP.' *East Anglian Daily Times*, 6 January 2006.

26 Suffolk Health Scruting Committee, 'Referral of the decisions of Suffolk East PCT.' Letter. 7 March 2006.

27 Barbara Eeles, 'Have your say on future of health care.' *Suffolk Free Press*, 18 August 2005.

28 *Modernising Health Care in West Suffolk: consultation, 1 August – 31 October 2005*. Bury St Edmunds: Suffolk West PCT, 2005.

the closure merely represented internal reorganisation and so did not, after all, require consultation.[29] It is difficult to see, however, how closure of so many beds – especially in tandem with the closure as well of 82 beds in satellite community hospitals – did not represent either a 'substantial variation in service' (under s.7 of the Health and Social Care Act 2001), or 'changes in the way services were provided' (under s.11 of the Act).

Likewise, 10 out of the 16 beds being consulted upon at Newmarket Hospital were closed prematurely in December 2005, before even the consultation process was concluded.[30] The PCT would claim that the closures were beyond its control, and were because of staff shortages. This was not necessarily taken at face value:

> The PCT claims '100 per cent honesty', in maintaining that the Newmarket closures are due to staff shortage beyond its control and nothing to do with cost-cutting... Yet the PCT itself has engineered the shortage. It encouraged staff to leave by letting it be known that the beds have no future. It then imposed a freeze on staff recruitment (including new bank or agency staff).[31]

Over in the East of Suffolk, the same thing was perceived to be happening. Closure plans, it was alleged, made it quite clear to staff that they had no future at some of the hospitals, hence some would leave. Accused of encouraging staff to leave and deliberately running down the hospitals, the Suffolk East PCTs would state that such allegations constituted 'malicious rumour'.[32]

Hints of pre-emptive decision-making continued. Having consulted on the GP out-of-hours service, it was decided to remove on-call doctors from Sudbury in February, nearly two months before the official Board meeting and before it had analysed all the consultation responses. The decision was taken ostensibly by SDOC (Suffolk Doctors on Call), but they were commissioned by the PCT to deliver the service.[33]

In Sudbury, an example of extreme pre-emption occurred. Of the 68 beds at Walnuttree Hospital, 36 never even made it into the consultation.

29 *Modernising healthcare in West Suffolk: additional information.* Bury St Edmunds: Suffolk West PCT, 2005, p.1.

30 Lisa Cleverdon, 'Hospital to cut beds over festive period.' *East Anglian Daily Times*, 6 December 2005.

31 Walnuttree Hospital Action Committee, 'NHS savings will be paid for in suffering.' *East Anglian Daily Times*, 31 December 2005.

32 Craig Robinson, 'Health care cutbacks "have caused deaths".' *East Anglian Daily Times*, 10 August 2005.

33 'On-call GPs quit town.' *Suffolk Free Press*, 23 February 2006. And: Rebecca Sheppard, 'Two towns will have no doctors based overnight.' *East Anglian Daily Times*, 18 March 2006.

They were closed permanently and informally before even the consultation process got off the ground in August. Shut temporarily for fire safety works in March 2005, the beds were simply spirited out of existence. They had gone off the map, even though legally such a major change to a local service should arguably have been consulted upon.[34]

Despite all these flaws in the consultation process, the Suffolk West PCT's Chairman would still maintain that correct procedures had been followed, attended by openness and transparency.[35]

This claim followed a sustained attack that had been launched on the PCT's Chief Executive by the South Suffolk MP, Tim Yeo. It illustrated just how bitter and serious the conflict between PCT and community had become during the consultation period:

> I much regret the trust's new Chief Executive...has obstructed the action committee's attempts to find a solution to the problem, to the extent of resorting on occasion to untrue statements and evasions when asked straightforward questions, and casting wholly unjustified aspersions on the integrity of people who are campaigning to protect our health service. Truth has, on occasion, flown out of the window during the course of the argument.[36]

It was all a far cry from cooperative working between the NHS and local communities, repeatedly envisaged by government policy documents.

Cutting up a PCT: consultation, outrage and anger

Another illustration of what the public perceived to be a sham consultation concerned the reorganisation of the PCTs in Suffolk that was taking place in 2006. It was not just the Suffolk public that was worried about the genuineness of the consultation; more generally, so too was the House of Commons Health Select Committee.[37]

In Suffolk, very strong feelings across the community favoured the creation of a Waveney and Great Yarmouth PCT. Waveney PCT was the only

34 *Response to Suffolk West Primary Care Trust's Consultation.* Sudbury: Walnuttree Hospital Action Committee, 2005, para 2.4.2.

35 Paul Holland, 'Yeo attacks health chief in furious Commons speech.' *Suffolk Free Press,* 26 January 2006.

36 Tim Yeo, MP. *Hansard.* House of Commons Debates, 24 January 2006, column 1405.

37 House of Commons Health Committee (2005) *Changes to Primary Care Trusts.* HC 646. London: HMSO, p.3.

Suffolk PCT in financial balance. It had worked with Great Yarmouth PCT closely to form a stable health-care system, and now wished for a combined Waveney and Great Yarmouth PCT. The vast majority of GPs and health-care professionals were strongly in favour of this option.[38]

By March, the director of clinical governance at Waveney PCT was prepared to speak out in favour of combining Waveney and Great Yarmouth PCTs, referring also to the support of the Suffolk Local Medical Committee and the Suffolk Local Pharmaceutical Committee.[39]

Notwithstanding this overwhelming opposition to the proposals for Waveney, the Board members of the Norfolk, Suffolk and Cambridgeshire Strategic Health Authority voted unanimously in favour of a Suffolk-wide PCT, and against the Waveney–Great Yarmouth option. A non-executive director of Waveney PCT pointed out that this decision went against the 'view of all GPs, clinicians, local residents, patient groups, staff and politicians'. The Chairman of the Waveney Practice Based Commissioning Board put it more bluntly:

> the feeling of GPs in Waveney is that this has not been a consultation exercise but merely a re-statement of central dogma from the SHA.[40]

At a public meeting on 20 February 2006, the project director of the SHA was reportedly 'visibly shaken' by the strength of feeling – to such an extent that the SHA members present promised a further public meeting before any decision was taken. Less than 48 hours later, the SHA took the decision to have one Suffolk-wide PCT, within which Waveney PCT would disappear. The feeling of powerlessness and frustration was summed up by one correspondent who had attended a consultation meeting:

> In short, these so called consultations were no more than a cynical pretence...[41]

Nonetheless, in the end there was a happy outcome on this occasion, but only at the last gasp. Perhaps because of its financial achievements, the

38 Dr A.N. Eastaugh and others, 'Centralised healthcare not the most efficient.' Letter. *East Anglian Daily Times*, 20 January 2006; Dr Annette Abott, Letter. *East Anglian Daily Times*, 20 January 2006. General practitioners continued to speak out publicly: Dr Bubb and others, 'Suffolk PCT would harm Waveney.' Letter. *East Anglian Daily Times*, 7 February 2006.

39 Govind Mohan, 'So much is riding on next week's meeting.' Letter. *East Anglian Daily Times*, 16 March 2006.

40 'Trusts to be cut. SHAs to merge.' *East Anglian Daily Times*, 6 April 2006.

41 John Brodribb, 'Public consultations are a cynical smokescreen.' Letter. *East Anglian Daily Times*, 28 February 2006.

Waveney PCT was eventually and unexpectedly rescued by the Secretary of State herself, when she overruled the SHA.[42]

Alienating and striking fear into local communities

The sense of bewilderment, anger, fear and helplessness in local communities, created by some PCTs and NHS trusts doing the bidding of central government, cannot be underestimated. Given that government policy is about involving local communities in decisions and about patient choice, this is a perverse outcome. It is disturbing how easily the trust and goodwill of local communities is sometimes destroyed.

For instance, in August 2005, the plight of Tetbury Hospital was highlighted by the Chairman of the Hospital Trust. Local people had saved the community hospital by raising £1.5 million, on the understanding that the NHS would commission services at the hospital. For the next 14 years, the community ran the hospital, raising a further £400,000 for capital projects, and an average of £100,000 per year for the last five years to subsidise the running costs. Then, suddenly, in August, the PCT announced that it would renege on its contract in respect of the inpatient beds, which represented 55 per cent of the hospital's income. As the Chairman concluded: 'some patient-led NHS!'[43]

Similar stories abound elsewhere. In Malmesbury, the friends of the hospital had paid for the X-ray unit. This didn't stop the unit being removed, together with the closure of several wards and the maternity unit.[44] Worse, local leagues of friends were now having to spend their hard-raised funds not on provision of local health services, but on fighting the local NHS bodies. The League for Hartismere Hospital in Eye, East Suffolk, bemoaned the fact that:

> Much work has been done over the past weeks, involving travel, taking advice from lawyers and using the services of health consultants to help us present our case. This does mean that the funds of the League of Friends are rather depleted and we believe whatever the Health Secretary's decision the fight will need to go on for which funds will be needed.[45]

42 'Battle to secure PCT is won.' *East Anglian Daily Times*, 17 May 2006.

43 Simon Preston, 'Our vanishing hospitals.' Letter. *Spectator*, 24 September 2005.

44 James Gray, MP for Wiltshire. *Hansard*, Westminster Hall, 2nd November 2005, column 273WH.

45 Eric Havers, 'Please help in our fight to save local hospital.' Letter. *East Anglian Daily Times*, 9 March 2006.

The extent to which local communities felt betrayed by the sudden, unaccountable decisions to close or severely run down about 100 community hospitals cannot be overemphasised. Not only had many community hospitals received, as at Tetbury, very substantial ongoing support from local people – but many had local communities to thank for their very origins. After the Second World War, they had been taken over by the NHS, but there was now real anger that the NHS was poised to destroy at breakneck speed these valuable and loved local health services. The following examples bear eloquent testimony.

Over the length and breadth of Suffolk, the shock, anger, fear and alienation of communities was well captured by the regional Press. Even allowing for Press licence, the headlines are telling, especially in newspapers with a reputation for generally sound reporting and not for sensationalism. For example, in June 2005, the *East Anglian Daily Times* had a full front page asking:

> WHAT IS GOING ON IN OUR HOSPITALS: WALNUTTREE HOSPITAL TO CLOSE; FELIXSTOWE UNDER THREAT, FOUR OTHERS BEING REVIEWED; SUFFOLK HEALTH SERVICES OVERSPEND BY £2000 AN HOUR.[46]

Less than a week later, the newspaper knew the answer to its question, when PCTs and NHS trusts across Suffolk announced swingeing cuts:

> AXE FALLS ON OUR HOSPITALS.[47]

Some months later, concern in Sudbury in West Suffolk was so great that the Chairman of the local action committee, Colin Spence, a county councillor and former Vice-Chairman of the PCT, spoke out. Not known locally to overstate the case, he was quoted as the source for the following headline:

> HEALTH – DRIFTING TOWARDS OBLIVION.[48]

Residents, in this case a retired local nurse, were quite clear about what was going on:

46 *East Anglian Daily Times*, 24 June 2005.

47 'Axe falls on our hospitals.' *East Anglian Daily Times*, 30 June 2005.

48 Barbara Eeles, *Suffolk Free Press*, 24 November 2005.

> I believe the [new] health centre will never be built and, if so, make no mistake about the outcome: old people, especially, will die prematurely for lack of professional care. But who cares?[49]

The same writer felt that bed closures would show the Secretary of State's 'complete contempt for the sick, the frightened and the deprived of this area'.[50] Similarly a former London District Nursing Officer pointed out that:

> It has been suggested that patients are best off in their own homes, but for the most part that means a very lonely existence as carers only have limited time allocated for each patient...[51]

The Principal Secretary of the Suffolk division of the British Medical Association spoke of how terrified the local community was about the changes being proposed:

> Those who are most afraid are those who live alone, those who are considered mentally ill, elderly carers with full responsibility for their loved one who may become demented, and working daughters trying to cope with ageing, sick parents as well as their own children.[52]

Dissolution of promises and trust in West Suffolk

The breaking of promises, withdrawal of assurances and changes of direction seemed all too common in the NHS. Measured changes in policy and planning were one thing; sudden, arbitrary change quite another.

For instance, in Sudbury, Suffolk, after 30 years of attempts to develop a new community hospital to replace the existing two hospitals, agreement had finally been reached in March 2005. Approval had been given by the PCT and all but gained from the strategic health authority. A Sudbury Health and Social Care Steering Group, with both PCT and lay members on it, was working well. Trust between the PCT and the local community had been established. This appeared to be what was envisaged by central government policy.

All this was destroyed overnight, when the PCT suddenly announced that there would be no new community hospital and the existing ones would

49 Philomena Spearpoint, 'Hospital closure is a disgrace.' Letter. *Suffolk Free Press*, 15 December 2005.

50 Philomena Spearpoint, 'Money to save hospitals.' Letter. *Suffolk Free Press*, 19 January 2006.

51 Mrs Patricia Harris, 'Community hospitals fulfil a vital role.' Letter. *East Anglian Daily Times*, 20 March 2006.

52 Mark Heath, 'Community "terror" over health plans.' *East Anglian Daily Times*, 5 January 2006.

close. By the end of June 2005, the PCT had proceeded to alienate several hundred people at a public meeting. It made what was perceived to be an unapologetic and uncompromising declaration. Diplomatic niceties were dispensed with. The new community hospital was dead in the water; it would not even remain as an option in the forthcoming consultation. The Walnuttree Hospital Action Committee would subsequently spell out the perceived consequences of such behaviour and broken promises. The Chief Executive:

> may wish to reflect that his two chief executive predecessors with responsibility for Sudbury...made many promises to the people of Sudbury. They have all been broken. He will also be aware that the PCT will not exist by June 2006 – so it will not be accountable when its assurances come to nothing. Taking all the above together [including the PCT's financial opacity, deficit and instability], it is obvious why any neutral and conscientious onlooker could only conclude that, from their perspective, Sudbury really will be bereft of health services, and is in great danger of becoming an NHS-free zone.[53]

A short chronology recording local reaction in Sudbury, West Suffolk, is instructive in understanding the degree to which a local community can feel betrayed when it comes to fundamental matters such as health. It was an understanding that, to the detriment of all concerned, seemed to elude Suffolk West PCT – which seemed to continue to be surprised and disappointed at the reaction its proposals received. It was a story repeated up and down the country. Many of its characteristics are all too familiar.

By January 2005, after three decades, the town had at last been assured that it would get a new community hospital. An attempt in late 2004 to close down Walnuttree Hospital on questionable fire safety grounds had been fought off. The *Suffolk Free Press* of 27 January 2005 showed on its front page a photograph of Walnuttree Hospital staff and supporters at a party, celebrating the saving of the current hospital until the new one was built. The £500 raised went to local charities.[54] The next day, a leading and longstanding local campaigner, Sylvia Byham, was quoted as saying that:

> Sudbury has been let down so many times and there has been a whole saga of events… I cannot allow myself to believe that this group of

53 Colin Spence, 'Even a neutral could see this means cuts.' Letter. *East Anglian Daily Times*, 19 December 2005.

54 'Victory party for hospital staff.' *Suffolk Free Press*, 27 January 2005.

> people [the PCT] can take us down yet another road with nothing at the end of it. They need to let the public know they mean business this time. There have been so many empty victories for the town and we need to make sure this is not another one.[55]

The PCT's Director of Clinical Services, Jonathan Williams, responded by referring to the positive mood of the steering group the PCT had set up and how local people would be kept informed about progress.[55] Come the end of March, the strategic health authority had all but approved the plans in outline; the PCT Board did so shortly afterwards. Mrs Byham again commented, still optimistically but as it turned out all too prophetically:

> It is nice to see common sense has prevailed thanks to the hard work of existing hospital staff and the people of Sudbury... We have to maintain support in the town to make sure nothing slips and that we get the facilities the town needs.[56]

By May, the outgoing Chief Executive, Tony Ranzetta, did not hold back:

> People are now looking to the future and are genuinely excited, as I am, of what the future holds for health services in Sudbury.[57]

The contrast with what followed was plain and scarcely believable. By the end of June, PCTs across Suffolk were announcing drastic cutbacks and closures. In Sudbury, the betrayal of the local community was reported widely. For instance, Michael Mitchell, a hospital porter who had led the campaign to Downing Street the previous year, said:

> We are disgusted with this because they must have known about this all along. There is no way health services across Suffolk will be able to cope with all these cuts, lives will be at risk. We fought closure all the way last time and we will fight even harder this time.[58]

A huge headline spelt out what working with the NHS in Sudbury had led to:

> BETRAYED.

The Town Clerk, Sue Brotherwood, would state: 'How can we believe anything they say?' An indication of the lack of transparency and trust was

55 Lisa Cleverdon, 'Hospital lobby bullish on win.' *Sudbury Mercury*, 28 January 2005.

56 Nicki Harvey, 'Hospital wins backing from health chiefs.' *Suffolk Free Press*, 31 March 2006.

57 Will Wright, 'Centre ready for July 2007.' *Sudbury Mercury*, 6 May 2005.

58 Patrick Lowman, 'Resign over debts crisis – bosses are urged.' *East Anglian Daily Times*, 24 June 2005.

explained by Tim Yeo, MP. The day before he heard the news about the closures, he had been in a meeting with the strategic health authority – which had given no indication of what was afoot. This was even though it was the SHA that, ultimately, had precipitated the about-turn.[59] The MP put it succinctly at a large public meeting held in Sudbury, referring to a:

> total collapse of confidence on the part of this local community in the health authorities [who] have lost all credence.[60]

Things deteriorated. Acting on behalf of the local community in West Suffolk, MPs Richard Spring and Tim Yeo met with the Suffolk West PCT in July. The words used to describe the nature of the meeting included 'furious', 'acrimonious', 'frank' and 'angry'.[61] Measured, cooperative working with local communities had been all but abrogated. It made a complete nonsense of government rhetoric about local community involvement. The iron fist had emerged.

Thus, at a meeting in Ipswich concerning widespread cuts to services in the East of Suffolk, 'tempers flared' at a 'highly-charged' meeting between local residents and the Suffolk East PCTs.[62] At a subsequent meeting also in Ipswich, anger was again the overwhelming theme.[63]

On it went into the autumn of 2005. Letters to the newspapers spoke of people's 'feeling of disbelief and helplessness about the future of health care on offer in the area'. And of how laughable it would all be if it 'were not so deadly' – since a 'small army of peripatetic nurses and other carers' would be required in a rural area to reproduce the services at Walnuttree Hospital.[64] Cynicism spread. Folllowing a meeting between the PCTs and district councils in Suffolk, the Deputy Mayor of Sudbury, Nigel Bennett, wrote:

> Interestingly, we were also told that there was a major breakdown in public trust in the Sudbury area because of past promises made. On this point, Mr Stonard [the Chief Executive] has got it right 100 per cent.[65]

59 Nicki Harvey, 'Betrayed.' *Suffolk Free Press*, 30 June 2005.

60 Dave Gooderham, 'Battle pledge to save hospital.' *East Anglian Daily Times*, 30 June 2005.

61 Benedict O'Connor, 'Sparks fly as MPs meet with health bosses.' *East Anglian Daily Times*, 12 July 2005.

62 Craig Robinson, 'Health care cutbacks "have caused deaths".' *East Anglian Daily Times*, 10 August 2005.

63 John Howard, 'People vent anger at NHS public meeting.' *East Anglian Daily Times*, 16 September 2005.

64 Peter Rowe, 'Be honest and admit it's a second rate system.' Letter. *Suffolk Free Press*, 1 September 2005.

65 Nigel Bennett, 'PCT must do as it promised.' Letter. *Suffolk Free Press*, 1 September 2005.

The gap – between the theory of cooperation and the reality of alienation and conflict – was summed up by the daughter of a former Sudbury GP. She wrote to the Press about the Walnuttree Hospital Action Committee (WHAC):

> My father...would have been devastated at the chaotic demise that the so-called bosses of our NHS have created... It is ludicrous – when you think about it – having to fight against the Primary Care Trust. What care? What trust?[66]

The Walnuttree Hospital Action Committee, in a large volume of correspondence and other communications, continued throughout a ten-month period to call on the PCT to pause, and to sit down and work with the local community and clinicians to find a way forward. For instance, following the publication of the government's White Paper in 2006, the Committee stated:

> We would all much rather work constructively with the PCT than continue in the current atmosphere of conflict and distrust. We therefore call on Suffolk West to respond positively by postponing its decision, so as to find a way forward in dialogue with the local community.[67]

In response, the PCT saw 'absolutely no reason' to postpone its plans.[68] This was despite an appeal from the local MP, Tim Yeo, pointing out that the PCT would gain enormous 'plaudits', could 'heal the conflict that the events of the last nine months have caused' – and that the community would give full backing to the PCT if it bid for the extra funding that might be available for new community hospital development.[69]

Lord Phillips of Sudbury summed up the wider principle. This was the detrimental effect of the helplessness felt by local residents and politicians in the face of decisions not only being dictated, but dictated from afar. This was 'dangerous because disconnectedness easily becomes resentment' – and democracy needed 'the allegiance of its citizenry'.[70] *An East Anglian Daily Times* editorial struck the same chord, setting out the consequences of

66 Mrs F. Willingham, 'Well done, WHAC, for caring for us.' Letter. *Suffolk Free Press*, 22 September 2005.

67 Colin Spence, 'Ministers pave way for U-turn.' Letter. *Suffolk Free Press*, 9 February 2006.

68 Dave Gooderham, 'Last-ditch pleas on health cuts rejected.' *East Anglian Daily Times*, 8 February 2006.

69 Tim Yeo, MP, 'Trust can do right thing.' *Sudbury Mercury*, 9 February 2006.

70 Lord Phillips of Sudbury, 'Time to stand up and fight for democracy.' *East Anglian Daily Times*, 18 January 2006.

pushing change through in the wrong way and under false pretences. It had been a:

> failure of communication from the very beginning: confusing for the man in the street, devoid of persuasive argument, and frustrating for health professionals... The picture has never been clear – a situation that breeds mistrust, cynicism and resentment. People are not stupid; they realised the proposed closures and cutbacks were about an underlying primary care debt of £20 million or so.[71]

By April 2006, the measure of desperation felt by local communities was evident in threats of legal action. Desperation, because judicial review by the law courts is a blunt tool of last resort. It can be used to challenge the decision-making process of the NHS (and other public bodies) – but is ill equipped to protect people's health directly. Nevertheless, following the decision in West Suffolk on 11 April 2006 to close all NHS community hospital beds, Warwick Hirst, Chairman of the Newmarket Health Forum, threatened just such legal action.[72]

The Chairman of the Walnuttree Hospital Action Committee was allowed to speak at the PCT Board's meeting, revealing the depth of feeling in the local community:

> Do not try and hoodwink the public that this nasty medicine you are delivering is all about modernisation when it is clear the real reason is a quick fix to cut budgets and raise capital. But short-term fixes do not deliver solutions in the long term. It is abundantly clear that those responsible for making the decisions have a shotgun to the head – but the people of Sudbury are the innocent victims. We have lost all faith in the PCT – the loss of beds will cause a devastating effect on the local community and big questions remain as to why.[73]

He would sum up by saying: 'Suffice it to say, what you are doing today is ripping the heart out of the community.'[74] Irony followed. The PCT was perceived blatantly to have broken assurances and promises. Having now voted to close all community hospital beds and ignore overwhelming local opinion about this, the PCT now talked about trust:

71 'Judgement day looms for NHS bosses.' *East Anglian Daily Times*, 21 January 2006.

72 Dave Gooderham, 'We'll see you in High Court.' *Sudbury Mercury*, 13 April 2006.

73 'Staff and patients unite against "nasty medicine".' *East Anglian Daily Times*, 12 April 2006.

74 Paul Holland, 'Decision "rips heart from community".' *Suffolk Free Press*, 13 April 2006.

> There has been a lot of mistrust in the past but I hope this PCT can allay those fears now.[75]

They appeared to be words only. Within a few weeks, all the reasons for the breakdown in trust were resurfacing afresh. They illustrated perfectly the seeming doublespeak and lack of transparency in the NHS and the reason why local communities are well advised not to treat statements and assurances at face value.

The further problems arose simply and in the following way. The PCT's decision on 11 April 2006 made clear that outpatient services would be retained in Sudbury. On 12 April, an explicit assurance was given at a public meeting that one of these services, the Talbot mental health unit, would remain open. By the end of May it was not functioning, because patients were, as a matter of policy, no longer being referred to it. Yet the PCT maintained that it was still 'open' and seemed almost exasperated at the fuss.[76] To the local community, this seemed simply disingenuous as the following exasperated letter suggests:

> The facts are these. The PCT and West Suffolk NHS Hospitals Trust undertook on 11th April not to close Sudbury outpatient clinics (other than audiology). Yet the Talbot Unit (mental health) has since been closed. The PCT commissioned it, the NHS Trust partly ran it, the Suffolk Mental Health Partnerships NHS Trust (SMHP) referred patients to it. All three trusts deny it is closed.
>
> However, the nurse who ran it has been redeployed. No patients now attend. Existing patients were told in May that they could no longer attend. The SHMP NHS Trust claims that such patients were discharged for clinical reasons. But at least three of these patients were in April told that they could no longer attend the clinic because it was closing. They were reduced to tears. The ambulance drivers, too, knew the clinic was being closed. In addition, equipment and furniture have been removed. In any language, this is a closed clinic…
>
> Decision-making of this nature goes to the very heart and integrity of a public service that holds our health in its hands. Cutting services is one thing. Doing it by stealth and concealment is quite another.[77]

75 'It's a question of trust, says health chief.' *Suffolk Free Press*, 13 April 2006.

76 Michael Stonard, 'Talbot unit: no policy to close it.' Letter. *Suffolk Free Press*, 8 June 2006.

77 Walnuttree Hospital Action Committee, 'When closed means closed.' Letter. *Suffolk Free Press*, 20 July 2006.

A request was made under the Freedom of Information Act for statistics relating to the Talbot Clinic. They disclosed that, by June 2006, the number patients attending had reduced to nought.

It was of little consolation to the local community in Sudbury that such discrepancies in perception were not peculiar to Suffolk. For instance, in south west London, two mental day hospitals were scheduled for closure but reprieved in mid June 2005, pending a consultation. However, a journalist, posing as the carer of a prospective patient, was told that no referrals were being taken, no patients were attending, and that staff were due to be redeployed. The South West London and St George's Mental Health Trust denied that either day hospital was closed to patients.[78]

The gap between the language of the NHS on the one hand, and public understanding on the other, could never have been more yawning.

In addition, back in Sudbury, the dietetic and nutrition clinic had also been withdrawn by the end of May, again contrary to assurances. The West Suffolk Hospitals NHS Trust stated that it had been withdrawn only temporarily because of staff shortages and would be reviewed. It did not mention that it had not filled the vacancies because of its financial problems. As a local campaigner put it: 'How could the PCT expect the people of Sudbury to trust them' when assurances were broken with such impunity?[79] Trust was further strained when emails were leaked to the local Press, revealing a clear intention to close the paediatric clinic in Sudbury, as well as referring to a future generally of minimal services in the town. All this was seemingly contrary to the assurances that had been given only two months earlier.[80] This leak had followed hard on the heels of a flat denial by the PCT that there was any 'active contemplation of closing other clinics'.[81]

Feeling helpless in the face of what it considered to be incremental closures by concealment and stealth, the Walnuttree Hospital Action Committee would appeal for local residents to 'Be our eyes and ears in fight for health services' – and to report the withdrawal of local clinics.[82]

With such irreconcilable views of the world, and with closed services remaining somehow 'open', the chances of meaningful dialogue between local community and NHS seemed as distant as ever. It was therefore no

78 Carron Taylor, 'We pose as carer – and expose NHS "closures".' *This is Local London,* 30 June 2006.

79 Paul Holland, 'Anger as clinic shuts.' *Suffolk Free Press,* 8 June 2006.

80 Paul Holland, 'Emails prompt health service fears.' *Suffolk Free Press,* 13 July 2006.

81 Colin Muge (PCT Chairman), 'Our answer to scaremongering.' Letter. *Suffolk Free Press,* 6 July 2006.

82 Paul Holland, 'Be our eyes and ears in fight for health services.' *Suffolk Free Press,* 22 June 2006.

surprise when a local resident, Frances Jackson, deemed by the NHS to be an 'expert' patient in managing her own long-term health condition, decided to bring a legal case against the PCT. She explained:

> I very much regret taking this action but feel that is the only thing left to do... I want to help myself and other patients with complex needs both now and in the future, and try to secure better health services in Sudbury... There is a heavy responsibility on my shoulders for taking this action, but I believe it is the right thing to do.[83]

The Walnuttree Hospital Action Committee echoed the sentiment, referring to the legal case as a cry for help.[84] In sum, it was all about trust and honesty, as the Suffolk County Council Health Scrutiny Committee put it, surprisingly bluntly. In its view, a key point was that the NHS had been nervous of putting the real options to the people of Suffolk. In fact more honesty might have avoided the undermining of public confidence, and the image of the NHS as a self-serving bureaucracy.[85]

And of course it was not just Suffolk. The NHS workforce director, Andrew Foster, admitted that there was a loss of confidence in the Department of Health at national level and a breakdown of trust. This had been brought about by a series of major policy changes without proper consultation.[86] Suffolk, East Anglia and indeed the country as a whole were arguably reaping the consequences of a highhandedness and arrogance that went to the very top.

Cutting the clinicians down to size

By 2006, New Labour was putting in place even greater centralisation by enlarging in size but reducing in number both primary care trusts and strategic health authorities (see above). This was despite the 2005 New Labour manifesto having continued to stress the importance of strengthening accountability. Increased centralisation is not normally the way to achieve this.[87]

83 'Frances, 60, why I'll fight on to save town's hospitals from axe.' *Suffolk Free Press*, 8 June 2006.

84 Walnuttree Hospital Action Committee, 'The state of our health services in Sudbury.' Notice. *Suffolk Free Press*, 8 June 2006.

85 *Interim Report on Committee Response to NHS Consultations, 1st November 2005.* H05/22. Ipswich: Suffolk County Council Health Scrutiny Committee, para 45.

86 John Carvel, 'Catcalls, barracking and laughter force Hewitt to abandon speech.' *Guardian*, 27 April 2006.

87 *Labour Party Manifesto 2005: Britain forward not back.* London: Labour Party, p.60.

New Labour's election manifesto had already in 2001 stated that it would 'decentralise power to give local primary care trusts control over 75 per cent of NHS funding'.[88] Yet four years later, in 2005, it appeared that primary care trusts had discretion over relatively little of their budget. In other words, while notionally it was their budget, in fact they spent most of it at central government's bidding. In 2001 also, reform was embodied in a policy document about 'shifting the balance of power'. It spoke of staff having a 'greater say in how services are delivered and resources are allocated' and of devolving 'decisions to frontline staff'. Staff would be engaged and empowered.[89]

In 2004, Tony Blair referred to NHS staff in the foreword of a document about 'putting people at the heart of public services'. By this time, NHS staff were in many places bewildered and groggy from the endless rounds of change, targets, new policies and reorganisations. Not to mention frustrated at the bureaucracy, rules, form-filling and gathering of statistics. Yet they were referred to by the Department of Health as 'dedicated, skilled and compassionate' and as helping to overhaul the system.[90]

By 2005, frontline staff were not only suffering from lack of power, resources and morale, but they were also losing their jobs. More than this, central government was also contemplating having all, or at least most NHS primary care trust staff in their hundreds and thousands, hived off into the independent sector.[91] No surprise then that the opposition shown by nurses to Patricia Hewitt at their 2006 annual congress was reported as the most strident in the Royal College of Nursing's 90-year history.[92]

Waving away the benighted clinicians of Suffolk

Down in Suffolk and elsewhere, experienced clinicians would speak out against the cuts being made, in particular about the loss of community hospital beds. It seemed that the more they protested, the more entrenched the PCTs became. It became difficult to see how this was about empowering and inspiring key members of the NHS workforce.

88 *Labour's Manifesto 2001: ambitions for Britain.* London: Labour Party, p.22.

89 *Shifting the Balance of Power within the NHS.* London: Department of Health, 2001, paras 10, 11, 19.

90 *Putting People at the Heart of Public Services.* London: Department of Health, 2004, para 6.

91 Sir Nigel Crisp, *Commissioning a Patient-led NHS.* Letter. 28 July 2005. London: Department of Health.

92 John Carvel, 'Catcalls, barracking and laughter force Hewitt to abandon speech.' *Guardian,* 27 April 2006.

For instance, out at Aldeburgh, a GP principal would maintain that the beds at the community hospital were always full, and should not be reduced in number.[93] By early November, doctors had more collectively registered their opposition, when the Suffolk division of the British Medical Association delivered a letter by hand to Patricia Hewitt. It stated that the division had 'little confidence' in those who had produced the proposals, and referred to the 'deep unrest and unfortunate distrust that is now pervading the county'.[94]

Suffolk West PCT seemed to give a decisive demonstration as to what it thought of its frontline clinicians. During the consultation process, it would dismiss its own general practitioners as disappointing and incapable of understanding consultation documents. The PCT would also appear to ignore the concerns of its own expert rehabilitation staff, physiotherapists and occupational therapists, who put forward detailed and substantial concerns. It did not even see fit to explain to its Board that key rehabilitation staff had opposed the proposals.[95]

This seemed all the more culpable because arguably 'the' key rehabilitation professional within the PCT, the physiotherapy service manager, had bravely spoken out in her professional journal – expressing concerns about the 'most vulnerable patients with complex needs and long-term conditions, some of whom also have mental health issues'.[96]

Five general practitioners from the Siam surgery in Sudbury outlined their grave concern at the closure of 68 beds at the Walnuttree Hospital. These beds were:

> an essential part of the medical and social care of our elderly, frail and chronically ill patients. Whereas some people could, with difficulty, be managed at home, there are many who even with increased community services could not be cared for properly other than in hospital.[97]

Seven general practitioners from Hardwicke House in Sudbury likewise signed a strongly worded letter to the effect that patient care would be

93 'Reducing beds "will cost more".' *East Anglian Daily Times*, 25 June 2005.

94 Rebecca Sheppard, '"Stop closures" doctors warn.' *East Anglian Daily Times*, 9 November 2005.

95 Michael Stonard (2006) *Modernising Health Care in West Suffolk: report for decision, 11th April 2006.* Bury St Edmunds: Suffolk West PCT.

96 R. Upton, 'Suffolk faces cuts in beds and jobs.' *Frontline*, 5 October 2005.

97 'Doctors voice "grave concern".' *East Anglian Daily Times*, 28 September 2005.

seriously affected by the proposals.[98] And a detailed letter, carrying heavy criticism of the PCT, was sent by the Long Melford practice. Among other things it drew attention to the lack of evidence base for the PCT's proposals, which would not meet the needs of patients.[99]

The general practitioners continued to voice their opposition right to the very end, when on 11 April 2006, the decision to close beds was made by the PCT. GPs responded by referring to the risk to care of the elderly and the fact that nursing home beds were not a satisfactory equivalent for community hospital beds.[100]

The PCT's reaction to such serious criticism from its key medical practitioners was not such as to suggest it would consider compromise. Its response was, to all appearances, to bury the criticism. It would attack the understanding of the doctors, and it would fail to draw the attention both of the public and of its own Board to their serious concerns.

First, the PCT would express itself 'deeply disappointed that the GPs at Hardwicke House have misunderstood the proposals'.[101]

Second, by mid-October – well after all those letters had been sent – it stated that the new model of care was being 'supported' by GPs.[102] This would on the face of it appear to be a misrepresentation.

Third, by April 2006, the report prepared for the PCT Board's final decision read so euphemistically as arguably to be plain misleading. It noted that 'there has been limited support' from GPs in the Sudbury and Newmarket areas.[103]

A respected, though now retired, Sudbury general practitioner, Dr McLauchlan, put it as follows. Agreeing that many patients could benefit from 'home care', nevertheless there were:

> many cases that need the regular attention and security that can only be provided in a hospital setting…an essential part of patient care and their rehabilitation. Ignoring these patients or trying to accommodate

98 Nicki Harvey, 'Doctors united in hospital fight.' *Suffolk Free Press*, 29 September 2005.

99 Letter. Long Melford Practice, 20 September 2005.

100 'Nursing home not hospital, say docs.' *Suffolk Free Press*, 13 April 2006.

101 'Town GPs express "serious worries" for patients.' *Suffolk Free Press*, 8 September 2006.

102 *Modernising Healthcare in West Suffolk: additional information.* Bury St Edmunds: Suffolk West PCT, 2005, p.1.

103 Michael Stonard (2006) *Modernising Health Care in West Suffolk: report for decision, Suffolk West Primary Care Trust Board, 11th April 2006.* Bury St Edmunds: Suffolk West PCT, para 9.6.

> them in far-off district hospitals, already over stretched and under-bedded, shows a complete lack of care, humanity and understanding of medical needs.[104]

Senior PCT staff would courageously speak out:

> We are absolutely furious, there is no way people will be getting adequate care if three hospitals lose wards, it is impossible. Lives will definitely be at risk...[105]

It all made no difference. In sum, Suffolk West PCT would, over the coming months, in effect act contrary to all these professional concerns and continue to threaten, and then finally decide, to close all its community hospital beds.

The PCTs in Suffolk were not alone. They were merely following a trend in disregarding the views of local clinicians. Thus, in North Yorkshire, it was reported in Parliament that:

> The local GPs are close to declaring a vote of no confidence in the chief executive of the PCT and are openly refusing to implement cuts in services that will put their patients at risk.[106]

In North Cumbria, GPs opposed the plan to close 118 community beds, which would leave elderly people in rural areas vulnerable and isolated. Nonetheless, that remained the plan.[107]

Lowering morale of the workers

Unison reported loss of morale, retention and recruitment problems and deterioration in service provision.[108] Stress-related illnesses were unsurprisingly being reported at the Sudbury hospitals.[109] In March 2006, a survey by the Healthcare Commission revealed worryingly low levels of job satisfaction and of positive feelings among staff in West Suffolk.[110]

104 Dr Alan E. McLauchan, 'Ignoring patient needs shows total lack of care.' Letter. *Suffolk Free Press*, 16 January 2006.

105 Patrick Lowman, 'Resign over debts crisis – bosses are urged.' *East Anglian Daily Times*, 24 June 2005.

106 Phil Willis, MP, Harrogate and Knaresborough. Hansard, House of Commons Debates, 25 July 2006, column 813.

107 Hazel Mollison, 'Community beds cuts will hit rural elderly.' *News & Star*, 6 January 2006.

108 Liz Hearnshaw, 'Health union in morale warning.' *East Anglian Daily Times*, 27 June 2005.

109 Dave Gooderham, 'Staff morale low at the hospital.' *Sudbury Mercury*, 2 September 2005.

110 Mark Heath, 'Staff exodus in NHS feared.' *East Anglian Daily Times*, 23 March 2006.

Yet central government's policy of 'creating a patient-led NHS' stated that there would be an emphasis on 'generating and developing a sense of pride, determination, momentum and pace in improving clinical services'.[111]

It had all happened before to an extent. In 1991, reforms added to the insecurity of staff, and to 'their alienation and to the feeling that they were being reduced in status to insignificant elements in the market mechanism'.[112] How much more insecure did staff feel when told in 2005 that within a year or two, some 250,000 PCT nurses and other staff would no longer be working for the NHS but would be effectively farmed out to private providers?[113]

By early May 2006, the Suffolk West PCT was praising its staff for enabling it to make savings. Nonetheless, by late May, it had taken on United Health, a private health-care provider, to carry out some financial accountancy and audit work at a reported cost of over £90,000. United Health was one of those private providers waiting in the wings to take over NHS primary care services. It seemed to bring closer the day when PCT staff might be 'rewarded' for their efforts by being forced to work in the private sector.[114] Even the PCT admitted that its drive for savings had only been sustained by putting all its staff under great pressure to cover vacancies and workload, brought about by a recruitment freeze and high vacancy level.[115] From embattled Felixstowe, it was put this way:

> The clinicians, who now keep the NHS in such high esteem, will become exploitable employees in the quest for profits for boards and shareholders as the incentive.[116]

All this seemed a long way from the NHS listening and giving power to its experienced, dedicated and skilled staff.

111 *Creating a Patient-led NHS.* London: Department of Health, March 2005, para 4.11.

112 Charles Webster (1998) *The National Health Service: a political history.* Oxford: Oxford University Press, p.197.

113 Sir Nigel Crisp, *Commissioning a Patient-led NHS.* Letter, 28 July 2005. London: Department of Health.

114 Peter Clifford, 'PCT questions are in need of answers.' Letter. *East Anglian Daily Times,* 6 June 2006.

115 Alison Taylor (2006) *Finance Report: PCT medium term financial strategy, 26th April 2006.* Bury St Edmunds: Suffolk West PCT, para 2.7.

116 Peter Mellor, 'Save Felixstowe Hospitals. Private quest hurts patient care.' *East Anglian Daily Times,* 17 August 2006.

9

Combing the Landscape for a Decision-maker

When decisions about local health services are being taken, particularly controversial ones, it can prove difficult to find the true decision-maker. Accountability has a habit of vanishing.

For all the talk of NHS bodies working with local communities, they would officially not be accountable to them. This was spelt out in a Department of Health document published in 2001, called *Shifting the Balance of Power.* Riddled with talk about devolving power to local people, and engaging and empowering local communities, the Annex to the document gave the game away. Spelling out the responsibilities of NHS bodies the document states baldly and bluntly: 'PCTs will be accountable to the Secretary of State through the strategic health authority.' Likewise NHS trusts. Likewise strategic health authorities. There was nothing about formal accountability to local communities.[1]

During 2005 and 2006, the Secretary of State would blame local NHS organisations for things going awry. Those local trusts quietly (but not too publicly, frequently or explicitly) blamed the government for setting whimsical and ever-changing targets, together with burdensome financial rules. And, as for the strategic health authorities, the go-betweens between the politicians and the frontline? They had all but donned cloaks of invisibility.

Down in West Suffolk, the local community would find itself at the centre of just such an accountability vacuum. The Suffolk West PCT was the frontline decision-maker, but would explain at a public meeting in June

1 *Shifting the Balance of Power within the NHS.* London: Department of Health, 2001.

2005 that a) it was answerable to the Secretary of State, and b) could not take major decisions without the approval of the strategic health authority. The Secretary of State, the SHA and the PCT would all come to deny ultimate responsibility for the proposals and decisions to take away people's health services. There seemed to be in effect no real decision-maker. What more effective way of stifling democracy, accountability, choice and the voice of a local community, if the decision-maker could not be identified?

One rung down from the Secretary of State in the great game of non-accountability come the strategic health authorities. Their role, in a nutshell, is described as to 'hold to account the local health service, build capacity and support performance'.[2] In many parts of the country, local people and their representatives would be hard pressed to see any of this occurring. The sole accountability of the SHAs was to the Secretary of State. The following exchange reported by one MP sums up the frustration:

> I had a most interesting experience in the summer when I visited something called the Avon, Gloucestershire and Wiltshire strategic health authority. It is unclear to me what a strategic health authority is. I said to the Chief Executive, 'What is it? What do you do?' and he said, 'Well we are strategic' and I said, 'Well, I'm glad about that'.[3]

In East Anglia, the Norfolk, Suffolk and Strategic Health Authority – attacked by an MP for its inaction – defended itself by describing its role as a mere 'postbox' between local NHS bodies and the Secretary of State.[4] Anger had mounted because, despite an acceptance that West Suffolk had received less than its fair funding allocation, it transpired that the SHA had never made representations to the Department of Health about this issue.[5]

In West Suffolk, the SHA's role turned out ultimately to be more shadowy than ever. It is true that in November 2004, it had shown itself meaningfully in public in West Suffolk. Its Director of Finance broke cover by braving an angry and heated public meeting in Sudbury attended by some 500 people. That night, on behalf of the Chief Executive, he partook of a promise made to the people of Sudbury about a new community hospital. In

2 Secretary of State for Health (2002) *Delivering the NHS Plan: next steps on investment, next steps on reform.* Cm 5503. London: HMSO, para 7.3.

3 James Gray, MP for North Wiltshire. *Hansard*, Westminster Hall, 2 November 2005, column 273WH.

4 Will Grahame-Clark, 'MP's anger at health bosses.' *East Anglian Daily Times*, 14 March 2006.

5 Tim Yeo, MP for South Suffolk. *Hansard*, House of Commons, 24 October 2005, column 490WA.

particular, the SHA stated that the PCT's financial deficit would not prevent the building of the new community hospital.

By May 2005, both the Chief Executive and Director of Finance of the SHA had departed. By June, the promise had been broken. The SHA's new Chief Executive, in correspondence with the Walnuttree Hospital Action Committee, simply stated that he was not able to comment on promises that may have been made in the past.[6]

At a public meeting in Sudbury in June 2005, the Suffolk West PCT had declared that it was the decision-maker, but could not act without approval of the SHA, which in turn acted on behalf of central government. This clearly begged the whole question as to who was really pulling the strings. The SHA from start to finish of the whole process would more or less deny all knowledge of everything. Yet it was in June that the SHA had sent in a team to the PCT, going through the books, and coming up with a financial recovery plan. Following a subsequent meeting with local MPs, Tim Yeo, MP, reported that the PCT conceded it was under the 'financial cosh' from the SHA.[7]

The SHA would deny that it was responsible for any specific proposals on closures, maintaining merely that it was instructing the PCT to manage its debts.[8] Yet reliable sources reported that the SHA had told PCTs in Suffolk to close the community hospitals. The hand of the SHA seemed to be everywhere. In October 2005, the Suffolk West PCT reported that it had to save more than it thought, because of new demands by the SHA.[9]

Suffolk West PCT found itself cut adrift, blamed by both central government and the local community for failures for which, ultimately, it should probably not have been blamed. After all, it had inherited a considerable overspend at its inception, and was anyway not in control of most its budget, such was the extent of the targets and rules set by central government. The PCT was in a hopeless position, in terms of policy and finance. It was charged with cutting services in its own name, but in reality at the bidding of

6 Alan Burns. *West Suffolk.* Letter, 19 October 2006. Cambridge: Norfolk, Sufolk and Cambridgeshire Strategic Health Authority.

7 Benedict O'Connor, 'PCT member reacts on return from holiday.' *East Anglian Daily Times,* 2 July 2005. And: Benedict O'Connor, 'Sparks fly as MPs meet with health bosses.' *East Anglian Daily Times,* 12 July 2005.

8 Benedict O'Connor, 'Major cutbacks in bid to save £7.4 m.' *East Anglian Daily Times,* 25 June 2005.

9 'Health trust still needing to make £6.6 million cutbacks.' *East Anglian Daily Times,* 1 September 2005.

central government. Worse, it had to cut services without admitting any associated detriment to patients.

In sum, the lack of decision-making accountability relating to the unpalatable closure of vital health services was well summed up by Boris Johnson, MP. Noting that the general election was now over and that the government was threatening community hospitals with closure:

> Did I say the Government? Forgive me: of course, the Government...denies all responsibility... It is, say ministers, entirely a decision for the local strategic health authority, or the primary care trust... These hospitals were by and large built and funded by local people. They have been loved and used by local people for generations. They were nationalised by the Labour government in 1948... It is not good enough for those national politicians now to say that they have no responsibility for whether those hospitals stay open... No one seems to be in charge. No one is accountable. It is infamous... Patricia Hewitt should recognise that she is presiding over a massacre of local hospitals, and that it is her job – and her job alone – to justify the actions of her appointees.[10]

Orchestrating the votes of PCT boards

Neither executive nor non-executive members of local NHS trust and primary care trust boards are directly accountable to the local community. The local community cannot vote them out of office.

Nevertheless, at times the local communities in Suffolk would wonder why the PCTs did not stand together with their local communities. A vain hope, but as one resident put it, at least if the PCTs fought for much-needed local services – such as the 'one-stop' health and social care centre in Saxmundham – the Chief Executive would have created something in which she 'could have enduring pride'.[11] Indeed, had local PCTs – or even government ministers – stood by local communities, they might well have had statues erected to them.[12] They would have become overnight heroes. Indeed, occasionally, PCTs aspire to this status. As when Bury PCT (in

10 Boris Johnson, 'Hewitt and her appointees are bad news for our hospitals and health.' *Daily Telegraph*, 13 October 2005.

11 John Carrington, 'PCT Chief Executive has thankless task.' Letter. *East Anglian Daily Times*, 19 October 2005.

12 Tim Yeo, MP. *Hansard*, House of Commons Debates, 24 January 2006, column 1409.

Lancashire) sided with the local community against the strategic health authority, which wanted to close a maternity unit at Fairfield Hospital.[13]

This did not happen in Suffolk. Nonetheless, the PCTs continued to refer to the potency of their non-executive Board members. Their role was described on the Suffolk West PCT's website as including acting as 'champions' for the needs, richness and diversity of the local community.

To the local community, high-flown words such as 'richness' and 'diversity' took on a very hollow ring. By voting through proposals which, on strong evidence, would discriminate against members of the community with more complex needs, the non-executive directors would – in the eyes of the community – forget their true role.

Suffolk West PCT had claimed that its decision, following consultation, would be by no means a foregone conclusion: 'the non-executive directors could vote this all out', said the Chief Executive.[14] Yet, when it came to the highly controversial decisions some eight months later, every single recommendation put forward by the Chief Executive was passed without a murmur by a vote of 11–0. Two minor, peripheral amendments were eventually put forward by one of the non-executive board members.[15] All this was despite a prior appeal directly to PCT Board members by the local MP, Tim Yeo:

> In 22 years as a Member of Parliament, I cannot recall any other issue which has provoked such a universally damning response... A heavy responsibility rests on you and your colleagues... It is clearly not the role of non-executive directors simply to rubber-stamp proposals... Thousands of families now look to you and your fellow non-executive directors to show the independence of judgement for which you were appointed.[16]

A more direct challenge was made by a local councillor, asking non-executive members to 'show a little muscle and stand up for what people want. They should get off their backsides and earn the £5000 they are paid.'[17] Following the PCT's decision, a county, district and parish councillor was more forthright, referring to the PCT Board's muteness and likeness to

13 'Health bosses reject unit closure.' *News.bbc.co.uk*, 3 May 2006.

14 Barbara Eeles, 'Cost effective and good for patients too.' *Suffolk Free Press*, 18 August 2006.

15 *Extraordinary Board Meeting Public, 11th April 2006.* Minutes. Bury St Edmunds: Suffolk West PCT.

16 Liz Hearnshaw, 'Eleventh hour bid to save beds.' *East Anglian Daily Times*, 3 January 2006.

17 Paul Holland, 'Health: we are relying on your vote.' *Suffolk Free Press*, 5 January 2006.

stuffed dummies.[18] Such a blunt letter illustrated the extreme sense of frustration in the local community at the apparent aloofness, inaccessibility and detachment of the non-executive members. This was not of course their fault directly. It was the way the system worked. They were not elected, they were appointed. Unlike local councillors, whose contact details are publicly available on the Internet, their contact details were not publicly available. It was difficult to get hold of them.

Nonetheless, the uncomplimentary letter drew a furious response from the PCT Board director who had tabled the two amendments at the meeting.[19] However, the amendments were minor when matched up with the original proposals, and did little to address the concerns of the local community. The fact that the non-executive director concerned had managed to convince himself that he was a local 'champion' was perhaps a telling comment on just how far the world of the PCT Board was from that of the local community.

In fairness, PCT Boards did not have any encouragement from the Prime Minister to show independence. In June 2006, he agreed with a captain of industry that recalcitrant board members, who might sympathise with staff concerned about drastic change, should be sacked.[20]

One former non-executive director of an NHS Trust in the north of England reflected on the powerlessness and futility of his role. This had included understanding very little of what was going on, nodding sagely, constantly cutting budgets, not asking awkward questions, maintaining consensus as a point of honour – and never disagreeing (this would have been 'bad behaviour'). On the whole, he had to be part of a happy family (the Board), whilst supervising an ongoing deterioration in services. In sum, the role had been akin to a child playing with a toy steering wheel in the back seat of a car, tooting, signalling and flashing lights on an imaginary journey. As the children (the non-executive directors) played in the back, the parents (the executives on the Board) were in control in the front.[21]

It seems therefore a vain hope of the Healthcare Commission that non-executive directors could help avoid the 'awful tragedy' at Stoke

18 Richard Kemp, 'How depressing.' Letter. *Suffolk Free Press*, 20 April 2006.

19 Dr Paul Rylott, 'Hospitals: I was our champion.' Letter. *Suffolk Free Press*, 27 April 2006.

20 John Carvel, 'Blundering ministers are making NHS patients suffer say consultants' leader.' *Guardian*, 7 June 2006.

21 Peter Barker, 'All work and no say.' *Guardian*, 5 July 2006.

Mandeville Hospital. The Buckinghamshire Hospitals NHS Trust had prioritised government targets on waiting lists and finance ahead of infection control. Nearly 40 patients died, and hundreds were infected with *Clostridium difficile*. The Commission stated that where the executive team is focused on day-to-day operational matters, 'non-executive directors had a duty to bring a balanced judgement to all the issues and choices faced by the organisation.'[22] A sensible recommendation, but arguably wishful thinking.

Despite the dire financial position, the panic-stricken cuts being implemented, and the conflict with local communities across Suffolk, resignations from NHS boards were thin on the ground. One notable exception was the resignation of the Vice-Chairman of the Suffolk West PCT Board, in protest at what was happening. This was in contrast to some other areas, such as Lincolnshire, where the Chief Executive of United Lincolnshire Hospitals NHS Trust stood down in November 2005, to be followed by the Chairwoman a few months later.[23]

A similar pattern of apparent non-accountability emerged when in 2006 the Chairman of the Norfolk, Suffolk and Cambridgeshire Strategic Health Authority was announced as the chair of a new, larger authority. This was despite the fact that he had in effect presided over, and allowed to develop, a deficit across the region that exceeded £90 million. His appointment, together with three of the existing non-executive directors, excited understandable criticism from John Gummer, MP. He was seeing his local health services in East Suffolk seriously cut as a result of the deficit, and yet senior figures were being rewarded for the debacle.[24]

In the East of Suffolk, the PCTs would refer to the 'robust challenge and consideration of proposals' by the Board. Yet six general practitioners from Saxmundham recalled the vote of the Suffolk East PCTs' Board some seven months earlier to veto a local 'one-stop shop' for health and social care:

> One of these directors, who was previously supportive some two months earlier, mumbled the execution proposal into his papers. Not one of the non-executive directors said a single word of 'robust challenge and consideration'.[25]

22 *Investigation into outbreaks of Clostridium difficile at Stoke Mandeville Hospital, Buckinghamshire.* London: Healthcare Commission, 2006, p.89.

23 'NHS Trust boss resigns her post.' *Sleaford Standard,* 8 March 2006.

24 Graham Dines, 'MP angry at choice of health chairman.' *East Anglian Daily Times,* 13 May 2006.

25 Drs Havard, Murphy, Evans, Hamblyn, Dunn and Oates, 'We must grasp the chance to air our views.' Letter. *East Anglian Daily Times,*10 November 2005.

Prominent members of the community had been appalled. Three, a local rector, Chairman of the town council and Chairman of the governors of a local primary school, wrote that the decision had been:

> stage-managed to produce the result the officers required. We feel that there has been behind-the-scenes briefing against this scheme for almost a year now.[26]

The Patient and Public Involvement Forum (PPIF) for the Suffolk Coastal area wrote an open letter to PCT Board members, pointing out the huge opposition to the most recent proposals for the East of Suffolk. It pleaded with them to vote according to their honest beliefs and reminded them that they did not have to approve every proposal on the table.[27]

All these pleas fell on deaf ears: on 25 January 2006, the Suffolk East PCTs passed the recommendations for the closure of the Bartlet and Hartismere Hospitals unanimously, as well as warning of yet more cuts to follow:

> FURY AS HOSPITALS CLOSED.[28]

However assiduously and critically Board members may have believed they were doing their job, this did not come over to the public. A resident of Leiston would conclude that PCT Boards were both subservient to, and protected by, the Secretary of State:

> doing exactly as Mrs Hewitt [Secretary of State] wishes and are all Teflon-coated by the Appointments Commission, hence their smugness when challenged by the public.[29]

Another resident referred to the PCT decision-makers as oblivious to the true effects of their decisions:

> if many of them had real first-hand experience of the likely effects of their decisions and the people they are 'dumping', they would find it hard to sleep at night. This issue affects future generations as well.[30]

26 Sarah Chambers, 'Stalwarts attack funding defeat.' *East Anglian Daily Times*, 11 November 2005.

27 Malcolm C.F. Briggs and others, 'Make the choices you honestly believe in.' Letter. *East Anglian Daily Times*, 25 January 2006.

28 *East Anglian Daily Times*, 26 January 2006.

29 Malcolm C.F. Briggs, 'Battle to retain health service must continue.' Letter. *East Anglian Daily Times*, 11 November 2005.

30 A.J.D. Mills, 'Health cuts will have long-term implications.' *East Anglian Daily Times*, 21 November 2005.

Keeping the non-accountability balloon airborne

The lack of accountability was omnipresent. Two more illustrations are as follows, one concerning exaggerated claims about financial matters. The other is an astonishing tale of how 17,000 expressions of protest were received by the Department of Health about Sudbury and promptly disappeared.

The first indicates a lack of accountability for factually incorrect information given to Parliament by the Secretary of State. When she was asked in Parliament about Walnuttree Hospital, she implied that the hospital was a hopeless case, not least because it had had £300,000 spent on fire safety works. A Freedom of Information Act request directed to the West Suffolk NHS Hospitals Trust established that the true figure was well under £100,000. The Secretary of State had been misinformed. She had then misled the House of Commons. A search for accountability and an apology were demanded by Tim Yeo, MP.[31] Neither ultimately were forthcoming.

Second, during the consultation process in West Suffolk, the local Sudbury community had not only sent in some 3000 responses to the PCT's consultation, but also sent 5500 letters and postcards to Patricia Hewitt, as well as an 11,500 signature petition. When, shortly before its final decision due to be taken in February 2006, the PCT was informed about these, it stated that it needed to see them in order to take account properly of local views.

The PCT accordingly took a swift and creditable decision to delay its decision by six weeks until 11 April. Much to its subsequent embarrassment and in a turn of events which can only be described as absurd, the Department of Health then refused to hand over either the petition or the letters.

The situation then became farcical. Having postponed by six weeks its all-important Board meeting, in order to take account of the 5500 letters sent to the Department of Health, the PCT now found the latter refusing to pass down the letters. As the *Suffolk Free Press* graphically put it on the front page:

> 5500: number of letters Department of Health received about threat to Sudbury hospitals; 65: number passed on to PCT decision-makers.[32]

31 Tim Yeo, MP. *Hansard*, House of Commons Debates, 24 January 2006, column 1406.

32 Paul Holland, '5500 number of letters.' *Suffolk Free Press*, 23 February 2006.

It had been buck passing by rote. Denied the letters, the PCT could scarcely criticise publicly Patricia Hewitt. Even so, the local Patient and Public Involvement Forum thought the PCT must have been privately furious at the Department of Health's attitude.[29]

The Department of Health then stated that it had now handed the petition to the PCT.[33] Nevertheless, the PCT's Board papers gave no recognition that this had ever happened.[34]

Unsurprisingly, the local Patient and Public Involvement Forum stated that this turn of events had rendered the consultation null and void, and that it was 'very undemocratic'.[35] This was a sentiment that the PCT had agreed with three days earlier when it said that it was not 'prepared to disenfranchise any consultees who had acted in good faith'.[36] By 11 April 2006, the day of the Board meeting, this sentiment had been set so far aside that not only had the letters not been received, but their very existence was not even alluded to.

So instead, as the NHS must always be seen to be in the right, the PCT blamed the local action committee, which it claimed had accepted responsibility for the 'error' of people sending their correspondence to the Secretary of State. The Walnuttree Hospital Action Committee responded:

> On behalf of the Action Committee I totally refute the Chairman of the Primary Care Trust's assertion – made in his letter to the Suffolk Free Press last week – that WHAC has accepted responsibility for errors in relation to correspondence sent to the Secretary of State rather than the PCT.
>
> This is simply not accurate. I know personally that all WHAC colleagues, including myself, who spent many hours meeting thousands of people, were categoric in advising people where they had to send their responses (i.e. to the PCT at the address on the consultation document).[37]

The whole episode was quite absurd. For the Department of Health not to have passed down the letters was inexplicable. It was the head office; why

33 Dave Gooderham, 'War of words over hospitals.' *East Anglian Daily Times*, 20 February 2006.

34 Michael Stonard (2006) *Modernising Health Care in West Suffolk: report for decision, Suffolk West Primary Care Trust Board, 11th April 2006*. Bury St Edmunds: Suffolk West PCT, para 15.3.

35 '5500: number of letters.' *Suffolk Free Press*, 23 February 2006.

36 Dave Gooderham, 'War of words over hospitals.' *East Anglian Daily Times*, 20 February 2006.

37 Colin Spence, 'Hospital jibe.' Letter. *Suffolk Free Press*, 2 March 2006.

had it not passed down the letters, postcards (and petition) to the relevant local office (Suffolk West PCT)? Even more remarkable, the Department had not even informed the PCT of the existence of the petition or the letters.[38] The PCT confirmed that it had not known of their existence. One way or another, it seemed to be confirmation that there was no longer a 'national' health service, let alone one that proceeded on vaguely democratic lines.

38 Mark Bulstrode, 'PCT decision delayed as objections go astray.' *East Anglian Daily Times*, 15 February 2006.

10

Rushing into Decisions and Reaping the Consequences

The pressure placed by central government and strategic health authorities on primary care trusts and NHS trusts to implement new policies, and to hit performance and financial targets, can be acute. It seems instant obedience and results are demanded. This puts immense pressure on local NHS bodies, which is augmented if some of those policies are themselves of doubtful substance or are cloaking hidden and sensitive agendas. It leads to rushed decision-making and a lack of transparency. And it all has to be sold to the public.

This can result in excessive use of emotive but empty language to try to explain new policies, both at national and local level. When more detail has to be mastered, and awkward cracks plastered over, then the language of euphemism takes hold. When that is itself inadequate, and 'less' has to be passed off as 'more', then the realms of doublethink or doublespeak are sometimes entered into. Misrepresentations may come into it. Evidence may be lacking or used highly selectively. And logic and facts are sometimes dispensed with.

The greater the unreasonable pressure from central government in terms of sudden demands and changing, contradictory policies, so the greater risk is there of corners being cut. Sometimes the pressures result in the floating of red herrings, to conceal underlying aims. Lastly, rushed and pressurised decision-making can lead NHS bodies to plan the sending in of imaginary armies – for instance, of peripatetic, community care staff. This in turn can lead to a bunker mentality on the part of NHS bodies, both to preserve the unreality and illusion of what they are proposing, and to protect themselves from criticism.

All this is by no means perpetrated intentionally. To local communities at the sharp end, NHS trusts and PCTs seem to act in such a manner unconsciously. In the skewed world of NHS management, shortcuts in decision-making, an involuntary reflex of disingenuousness, and loss of judgement appear to be endemic.

Overall, the extent to which the NHS speaks a different language was well described by Peter Rainsford, Chair of the Campaign to Save Wells Hospital, in Wells-next-the-Sea:

> There were a lot of very cross people and a lot of raw energy, but it was a question of channelling that raw energy. We needed a leader to focus the campaign. We needed local MPs, GPs and we needed the media. We also needed an interpreter because the NHS doesn't speak English.[1]

In Suffolk, the view generally taken by the Walnuttree Hospital Action Committee (WHAC) was that the shortcuts in decision-making that appeared to be taken were almost certainly unwitting. In its view, they were brought about by too much pressure and eagerness to please central goverment. This caused understandable lapses of judgement – although the consequences for local people were no less serious. But not all onlookers were so charitable. Using Parliamentary privilege, Tim Yeo, MP, referred to the PCT's tendency to throw truth to the wind – or at least out of the window.[2]

Tuning up the policies: song of the nightingale

Policies have to be made to sound good. So we find the New Labour 2001 manifesto referring to 'world class public services'.[3] To become world class, it has also to be visionary. For instance, when explaining plans for greater centralisation – by reducing the number of NHS primary care trusts – the Norfolk, Suffolk and Cambridgeshire Strategic Health Authority claimed that government had 'captured and shared this vision in its cornerstone document, *Creating a Patient-led NHS*'.

1 Mark Gould, 'No closure on campaigns to save community hospitals.' *Health Service Journal*, 23 February 2006.

2 Tim Yeo, MP. *Hansard*, House of Commons Debates, 24 January 2006, column 1405.

3 *Labour's Manifesto 2001: ambitions for Britain.* London: Labour Party.

Wariness is required of cornerstones and of the capturing and sharing of visions – especially when they are followed by words such as 'reality', 'shared aspiration', together with everything that would be 'new': standards of care, skills, freedoms, incentives and, of course, systems. This document talked of a wider range of services in community settings.[4] Such wariness is vital, given that at the time the SHA was allowing its PCTs in Suffolk to try to implement a wide range of cutbacks.

Brightness and jollity should also be approached with caution. As Libby Purves found in Suffolk, the cyberworld of the websites of PCTs is 'bright and jolly', with 'babies smiling at grandmothers' and consultation is about 'changing for the better' (the mantra adopted for cutbacks to services in the East of Suffolk). The scriptwriters were:

> plainly feeling good. Their cyberworld is a far cry from the timeless aches and staggerings of humanity; like Keats's nightingale, they live apart from the weariness, the fever and the fret of this sad world where palsy shakes a few sad last grey hairs and men must sit and hear each other groan… From PCT websites you would never guess at the depth, breadth and despair of NHS recession…the glossy PCT websites look more and more like skeins of stardust thrown over real anxiety and pain.

What was being concealed under the stardust? The fact that 22 years ago, the writer of the article had a cottage hospital, GPs who came out at night, an NHS dentist within cycling distance and a maternity home and mental hospital ten miles away. Now the latter two were shut, and out-of-hours access was restricted – if you overcame the evasions of NHS Direct telephone service – to a tired, cross locum. To top it all, the cottage hospitals were now being axed.[5]

The PCTs, too, would at local level make use of emotive language. In West Suffolk, good, solid hospitals with dedicated staff once provided real care and recuperation. But now, the new airy health centres being proposed – with no beds, no consultants and unspecified staff and facilities – would be places where the new model of care would 'develop and thrive'. They would be 'dynamic'.[6]

4 NSCSHA (2005) *Consultation on new Primary Care Trusts arrangements in Norfolk, Suffolk and Cambridgeshire: ensuring a patient-led NHS.* Cambridge: NSCSHA, pp.4–5.

5 Libby Purves, 'Health alert: infectious ideas.' *The Times*, 24 January 2006.

6 Suffolk West PCT (2005) *Modernising Health Care in West Suffolk: consultation, 1 August – 31 October 2005.* Bury St Edmunds: Suffolk West PCT, p.7.

These were the sorts of emotive and positive terms designed to make the reader of a consultation document think it will all be for the best, even though the document in question gave absolutely no idea about how this was to happen. The Suffolk West PCT, citing little evidence, would also attempt to reduce the whole affair to a trivial game of tag, calling it a game of 'catch-up' with the rest of the country. The game would involve closing its community hospital beds as well as removing other services from Sudbury.[7]

But the PCTs hadn't necessarily aligned their stories. The Suffolk East PCTs explained that far from catching up, the changes were happening in Suffolk at 'a faster pace' than elsewhere, because of the 'particular financial challenges'.[8] More sweeping statements by the PCTs in Suffolk came in the form of claims about what a modern health service should look like. The PCTs in the East would imply that community hospital beds were a thing of the past, and that in other parts of the country strong community services meant they were not needed.[9]

Either way, the PCTs in Suffolk were not giving the full picture. Not least, because there was evidence and reports of new community hospitals being built in some areas, with beds. For example, a new rehabilitation wing with beds was being built for the community hospital at Halstead – just down the road in Essex.[10] Further illustration of just how misleading such statements were came in the form of the government's White Paper of 2006, which supported community hospitals and their beds.[11]

In the West, the PCT would not be delivering ordinary 'intermediate care'. It would be 'enhanced', whatever that was supposed to mean. Probably no more than to convince local people they would be getting something special. In fact, 'enhanced' meant nothing, since there has to be something to enhance. In Sudbury, Suffolk, there was no pre-existing intermediate care to enhance; and the intermediate care on offer was anyway of an apparently standard, not an 'enhanced', variety.[12]

7 Benedict O'Connor, 'NHS boss spells out why health cuts are needed.' *East Anglian Daily Times*, 18 August 2005.

8 *Changing for the Better: next steps.* Ipswich: Suffolk East PCTs, 2005.

9 'Trust outlines health care changes.' *East Anglian Daily Times*, 10 November 2005.

10 *Halstead Gazette*, 26 August 2005.

11 Secretary of State for Health (2006) *Our Health, Our Care, Our Say: a new direction for community services.* Cm 6737. London: HMSO, para 6.40.

12 *Modernising Health Care in West Suffolk: consultation, 1 August – 31 October 2005.* Bury St Edmunds: Suffolk West PCT, 2005, p.7.

The changes were, the public was told, all being based on 'expert medical evidence' and 'sound financial judgement' – 'with the interests of the people of West Suffolk at heart'.[13] But it was unclear just where the 'expert medical evidence' was that supported the extreme form of intermediate care being proposed by the PCT (see Chapter 13). And the local community couldn't see that the sound financial judgement was anything more than the uncontroversial premiss that it is always cheap to provide nothing.

Perhaps, above all, the word 'modernisation' was the one that was meant to take the public with it. Both nationally and locally, it was modernisation that seemed to be the key word. Nationally, New Labour would talk about the need for change and modernisation to justify its glittering new policies of patient choice, opening up the NHS to competition the marketplace and the private sector. Hand in hand with modernisation, came the charge that not only was the current health service 'old-fashioned' but it wasn't working. What it did not do, for example, was analyse why there had been problems – for example, because there had been decades of relative under-investment.[14]

Health mantras on the wing: a daily chorus

Mantras, too, have had their place in the bold new world of New Labour's NHS. One of these has been along the lines of provision of 'patient-centred care – the right care, in the right place, at the right time'. In particular such a commitment must be 'above all, honoured, in the delivery of care for older people'.[15] Local PCTs took it up, as they consulted on widespread cuts and closures, which most of all would affect older people. In West Suffolk the 'vision' was that people should receive not only the right care, in the right place at the right time, but also have it delivered by the right person.[16]

Such mantras are of course inadequate substitutes for true substance and evidence. This particular one is anyway redundant and otiose, since even to

13 Benedict O'Connor, 'NHS boss spells out why health cuts are needed.' *East Anglian Daily Times*, 18 August 2005.

14 Allyson Pollock (2005) *NHS plc: the privatisation of our health care.* London: Verso, p.36.

15 Secretary of State for Health (2002) *Delivering the NHS Plan: next steps on investment, next steps on reform.* Cm 5503. London: HMSO, para 8.5.

16 *Modernising Health Care in West Suffolk: consultation, 1 August – 31 October 2005.* Bury St Edmunds: Suffolk West PCT.

contemplate doing the opposite – to provide the wrong care, in the wrong place, at the wrong time, by the wrong people – would be absurd.

Another has been that, no matter how serious the cutbacks in services being made, 'patient care will not suffer'. Of course sometimes people do not get the mantra right. In January 2006, the Chief Executive of the Royal Free Hospital, was reported as saying that the cuts he was implementing could harm patient care. His spokeswoman had described the position as 'grim'. By the end of April, he was back on track, talking about the marvels of efficiency savings and how patients would benefit.[17]

Even more bravely, a chief executive in Leicestershire – in the face of overall savings to be made locally of £62 million – could still maintain that he 'remained committed to ensuring that health care services remain of the highest quality'.[18]

Likewise in Southampton where, in June 2006, it was announced that 564 jobs and 140 beds were to be lost – following 600 posts and 109 beds lost the previous year. This was toward the making of £26 million savings. Nonetheless, the inevitable reassuring words from the chief executive followed. It was all about improving services for patients. It would even be exciting for staff.[19]

In Suffolk, the new chairman of Ipswich Hospital NHS Trust – facing a deficit of £12 million (to be revealed three weeks later as in fact £16.7 million) – would talk of 're-energisation', 'efficiency' and 'cost reduction'. Most importantly, the people of east Suffolk had nothing to fear.[20] One of his senior consultants was more straightforward. He referred to staff being fed up and unable to provide a service, and the whole situation as being very worrying. Another recently retired consultant spoke of 'disastrous strains'. Even the hospital spokeswoman felt forced to admit to 'difficult circumstances'.[21]

Sometimes, even PCT chairmen allow a little reality to creep into their statements. In the wake of plans to close rehabilitation wards at Evesham hospital, replace a five bed Macmillan (palliative care) unit, and possibly to cut school nurses, sexual health clinics and out-of-hours GP surgeries, the

17 Ellen Widdup, 'Wards shut to save NHS cash.' *Evening Standard,* 31 January 2006. And: 'NHS faces up to dawn of a new era.' *News.bbc.co.uk,* 28 April 2006.

18 Jenny Hardcastle, 'Jobs at risk under £62m health cuts.' *Leicester Mercury,* 15 June 2006.

19 Jenny Makin, 'Job cuts will lead to a better service.' *Southern Daily Echo,* 28 June 2006.

20 Graham Dines, 'Healthy outlook for ailing trust.' *East Anglian Daily Times,* 4 July 2006.

21 Mark Bulstrode, 'Surgeon says morale is down at hospital.' *East Anglian Daily Times,* 12 August 2006.

chairman of South Worcestershire PCT did refer to a 'very uncomfortable programme of cost reductions' – given the debt of £12.8 million.[22]

But, by and large, the line is toed. A period of chaos occurred at West Suffolk Hospital in Bury St Edmunds in the middle of August 2006. This involved nine-hour accident and emergency waits, queuing ambulances unable to unload patients, and some patients suddenly taken miles away to Cambridge and Ipswich Hospitals. The strategic health authority nevertheless rose impeccably to the occasion:

> We are aware that West Suffolk Hospital has experienced exceptional attendance at their A&E department in the last few weeks. Together with the ambulance service and other neighbouring hospitals, they have demonstrated how effectively the NHS works.[23]

So, bodies were evidently past masters of wishful thinking and disingenuous statements to the point of absurdity. Unfortunately, local councils did not lag behind as they took their cue from the NHS, both setting about cutting services with a will and managing to deny it. For instance, Suffolk County Council, announcing possible widespread closures of its day centres, and the cutting down of its specialist hospital discharge team, could nevertheless announce that it was about 'to develop and expand' its services. This was against the background of a £24 million deficit, of which some £15 million was being cut in adult social care.[24]

Similarly, when the Sandwell and West Birmingham Hospitals NHS Trust planned to reduce its 7500 workforce by 800 jobs, it promised that the cuts would not overstretch staff providing frontline care.[25] But, as Dr Malone, general secretary of the RCN, put it:

> NHS deficits are hitting patients services; to claim otherwise is simply wrong. These are real services for real people with real illnesses, and we have got to stop treating them as statistics on a balance sheet.[26]

At least former health ministers such as Frank Dobson, if not the incumbent ones, could see the real world:

22 'Wards to close in £12m cuts.' *News.bbc.co.uk*, 9 June 2006.

23 Will Clarke, 'Hospital "already streteched to limit" warning.' *East Anglian Daily Times*, 18 August 2006.

24 'Council to review provision of adult care.' Press release. Suffolk County Council, 8 August 2006.

25 'Care pledge as NHS jobs axed.' *East Anglian Daily Times*, 14 April 2006.

26 John Carvel, 'NHS cuts hit cancer care for children.' *Guardian*, 24 April 2006.

> I wish ministers would give up the stupid pretence that getting rid of hundreds of staff will not damage patient care.[27]

The public, too, is not so easily taken in. For instance, after the Suffolk East PCTs had voted for a long list of cuts to services, a correspondent stated sarcastically that the Chief Executive had promised to continue to explain:

> until we get her message, that savage cuts are good for us and that NHS users must accept this.[28]

Dispensing glad tidings and euphemism

When awkward detail has to be papered over, the language of euphemism plays an important role. At an extreme, it turns into doublethink or double-speak. For instance, Patricia Hewitt felt able to refer to the NHS having had its best year yet – in the midst of cuts, closures, deficits and redundancies.[29]

Suffolk West PCT, too, would display the art of euphemism. After the three main general medical practices had raised fundamental doubts about the PCT's proposals, the PCT nevertheless reported to the PCT Board that there was 'limited support' from those general practitioners.[30] This was unfathomable. When one of the Sudbury general practices wrote to the PCT in September, referring to its 'dire concerns', it asked the Chief Executive to bring these concerns to the notice of the Trust Board.[31] A PCT spokeswoman said at the time that the concerns would indeed be put to the Board.[32] The notion of 'dire concerns' simply does not equate with the term 'limited support'.

Likewise, the term 'limited support' was inappropriate in relation to a second letter sent by another general practice in the Sudbury area. This letter had spoken of how insubstantial the PCT's claim to be improving services was, dismissed the wonderful soundbite of the mantra of the right care, in the right place, at the right time – and referred to the extreme unlikelihood

27 John Carvel, 'NHS hospital redundancies gather pace.' *Guardian*, 23 March 2006.

28 D. Ardizzone, 'Weasel words when matched with reality.' Letter. *East Anglian Daily Times*, 6 February 2006.

29 'Health secretary's comment draws criticism from nurses.' *East Anglian Daily Times*, 24 April 2006.

30 Michael Stonard (2006) *Modernising Health Care in West Suffolk: report for decision, Suffolk West Primary Care Trust Board, 11th April 2006.* Bury St Edmunds: Suffolk West PCT, para 9.6.

31 Drs Donnelly, Kemp, Taylor, O'Neill and Ahmed, 'Sudbury hospital is essential.' Letter. *Suffolk Free Press*, 29 September 2005.

32 Nicki Harvey, 'Doctors united in hospital fight.' *Suffolk Free Press*, 29 September 2005.

of care in the home meeting the needs of people who currently needed to occupy community hospital beds.[33]

More euphemism was used to describe aspects of the consultation process undertaken by Suffolk West PCT, including the roadshows it held. At Newmarket, 9 people attended, at Mildenhall 12, and at Ixworth 25. At Sudbury, 100 attended, but this was probably only because the local action committee decided, unilaterally, to publicise the event and direct people to it in the local church. All this would not however stop the PCT referring to the roadshows euphemistically as 'quite successful'.

A former non-executive director of the PCT, now living in the real world, was rather more accurate, referring to the Newmarket event as 'dismal'. In the same vein, after two months of the consultation period had run, only 152 replies had been received. Yet the PCT could still refer to the consultation as 'encouraging', although the Chief Executive did concede that it had not been a 'runaway success'.[34]

Behind the euphemism lay an altogether different story. By the end of the consultation process, another two months later, the replies to Suffolk West PCT's consultation had rocketed to several thousand. This was in large part due directly to the extensive efforts not of the PCT but of the local action committees in Sudbury and Newmarket. In Sudbury, the committee was out on the streets for many weeks, talking to people and giving out consultation documents to be filled in.[35]

The MP, Tim Yeo, continued to urge people to respond[36] and a public meeting was held, at which the Walnuttree Hospital Action Committee urged the importance of responding.[37] The Sudbury Mayor, Lesley Ford-Platt, too would make a last-minute appeal to the town to respond.[38]

The PCT would seek to take credit nonetheless, stating that the fact of having received so many responses meant that the 'general public do not

33 Letter. Long Melford Practice, 20 September 2005.

34 Benedict O'Connor, '£20m health process not "runaway success".' *East Anglian Daily Times,* 3 October 2005.

35 Benedict O'Connor, 'MP: speak out over health cut proposals.' *East Anglian Daily Times,* 17 October 2005.

36 'Last-ditch bid to save Walnuttree.' *East Anglian Daily Times,* 14 November 2005.

37 'Final effort to safeguard Walnuttree.' *East Anglian Daily Times,* 15 November 2005.

38 'Vital that people make their feelings known.' *East Anglian Daily Times,* 3 December 2005.

perceive the consultation as a farce and they have responded in their thousands'.[39] But, in short, as the Mayor put it:

> the only reason [the PCT] has received so many responses is that others took the trouble and the expense to provide the required copies, so all those who wished could have the opportunity to make their views known.[40]

Further evidence of the PCT's apparently limited expectations was revealed by its lack of preparedness for receiving such a large volume of responses. It was forced to postpone its decision by a month in order to analyse them.

The extent to which the PCT would try to take credit for all the efforts of local people became clear later on. It had launched the consultation in the summer holidays, and been forced to extend the timescale and to publish further information, essentially because of the demands of the Health Scrutiny Committee and possibly the Walnuttree Hospital Action Committee.[41] To all appearances it had been forced into this. But the PCT would now claim that it had:

> bent over backwards to ensure that, firstly, everyone had more than ample opportunity to give their views in response to the consultation and, secondly, we have sufficient time to analyse all of the feedback.[42]

Dealing in doublethink

George Orwell famously described the art of doublethink. Part of the definition is as follows:

> Doublethink means the power of holding two contradictory beliefs in one's mind simultaneously, and accepting both of them. The Party intellectual...knows that he is playing tricks with reality; but by the exercise of doublethink he also satisfies himself that reality is not violated. The process has to be conscious, or it would not be carried out with sufficient precision, but it also has to be unconscious, or it would bring with it a feeling of falsity and hence of guilt...the essential act is

39 Dave Gooderham, 'Last-minute effort to keep hospitals open.' *East Anglian Daily Times*, 12 December 2005.

40 Lesley Ford-Platt, 'Get your facts right first and then speak.' Letter. *East Anglian Daily Times*, 20 December 2005.

41 *Interim Report on Committee Response to NHS Consultations*, 1 November 2005. H05/22. Ipswich: Suffolk County Council Health Scrutiny Committee.

42 Dave Gooderham, 'War of words over hospitals.' *East Anglian Daily Times*, 20 February 2006.

> to use conscious deception while retaining the firmness of purpose that goes with complete honesty. To tell deliberate lies while genuinely believing in them, to forget any fact that has become inconvenient, and then, when it becomes necessary again, to draw it back from oblivion for just so long as it is needed, to deny the existence of objective reality and all the while to take account of the reality which one denies...it is a vast system of mental cheating.[43]

Without overplaying the parallel, it is an instructive comparison to make with some of what has happened in the NHS. It does seem – so schooled are ministers, NHS trusts and PCTs in coming up with convincing, infallible explanation – that they will say things neither consistent with the facts nor with what they may have said a week or month ago. Most importantly, they appear genuinely to believe it. It was the Walnuttree Hospital Action Committee's view that the doublethink or doublespeak did not necessarily equate to bad faith in West Suffolk. The PCT really did seem to believe it all. On the other hand, the Suffolk County Council Health Scrutiny Committee was not so charitable, referring to a lack of honesty in the way in which the Suffolk PCTs put forward their proposals.[44]

For example, the word modernisation came to Suffolk. It was this word that the PCTs used so heavily and emotively to explain that cutting back vital local community hospital beds was the way forward. They were 'old-fashioned' and so would be swept away for people's own good. The problem was the PCT had been going to build what it had described as a modern new community hospital in Sudbury to meet the needs of the local population for decades to come. This had also been in furtherance of its long-term intermediate care strategy.[45]

In June 2005, it abandoned the hospital because 'community hospitals tend to be used as part of an old fashioned model of care that often caters more for the social aspects of care occasionally required by older people'.[46] The only thing that could possibly account for this complete change of tack was that the strategic health authority had demanded that the PCT make financial cutbacks. The word modernisation was clearly an elastic term. So

43 George Orwell [1949] (2003) *Nineteen Eighty Four.* London: Penguin Books, p.244.

44 *Interim Report on Committee Response to NHS Consultations,* 1 November 2005. H05/22. Ipswich: Suffolk County Council Health Scrutiny Committee, para 45.

45 *Outline Business Case for the Development of Sudbury Health and Social Care Centre.* March 2005. Bury St Edmunds: Suffolk West PCT, para 1.1.

46 Mike Stonard (2005) *Proposed Local Delivery and Financial Recovery Plan, 29th June 2005.* Bury St Edmunds: Suffolk West PCT, appendix 3, para 15.

elastic that the PCT's financial recovery plan would fly directly in the face of the government's White Paper of six months later, praising community hospital beds.[47] More importantly it flatly contradicted what it had been saying but a month before. In effect, what had been cracked up as a modern hospital at the beginning of June 2005, was derided as old-fashioned by the end of June 2005. This was an exercise in the true art of doublethink or doublespeak.

Likewise, the reason for the modernisation was both financial and it wasn't financial. The PCT was overspent by some £20 million. It continued to claim that finance was not the reason for the changes and cuts to Suffolk health services: 'It is absolutely not the case that the PCT is using service modernisation to hide cuts in services'.[48] But in the same breath, it would make quite clear that the reason for the abrupt changes and cuts to services was precisely to do with money:

> We are reviewing all expenditure and services. Nothing is excluded. The PCT is spending more money than it receives and is building up debts and we have to get the situation back under control.[49]

It was unsurprising that local elected councillors, such as the Mayor of Sudbury, were unconvinced by such ambiguity. Huge financial debt, sudden demands from central government for it to be wiped out, and equally sudden changes and cuts to local services ensured this scepticism would flourish. In sheer bemusement, they would refer to the Chief Executive as acting like an:

> accountant, just adding up the figures with no regard for what is best for our town and future generations.[50]

In Suffolk, the PCTs must have been convinced about what they were claiming, and really believed they were offering something better. But the local communities involved would find this unbelievable. Their local services were threatened with closure, and in their place would come services that they had every reason to believe would be inappropriate and under-resourced. The doublethink, the doublespeak, wasn't working.

Over in the East of Suffolk, the cutbacks were called *Changing for the Better*. If there is one thing that alienates local communities more than having

47 Secretary of State for Health (2006) *Our Health, Our Care, Our Say: a new direction for community services*. Cm 6737. London: HMSO, para 6.40.

48 Dave Gooderham, 'Health cuts plan "flawed".' *East Anglian Daily Times*, 31 October 2006.

49 Patrick Lowman, 'Resign over debts crisis – bosses are urged.' *East Anglian Daily Times*, 24 June 2005.

50 'It's up to you to have a say.' *Suffolk Free Press*, 15 September 2005.

their services taken away from them, it is if they believe a deceptive veneer has been overlaid. As the Save our Felixstowe Hospitals Action Group put it:

> we are incensed that they are calling [their plans] *Changing for the Better.* They are cuts, and cuts will lead to problems and a poorer service.[51]

This theme was constant: a considered letter to the *Suffolk Free Press* from a local resident concluded:

> Why, oh why, can't they be honest and admit that they can only offer a second-rate system of healthcare, being the puppets of Whitehall. Then, we could at least admire them for being honest.[52]

The Walnuttree Hospital Action Committee lamented that it was 'bad enough' that services should be removed. But:

> not to explain this – and instead to pretend that it is all about improvement and modernisation – is truly unforgivable. It shows utter contempt for us all and is an abuse of power.[53]

The doublethink seemed to continue. In May 2006, the West Suffolk Hospitals NHS Trust denied that a unit for people with mental health problems in Sudbury was closing – 'as long as patients are referred to the unit'.[54] However, it did not point out that there was actually a policy not to refer patients to the unit.[55] So it was closure – and it was not closure.

Closely linked to doublethink is the rewriting or altering of history, also explored by George Orwell. For instance, in Sudbury, 36 beds simply ceased to exist. In August 2005, the PCT stated that it proposed to close the 32 beds at Walnuttree Hospital.[56] Yet there were 68; it was just that 36 had been temporarily closed for fire safety works in March 2005, a few months earlier. They had not been reopened, for the simple reason that the PCT had brought the works to a halt. They had never been formally closed. Nevertheless, the PCT now ignored their existence. It was as if they had never been –

51 'Meeting aims to put case to keep hospital.' *East Anglian Daily Times*, 26 August 2005.

52 Peter Rowe, 'Be honest and admit it's a second rate system.' *Suffolk Free Press*, 1 September 2005.

53 Walnuttree Hospital Action Committee, 'Most vulnerable under attack.' *Suffolk Free Press*, 15 September 2005.

54 'Town mental health unit "will not close".' *Suffolk Free Press*, 18 May 2006.

55 Peter Clifford, 'Talbot unit poser.' Letter. *Suffolk Free Press*, 1 June 2006.

56 *Modernising Health Care in West Suffolk: consultation, 1 August – 31 October 2005*. Bury St Edmunds: Suffolk West PCT, 2005.

with the outcome that the proposed closures sounded less drastic than they really were (i.e. 32 rather than 68 beds).

How many red herrings swim in the wood?

Faced with a wish to close down services, but unable to think of compelling reasons for doing so, the NHS sometimes resorts to what turn out to be red herrings. Of these health and safety takes pole position, sometimes used to justify temporary, at other times permanent, closure of hospitals.

Occasionally, given persistent local residents and skilful lawyers, the NHS or local councils are caught out. In one such legal case, the council argued for closure of a care home on health and safety grounds. However, the evidence and documentation pointed to finance and strategy as the true reason for closure. The council's decision was therefore held to be unlawful because misleading reasons had been given.[57]

Kingston PCT:

> announced, totally out of the blue that it wanted to close Surbiton Hospital. We were told not to worry and that that would be temporary. A new survey had been received on the roof and, because of one little leak in one room, the trust thought that there was a case for closing the hospital. The survey found that to replace the roof entirely, which apparently was the only option that could be considered, would cost £300,000 and bust the budget. Health and safety required that all the elderly patients in the hospital were moved out. Some had been there for years. The outpatient facilities were also closed. One can imagine the local uproar. When people asked when the hospital would reopen, the PCT could not answer. There was no plan and no strategic approach.[58]

In the New Forest:

> Fenwick hospital was 'temporarily closed' because of a shortage of staff leading to health and safety concerns. Once that was rectified, did it reopen? Not likely.[59]

57 *R (Madden) v Bury Metropolitan Borough Council* [2002] EWHC 1882 Admin, High Court, para 58.

58 Edward Davey, MP for Kingston and Surbiton. *Hansard*, Westminster Hall, 2 November 2005, column 265WH.

59 Dr Julian Lewis, MP for New Forest, East. *Hansard*, 2nd November 2005, column 265WH.

At Wells-next-the-Sea, the PCT closed the beds 'temporarily' immediately prior to Christmas 2004, but with no plans to reopen them. A vigorous local campaign followed, a charitable trust was formed and plans laid to reopen the beds.[60] Two rehabilitation wards were to be shut at Altrincham General Hospital because, according to Trafford Healthcare Trust, patient safety meant it had no choice. It did also admit that closure would help it manage its £9 million deficit.[61]

Such closures, on grounds of safety because of lack of staff, are widely understood locally as often stemming from deliberate, but unstated, policies of closure by stealth or death by a thousand cuts. Safety also seems the favoured ground on which to anticipate the result of reviews or consultations. So, for instance, the closure in August 2006 of the accident and emergency department in Cockermouth was seen by the local MP as a policy of closure, 'a little bit here and there until there are no services left'. This was made worse by the fact that the closure took place, even before the results of a review of local services had been made known.[62]

Another minor injuries unit in Bridlington, Yorkshire, was to be closed overnight from Sepetmber 2006, owing to staff shortages. The local Mayor was in no doubt that the real agenda was to close the hospital altogether.[63]

When ten beds were closed at Newmarket Hospital by Suffolk West PCT in December 2005, even before the consultation process was complete, the PCT stated that it was because of staff shortages beyond its control, and that it was trying to be '100 per cent honest'. However, it claimed that it would not be safe to keep the beds open.[64] The PCT did not explain that the reason for the staff shortages was because of a recruitment freeze imposed by the PCT.

On an altogether larger scale, Sudbury had already had experience of health and safety issues in late 2004. At this time, the two Sudbury community hospitals had been operated by an acute trust, the West Suffolk Hospitals NHS Trust. A major obstacle to it achieving the status of a Foundation Hospital was its financial spending. A new chief executive had been

60 Mark Gould, 'No closure on campaigns to save community hospitals.' *Health Service Journal*, 23 February 2006.

61 Caroline Jack, 'Axed wards win reprieve.' *Manchester Metro News*, 21 August 2006.

62 Gemma Fraser, 'Closure of injury unit is thin end of wedge.' *News & Star*, 4 August 2006.

63 Alex Wood, 'Anger as Trust cuts hospital centre's hours.' *Yorkshire Post*, 16 August 2006.

64 Lisa Cleverdon, 'Hospital to cut beds over festive period.' *East Anglian Daily Times*, 6 December 2005.

appointed during 2004. The Trust was determined to achieve 'foundation hospital' status (something it would fail to do).

In October 2004, the Trust made clear that Walnuttree Hospital, one of the two community hospitals in Sudbury, would have to close. This was due to fire safety issues, not finances, the Trust claimed. Nevertheless, the local community could not but help equate the sudden, proposed closure with the £4 million deficit that had to be shed by the NHS Trust. It was for example alleged that health and safety was being used spuriously and prematurely to justify a decision taken for other reasons.[65] There was local uproar, a huge public meeting and a 10,000 signature petition.

A meeting with the Fire Service in late November 2005 subsequently revealed that the fire safety issue was manageable, and at far less cost than the NHS Trust had been arguing. It was agreed that fire safety works costing something over £200,000 and no more than £300,000 (as opposed to the several million pounds the Trust had been citing) would be carried out to make the hospital serviceable on both ground floor and first floor until the end of 2007.

The whole episode was instructive. It followed the all too familiar pattern of a highly suspicious local community on the one hand and an NHS trust or primary care trust protesting its innocence on the other. The Trust claimed that it had no hidden agenda to close the hospital and save money, but that it was acting in good faith for patient safety. The local community was sceptical. In the past, the Trust had taken advice from the Fire Service, which ultimately was responsible for enforcing fire safety. On this occasion, the Trust had gone to an independent consultancy which produced an alarmist report. The Trust then took up the cry of alarm itself. It went on to argue that its proposals were not only to safeguard patients but also to protect its own Board from manslaughter charges which would surely follow if there were a fatal fire at the hospital. This argument attracted suitably lurid and alarmist headlines in the local Press: 'DEATH TRAP'.[66]

This was a curious statement to make because at the time it was made, the Trust was in compliance with existing safety obligations and had the requisite fire safety certificate. This would, all other things being equal, preclude the bringing of manslaughter charges or health and safety prosecution. An executive member of Suffolk County Council, Kathy Pollard, was in

65 Will Wright, 'Hospital fire risk dismissed.' *Sudbury Mercury*, 12 November 2004.

66 Will Wright. *Sudbury Mercury*, 26 November 2005.

no doubt that the Trust's Board had been presented with information in an 'unbalanced' way:

> Board members should have been made aware…that although they could be liable to manslaughter charges if there were loss of life due to fire at Walnuttree Hospital, they would not be blamed as long as reasonable steps had been taken to comply with fire safety recommendations.[67]

The Trust's apparent overstating of the risks was further unfortunate, not least because such alarm about fire safety can attract arsonists. Night security at the hospital was stepped up. As the local community had predicted, the alarmist safety arguments and the financial implications argued by the Trust turned out to lack substance. The Fire Service eventually came to the rescue once it had been consulted, and put the matter in perspective, safety-wise, legally and financially. As the county councillor, who had involved the Fire Service, summed up:

> The costings and the amount of work needed has been inflated when in the opinion of our own fire experts there are much cheaper options.[68]

Overall, the apparently flimsy logic of the West Suffolk NHS Trust's position was best illustrated in late November 2004. By this time, it had already started to run down the hospital, by reducing admissions in advance of its anticipated decision to close. And, as already noted, it was talking feverishly about manslaughter charges. However, at the beginning of December, the acute hospital in Bury St Edmunds was nearly full, as it was on 'red alert'. Suddenly, the fire safety, manslaughter charges and everything else were forgotten. Ambulance loads of patients began to arrive at Walnuttree Hospital. The 68 beds were soon full again.[69]

The NHS Trust would still maintain that it had acted reasonably and only with the safety of patients and staff in mind. It represented the whole episode as responsible decision-making:

> Early indications were that there might be a significant fire safety risk and at that time it was good management practice to talk about contin-

67 Will Wright, 'MP's inquiry demand.' *Sudbury Mercury*, 31 December 2004.

68 Patrick Lowman, 'Work on threatened hospital "overstated",' *East Anglian Daily Times*, 29 November 2004.

69 Will Wright, 'Council: fire report wrong.' *Sudbury Mercury*, 3 December 2004.

> gencies and staff and patients needed to be involved in that, which is why we were open and honest.[70]

At best, even accepting the Trust's claim of good faith, it seemed to have acted rashly and prematurely by making rushed and excessive proposals, before the facts and the finances had been established. In retrospect its actions were highly damaging. It was seen to have begun the erosion of both local services and the local community's trust in the NHS – trust that the following year would wash away altogether.

Thus, in 2004, the cloak for closure had come in the form of health and safety; in 2006, it would take the guise of an improved model of care put forward by the PCT. The community would remain unconvinced, believing that it all boiled down to much the same thing: trying to save money at the cost in health and welfare to elderly, chronically sick and disabled people.

In fact, in May 2006, the local NHS was once again to introduce the fire safety issue, and to do it in such a way as to raise doubts. This time around, the Suffolk West PCT claimed that Walnuttree Hospital would have to close in December 2007 because of a fire notice to that effect.[71] What it omitted to mention was that in May 2006, the extant fire notice was based on the risk to both ground and first floors. Now that the first floor was shut, the risk was less, and a new risk assessment and fire notice would be required to ascertain the risk and the practical implications. But the PCT had not waited for this, and was prepared apparently to use the fire safety concerns to bolster what were perceived to be threats against the local community.[72]

Down in the bunker: sending in the imaginary armies

Akin to ignoring or selectively using evidence is an indulgence in wishful thinking. This is an alarming tendency of both central government and local NHS bodies. When attempting to save money and shift services out into the community and into people's homes, they readily resort to the deployment of imaginary armies of health-care staff and carers. At the same time, they tend often to oversimplify the problems and obstacles that exist. This is a dangerous combination.

70 Benedict O'Connor, 'Saved: Walnuttree Hospital will stay open after campaign victory.' *East Anglian Daily Times*, 11 December 2004.

71 Paul Holland, 'Health chiefs' threat to delay town plans.' *Suffolk Free Press*, 25 May 2006.

72 Walnuttree Hospital Action Committee, 'The state of our health services in Sudbury.' *Suffolk Free Press*, 8 June 2006.

For example, at central government level, as they look out over South London from their fortresses in Whitehall (Richmond House), at the Elephant and Castle (Skipton House) and at Waterloo (Wellington House), civil servants and consultants summon up magnificent visions of care in the community.

The visions are suitably all dressed up of course in the language of choice, individual planning, independence and so on. Such words trip easily off the tongue and onto paper, but not perhaps into local reality. Bunkers, fortresses, other planets, parallel worlds, they all come to much the same thing in describing the detachment of NHS decision-makers. Referring to the Secretary of State's wish to 'make it as easy to access NHS treatment as it is to get a pint of milk', the shadow health minister could only point out:

> Well, back on Planet Earth we know what is really going on. I know what is happening in my own constituency, where services and wards are being shut at Brookfields community hospital in Cambridge; the young people's mental health service is being shut down and the PCT is refusing to fund the hospice at home services. That is what is happening on Planet Earth. The Secretary of State should come back to Planet Earth.[73]

Similarly, in response to Patricia Hewitt's policy of making more use of community hospitals, another MP could not understand how this squared with the closure of swathes of community hospitals:

> I thank the Secretary of State for her statement. It is always fascinating to step with her into the parallel world that she inhabits, where shiny new hospitals are delivered to a glad and happy local population.[74]

We find, for example, the *National Service Framework for Long-term Conditions* producing a whole 'standard' on the provision of equipment and adaptations in people's own homes. This at a time when, throughout England, the system of adapting people's homes through disabled facilities grants (under the Housing Grants, Construction and Regeneration Act 1996) is in disarray and on its knees through underfunding.[75] And local social services authorities, major providers of daily living equipment, were busy throughout 2005

73 Andrew Lansley, MP, South Cambridgeshire. *Hansard*, House of Commons Debates, 5 July 2006, column 819.

74 Steve Webb, MP, Northavon. *Hansard*, House of Commons Debates, 5 July 2006, column 821.

75 *Reviewing the Disabled Facilities Grant Programme.* London: Office of the Deputy Prime Minister, 2005, p.6.

and 2006 tightening up their eligibility criteria, so as to limit provision of equipment and other services. Given this state of affairs, it was unsurprising that the National Service Framework signally failed to indicate where the funding was coming from, under what legislation, and through which statutory provider.[76]

In 2005 and 2006 there was a wholesale assault on community hospitals. By those dates, central government had already been presiding over an unfair system of denying continuing NHS health care to older people. Yet this did not stop it talking about the joys of choosing from four or five different health-care providers. Each patient would have 'access to their own personal Healthspace on the internet, where they can see their care records and note their individual preferences about their care'.[77] For increasing numbers of older people, however, their health care was likely to stop at the 'virtual'.

Not so fanciful a claim. As a resident of Suffolk would put it commonsensically, local hospitals and beds were being closed down (for want of a few million pounds), whereas between £6.2 and £20 billion was being spent on a flawed NHS computer network.[78] True, a National Audit Office report in June 2006 basically approved the national NHS computer project. However, leaked information from a senior source within the project in August suggested that it was grossly flawed. As one MP on the Parliamentary Health Select Committee pointed out, the billion pounds spent already could have been used to run ten district general hospitals a year. To date only 12 of England's 176 major hospitals had implemented even the most basic part of the new system.[79]

In Suffolk, still a significantly rural area, it did not take highly paid experts, NHS managers or otherwise, to realise that imaginary health professionals roving the countryside would not be delivering health care. As one East Suffolk resident put it plainly and simply:

> There is also the pressure on medical staff to be considered. They are trained to care for patients, not to drive around the countryside to

76 *The National Service Framework for Long-term Conditions.* London: Department of Health, 2005, Quality Requirement 7.

77 *Putting People at the Heart of Public Services.* London: Department of Health, 2004, para 12.

78 Peter Norton, 'Cash for computers but none for beds.' Letter. *East Anglian Daily Times*, 27 June 2006.

79 Jamie Doward, 'NHS computer system "won't work".' *The Observer*, 6 August 2006.

> remote villages. It is obvious that their skills are put to best use, for effect and economy, when they are based in a central location.[80]

Indeed, in West Suffolk, a 2003 report commissioned by Suffolk West PCT itself identified that a basic rehabilitation service was not being provided five days a week, because of a shortfall in therapy services in the Newmarket, Bury St Edmunds and Sudbury hospitals.[81] Since that date, no extra therapists had been recruited. In its proposals, the PCT appeared not to consider the implications that if it was already short of therapists when they were hospital-based, then changing to a peripatetic system in a rural area would undoubtedly exacerbate the shortfall. This was an especially notable omission because its own public health doctors had been carrying out a study which precisely identified the extra costs of providing dispersed services in a rural area.[82]

Thus, it was reported that the Suffolk West PCT apparently intended that the equivalent of fleets of nurses should stalk the roads and lanes of Suffolk.[83] This, all at a time when it had a large deficit and a recruitment freeze, and notwithstanding that such peripatetic staff would be more resource intensive than when based at a community hospital. The worries seemed by no means academic. On Christmas Eve 2005, the *East Anglian Daily Times* led with the headline: 'ONE CARER TO 500 PATIENTS'. The union Amicus had revealed that within Suffolk a health visitor had a caseload of more than 500 patients. While defending their proposals for care in the community, the PCTs in Suffolk did not deny the claim.[84]

It was not just staff either. The Suffolk West PCT stated categorically that rehabilitation equipment could be taken in and out of people's homes.[85] This was, and is, simply not the case. It was imagined portability. The position is in fact that some equipment, crucial for rehabilitation, is not portable. For example, physiotherapists regularly use a range of heavy, generally non-portable equipment including plinths, parallel bars, sit to stand hoists, tilt tables etc. Some equipment may to a degree be portable, but

80 Richard Atkins, 'How can closures improve patient care?' Letter. *East Anglian Daily Times*, 16 September 2005.

81 *Developing New Models of Intermediate Care*. London: Secta, 2003, para 9.

82 Padmanabhan Badrinath and others (2006), 'Characteristics of primary care trusts in financial deficit and surplus: a comparative study in the English NHS.' *BMC Health Services Research 6*, 64.

83 Ross Clark, 'Botched operation.' *Daily Telegraph*, 12 March 2006.

84 Craig Robinson, 'One carer to 500 patients.' *East Anglian Daily Times*, 24 December 2005.

85 Modernising Healthcare in West Suffolk: additional information. Bury St Edmunds: Suffolk West PCT, 2005, p.27.

has severe limitations. For instance, some plinths are portable but non-adjustable, but in any case are not intended to be constantly carried, assembled and disassembled on a daily basis. And portable parallel bars are too unstable for use with many patients. Apart from the impracticality or impossibility of carrying such equipment around, space is also required to use it and to conduct the rehabilitation required. Many patients' homes will contain insufficient space or be otherwise unsuitable. The PCT explained none of this. The reason appeared to be that it wanted to present a black and white picture; the awkward detail didn't come into it. It wished to remain in an imaginary world of wishful thinking.

To the extent that the PCT expected the county council social services department to provide support to people who would now be in their own homes rather than recovering in hospital, the same fiction was apparent. Although in principle the county council had special services to assist with hospital discharge, they would be time-limited and in any case not always available. Longer-term ready availability of carers in areas such as Suffolk, particularly in more rural areas, is a well-known problem – as local residents repeatedly pointed out in public meeting after public meeting across the county in late 2005.

The noises coming from the PCTs were reassuring about social care capacity. This was unsurprising because they would not have to provide the care. At least in the East of Suffolk, the Professional Executive Committee (PEC) of the PCTs spoke up about both health and social care capacity. Although supportive of the changes in principle, it had continuing concerns about the ability of both health care and social care teams to deliver the additional level of care required in the community.[86]

The equivalent committee for the Suffolk West PCT was either not so bold or not so searching. At the equivalent decision-making meeting in the West, its Chairman went out of his way to laud the new model of care and express no doubts at all.[87] It should be noted, although the PEC Chairman did not explain this, that the local GPs in Sudbury and Newmarket, whose clinical concerns the PEC was in some sense meant to be representing, believed the opposite.

Thus, when a woman with partial paralysis was discharged home from Ipswich hospital, rather than to a community hospital, she had been told by social services that there was a shortage of care workers and they could not

86 *Minutes of the Suffolk East PCTs Combined Board Meeting*, 25 January 2006. Ipswich: Suffolk East PCTs.

87 'Thousands of beds at home.' *Suffolk Free Press*, 13 April 2006.

help. Her daughter and husband looked after her, but he was now 'shattered'. Once it was highlighted in the Press, Suffolk County Council put it down to a misunderstanding. But even the Suffolk East PCTs admitted that the timescales required to build up sufficient care in the community were 'challenging'.[88]

As Libby Purves writing in *The Times* observed, receiving care at home 'when you live alone in a cottage up a track, with a five-hundredth share of a health visitor and no bell to ring if you can't breathe at 3am, is not convincing'.[89] And not just cottages in country lanes. Thus, one Felixstowe resident responded to the suggestion that:

> more patient after-care would be provided at home. But by who and from where? What about during the night? In Felixstowe there is only one road access to Ipswich and the consequences of a major road closure would be unthinkable.[90]

From the East of Suffolk, where the Bartlet Hospital – which had always provided excellent care – was threatened with closure, came warnings of what alternative care in the community entailed for people in, for example, sheltered accommodation:

> Frail, elderly people condemned to early bedtimes each night because of the sheer volume of work allotted to their carers. Frail elderly people left in bed until lunchtime because for various reasons their carers have not turned up.[91]

In sum, the Walnuttree Hospital Action Committee would write in despair about what it perceived to be the bunker mentality of the Suffolk West PCT:

> Detached from reality and disengaged from the local community it is meant to be serving, the PCT now occupies a world where it has convinced itself that black is white and less is more – and that consultation means a) not listening to people, b) disregarding the evidence (even when the latter is put forward by its own clinicians), c) making personal attacks on representatives of the local community…unless the

88 David Green, 'Carer found after we reveal woman's plight.' *East Anglian Daily Times*, 29 December 2005.

89 Libby Purves, 'Health alert: infectious ideas.' *The Times*, 24 January 2006.

90 Peter Clark, 'Inquiry must be held into health care debt.' Letter. *East Anglian Daily Times*, 7 September 2005.

91 Mrs Doreen Lambert, 'Community care can't ever equal Bartlet.' Letter. *East Anglian Daily Times*, 20 February 2006.

> PCT now plucks up the courage to emerge from its bunker, its proposals will lead to increased disability, suffering, illness and death among elderly and vulnerable people in the Sudbury area.[92]

One last example illustrates how Suffolk West PCT's financial position led it into a theoretical and imaginary, rather than realistic, plan to deliver services. The closure of Walnuttree Hospital was, according to the PCT, in order to provide alternative care services closer to home. Some of the care provided at Walnuttree is palliative in nature. So, in June 2006, St Nicholas Hospice required financial assistance to provide palliative care in people's own homes. The PCT refused to support the scheme, explaining:

> In principle, Suffolk West PCT is in favour of all models of care that move towards increasing support to patients at home...

But it was unable to provide that support, as the hospice explained:

> We have negotiated with the PCT and asked them to come on board as a financial partner but they cannot because of their financial deficit and couldn't even commit in the next few years.[93]

Shutting out the overspill and the dying

Akin to conjuring up imaginary services is shutting out real services from the equation. One example of this was of a question apparently not asked by the Suffolk West PCT, and therefore not even answered with or without evidence. This concerned the regular use of community hospitals by acute hospitals for the purpose of 'overspill'.

Throughout winter and sometimes in summer, the local acute hospital, West Suffolk Hospital, had been often on Red Alert, sometimes on Black Alert.[94] This signified real pressure on beds, which had traditionally been relieved by using the community hospital beds at Sudbury and Newmarket. In October 2005, local GPs in Suffolk warned of the crisis that would occur in the case of an influenza epidemic or other event – if there were no

92 Walnuttree Hospital Action Committee, 'Emerge from the health bunker.' Letter. *Suffolk Free Press*, 26 January 2006.

93 Dave Gooderham, 'No cash for 24-hour home care scheme.' *East Anglian Daily Times*, 10 June 2006.

94 Walnuttree Hospital Action Committee, '"Red alert beds" crisis could loom.' Letter. *Suffolk Free Press*, 20 October 2005.

community hospital beds and beds were being closed at the acute hospitals as well.[95]

County councillors and Unison raised the same issues, and the danger of the acute hospital lacking the capacity to deal with major outbreaks of illness.[96] At one of the Suffolk West PCT's roadshows, the PCT was quoted as replying that operations would be cancelled at the acute hospital in order to manage the patients who previously could have been decanted to the community hospitals.[97]

Nonetheless, the matter of this overspill function was mentioned neither in the PCT's consultation document, nor in the report for the meeting at which final closure decisions were taken. In other words, this highly relevant issue appeared not to have been formally brought to the Board's attention.

It did not even take a hard winter or an influenza outbreak to expose the fragility of the policy of large-scale bed closures. In mid-August 2006 bed availability at West Suffolk Hospital in Bury St Edmunds meant nine-hour waits for A&E patients, queuing ambulances unable to take patients into the hospital, and some patients being taken miles away either to Addenbrook's Hospital in Cambridge or to Ipswich Hospital.[98]

Likewise, the use of community hospital beds for palliative care, where that is not appropriate in the acute hospital or in people's own homes, was also not addressed by the PCT in either its consultation document or its final report. The evidence about it was therefore not collated or examined.

95 Sarah Chambers, 'If people become ill we've got a crisis.' *East Anglian Daily Times*, 14 October 2005.

96 Liz Hearnshaw, 'Winter hospital worry over beds.' *East Anglian Daily Times*, 9 September 2005.

97 Jill Fisher, 'Beds needed if flu breaks out.' Letter. *Suffolk Free Press*, 13 October 2005.

98 Will Clarke, 'Hospital "already stretched to limit" warning.' *East Anglian Daily Times*, 18 August 2006.

11

Discarding the Chaff: the Shedding of NHS Responsibilities

There has always been a lack of universality and comprehensiveness in the NHS. This is unsurprising, since the terms are both relative and ambitious.

Variability of service can affect all types of patient of all ages, and has done since the inception of the NHS. In recent years, for instance, hospital accident and emergency department delays have probably been fairly indiscriminate. Similarly, the availability of treatments for cancer can vary depending, for example, on the particular approach of a local NHS Trust, but not on age. So, potentially lifesaving treatment may be denied to a woman in need of a breast cancer drug or a ten-year-old girl with leukaemia.

Nevertheless, there is, and has always been, a temptation either not to include, or sometimes to jettison, certain services on the fringe. For instance, at the outset of the NHS it was recognised that achieving a universal NHS dentistry service might take time. It would now appear that, 60 years later, the government has given up the fight on this one as NHS dentistry appears to be in terminal recession – despite the inevitable government claims to the contrary.

A 2006 booklet issued by the Department of Health states confidently that 'NHS dentistry is changing to provide better access to high quality services.'[1] Nonetheless, by early 2006, less than one in six Yorkshire dentists

1 *What You Need to Know About Changes to NHS Dentistry in England.* London: Department of Health, 2006.

was accepting new NHS patients, and the *Yorkshire Post* had been driven to run a 'Stop The Rot' campaign.[2]

In April 2006, with the introduction of a new dental contract – to be operated by already cash-strapped PCTs – it was reported that across Suffolk (particularly in the East), significant numbers of dentists would opt not to provide dental care on the NHS.[3] Likewise, general ophthalmic services were during the 1990s effectively jettisoned by the NHS and thrust into the high street.

A degree of visibility has attended the fate of NHS dental and optical services and perhaps a degree of equity in that the exclusions are generally across the board. Nevertheless, there have always been more covert and discriminatory exclusions from services.

The history of the NHS suggests that vulnerable groups – older people generally, people (of all ages) with learning disabilities, physical disabilities, serious sensory impairments or mental health problems – have always been prone to losing out. There is a perversity that they should in some sense be excluded or discriminated against by a national health service, given their large numbers (e.g. in the case of older people) and the fact that they arguably have the greatest needs.

Examples can be seen in respect of specific services for particular groups of people. For instance, over the last 40 years, numerous reports have been published indicating inadequate provision, in relation to disability equipment services, wheelchair services, rehabilitation services, services for people with various disabilities, incontinence services – and so on.

At least there is then no danger of harking back to a golden age, when all needs were met. Nevertheless, one disturbing feature of current practice (and arguably policy) appears to be that people are being excluded, in discriminatory fashion, from provision not just passively by omission, but actively. The most common way of kicking services for these groups into the long grass and out of sight has been to talk about 'care in the community'. Nevertheless, when an 'expert patient' with a long-term condition sought to bring a judicial review case in Suffolk, the issue of discrimination was rightly raised by the local community that supported her. The PCT had been urging the community to accept the outpatient services on offer but to forget the inpatient beds. But the local action committee responded as follows:

2 Jayne Dowle, 'Something rotten in the state of NHS dentistry.' *Yorkshire Post*, 2 March 2006.

3 'Blow for patients as dentists go private.' *East Anglian Daily Times*, 1 April 2006.

> The absence of community hospital beds will mean that some of the most vulnerable members of our community will not get the care and rehabilitation they need. They will effectively be abandoned. We cannot allow this to happen. To do so would be discriminatory, cowardly and wrong.[4]

One key problem is perceived to be that of an ageing population. Central government appears to have tried to grapple with the issue only piecemeal, tangentially and often in a negative fashion. For instance, legislation and guidance bears the hallmarks of having been introduced to reduce hospital costs, and only secondarily with the welfare of older people in mind. The issue is not new. Even in the 1970s, with a smaller elderly population than now, central government was shying away from the implications of expanding community services to meet the needs of older people. At the time, a discussion document, called *Happier Old Age: a discussion document on elderly people in our society*, was published in 1978, but an expected White Paper never materialised.[5]

New Labour has been infatuated with targets, indicators and statistics. It has shown every desire to open up the NHS to market forces and to subject it to tests of business viability. All this may put more vulnerable and needy groups of people at even greater risk of being sidelined. This is because it tends to reduce patients to units that can be neatly measured and processed on the basis of 'contestability' and competition (between public and private sector). This being so, there seems already to be an overwhelming temptation to avoid including those patients who do not deliver easy and clear returns. They are too complex, too expensive to care for and, in the case of older people, there are thought to be simply too many of them. Central government, together with local NHS trusts, appears to have woken up to the fact that even cheaper than providing inadequate health services for these groups of people would be to provide no services at all. This may seem to be an extreme assertion but there are sufficient examples to suggest that it carries some substance.

Such brushing away of people from a universal health service can be seen in various guises. Some examples come on the back of legislation and properly debated government policy; others are implemented more quietly

4 Walnuttree Hospital Action Committee, 'The state of our health services in Sudbury.' Notice. *Suffolk Free Press*, 8 June 2006.

5 Charles Webster (1996) *The Health Services Since the War*. Volume 2. London: HMSO, p.658.

through the back door. For instance, in 2003, central government turned its attention to discharging people quickly from acute hospitals, particularly older people. It issued explicit legislation and guidance. Although this policy had an unattractive flipside, at least there was arguably a degree of transparency.

Nevertheless, not all such policies are visible. For instance, the provision of what is known as 'NHS continuing health care' has been notorious for the underhand manner in which the NHS has attempted precisely to deny it to elderly, vulnerable people. The reason? The high financial and political stakes (see Chapter 12).

When the NHS sheds responsibilities, publicly or covertly, the question arises about how people will be supported elsewhere if at all. Here is the rub. It appears to be an almost invariable rule of thumb that when such policies are implemented, there are two underlying categories of motivation. The first, on the surface at least, is genuinely to implement new and better models of care for vulnerable groups of people. The second is to save money, which means that, all too often, the policy is implemented – arguably foreseeably in many cases – improperly. The alternative support tends not to be forthcoming. For example, community care – perhaps better named care in the community – has been seriously afflicted in this respect, whether provided by the NHS or by local councils in the form of social care services which can be charged for.

Tilling of the arid common land: joint working in health and social care

'Joint working' is the jargon for increased cooperation at local level, in particular between PCTs and NHS Trusts on the one hand and local social services councils on the other. Central government advocates it incessantly year after year. On top of a number of scattered legislative provisions making it possible, further legislation was passed in the form of the Health Act 1999 to encourage and facilitate joint working still further, including pooled budgets.

Once again, the policy on its face has much to commend it. There has been a history of people falling through the net between the NHS and local council care, when it has been unclear whether the service in question should be regarded as 'health care' or as 'social care'. Nobody would argue that the NHS and local councils should work cooperatively at local level in order to clarify local responsibilities.

However, joint working seems to have developed a distinctly dark side, with serious ramifications for users of services. First, it sometimes involves an almost one way movement of services from the NHS to local councils (where those services can be charged for, always assuming they are provided at all).

Second, the kindly, ordered world of the NHS and local councils, benevolently cooperating and looking after our interests, is by no means the rule – although clearly some areas do better than others. To the detriment of patients, NHS bodies and local councils will sometimes argue tooth and nail over all manner of service. In times of financial crisis, the arguments escalate. From a special bed (e.g. multi-adjustable and pressure relieving) to a bath. From a care home placement to equipment and services for a terminally ill person dying at home. And from essential passive leg movement, to assist a paraplegic person maintain sitting posture, to essential assistance for a mother with the tracheotomy care for her three-year-old child – it is all the same to them. Nothing is sacred; they will argue over them all. Even if they finally decide who should shoulder responsibility in principle, the responsible party may simply refuse to fund it. This occurred in the tracheotomy case, when the High Court ruled that it was a health care issue but the PCT refused anyway to increase the assistance that it was providing.[6]

The 'continuing NHS health care' saga (see Chapter 12) is a glaring example of this ugly trend, as PCTs bend over backwards to avoid paying for people's health care needs. In any case, when financial pressures bite, joint working rapidly unravels and hostilities soon break out.

For instance, Suffolk West PCT had always maintained that it was working closely with Suffolk County Council over the PCT's proposals for closing down scores of NHS beds in the county. Nonetheless, in July 2006, it transpired that a legal dispute had developed. The PCT was attempting to claw back some £1.8 million that it had given the council over the past two years to facilitate more rapid hospital discharge. It was also now withholding a further £957,000, which the council had been expecting to receive.[7] All at a time when the county council was on its financial knees and having to save £24 million, including £15 million from the social care budget. This included cutting back its 'Home First' service, specifically designed to put people back on their feet in the twelve weeks following hospital discharge.[8]

6 *R(T) v Haringey London Borough Council* [2005] EWHC 2235 (Admin), High Court.

7 Graham Dines, 'Trusts demand £2m back from county.' *East Anglian Daily Times*, 8 July 2006.

8 'Council to review provision of adult care.' Press release. Ipswich: Suffolk County Council, August 2006.

In this respect, Suffolk West PCT was of course merely partaking of the national trend. A 2006 survey showed over 35 per cent of local authorities being affected by the NHS locally withdrawing from jointly funded services. In addition, 40 per cent of authorities were affected by the referral of cases that appeared properly to be an NHS, rather than a social services, responsibility.[9] Thus, in Wiltshire, significant cuts to social care budgets were required. This was mainly because of what the well-respected former director of social services referred to as cost shunting by the NHS. He had resigned, effectively in protest.[10]

The great rebranding: health care into social care

The aim and upshot of some government policies is thus not just to shed NHS responsibilities, but also to re-brand health care as social care. This has the happy outcome not only of reducing the workload on the NHS and transferring the more complicated and 'messy' care to local councils, but also of allowing people to be charged for the 'social care' services they may receive.

As far as older patients currently using the community hospitals in Suffolk were concerned, Suffolk West PCT, in common with many other PCTs, tried this approach. This is unsurprising. It was and is happening all over the country. The PCT would argue, for instance, that community hospital patients had basically social care rather than health care needs. The fact that cogent evidence for this was lacking didn't seem to matter (see Chapter 13).

Likewise, it argued that there would not be major implications for the local council's social services if it were to take on these patients.[11] The council leader, unsurprisingly,[12] was not convinced, referring to a total collapse of local health services. It all seemed contrary to the law of physics that matter can't just disappear. But patients' needs apparently would disappear – off the NHS radar screen, but not on to that of local council social care.

9 *The impact of NHS trust financial deficits on English local authorities.* London: Local Government Association, 2006.

10 'Wiltshire boss quits over cuts in services.' *Community Care,* 4–10 May 2006.

11 *Modernising Healthcare in West Suffolk: additional information.* Bury St Edmunds: Suffolk West PCT, 2005, p.16.

12 'County Warns of Fears of a Total Collapse of Local Health Services.' Press release, 9 September 2005. Ipswich: Suffolk County Council.

The Chief Executive of the Suffolk East PCTs would argue that it was not the role of the NHS to provide 'social care' and that they would be returning to providing 'core services'.[13] Such an argument was difficult to follow because it appeared to carry with it the implication that in the past the NHS had been providing social care in community hospitals, even though the patients were there on the recommendation of medical consultants and general practitioners.

The argument was anyway not consistent, because the PCTs in Suffolk would alternatively argue that such patients still had health-care needs after all, but that they would be met in people's own homes. They would state, for instance, that 'people prefer to be at home and they progress more quickly at home'.[14] In itself this was not wrong; but it painted only half the picture. It presupposed that everybody had the sort of needs and the sort of home environment that were conducive to rehabilitation and recuperation in that setting. And this is of course not the case, as national evidence, the government's White Paper, and indeed Suffolk West's own rules and criteria made clear (see Chapter 13).

Shedding people with learning disabilities and mental health problems

A longstanding plank of government policy, care in the community for people with learning disabilities, has proved elusive. It provides another stark illustration of the gap between government aspiration and reality, and the detrimental consequences of such a gap.

By 1958, government was talking about preventing illness, shifting away from hospital and institutional treatment and increasing efficiency in those longstay institutions – similar to what central government is still saying in 2006. The Mental Health Act 1959 was intended to signal the beginning of a long and continuing move of patients with mental disorder (including mental health problems and learning disabilities) out of long-stay hospitals. Clearly, there was a pressing reason for such changes; the inappropriate incarceration of people labelled as insane, lunatic or moral degenerates was clearly unacceptable. By 1971, a White Paper, *Better Services for the*

13 Sarah Chambers, 'Packed meeting warned of cuts to care,' *East Anglian Daily Times*, 17 September 2005.

14 Nicki Harvey, 'Betrayed.' *Suffolk Free Press*, 30 June 2005.

Mentally Handicapped, had been published with the objective of minimising long-term hospital care in favour of care in the community.[15]

Nevertheless, it was still a long march. Another White Paper issued in 2001, called *Valuing People*, spoke of choice, opportunity and independence. It called on the creation of local partnership boards to organise services for people with learning disabilities.[16] Local social services authorities (i.e. local councils) were to have the lead. People with learning disabilities should not remain in long-stay NHS institutions. In 2006, another White Paper renewed this last call.[17]

Not everybody of course is convinced that such all or nothing approaches are right; sometimes, for instance, the parents of people with severe learning disabilities fight hard campaigns against the assumption that under-funded, ill-defined 'care in the community' is best for everybody. The courts stepped in on one occasion, when it was proposed to hand a community of people with learning disabilities wholesale over to social services from the NHS without proper individual assessment of these people's needs.[18] Nevertheless, in addition, even where such transfer is appropriate, local councils struggle financially to pick up what in some cases represents extremely expensive care. Ironically, in the aforementioned legal case, even after the legal proceedings were concluded and the hospital was due to close, nothing happened. This was because the Sutton and Merton PCT required some £15 million to close the hospital – but had only £1 million available.[19]

For instance, in 2006, the Association of Directors of Social Services had drawn attention to this, pointing out there was now a significant increase in the number of people with learning disabilities in society. Their life expectancy had increased, and local authority expenditure had increased steeply while NHS expenditure had not increased and may have decreased. It expressed alarm and stated that the impact was not sustainable.[20]

15 Charles Webster (1996). *The Health Services Since the War.* Volume 2. London: HMSO.

16 Secretary of State for Health (2001) *Valuing People: a new strategy for learning disability for the 21st century.* Cm 6700. London: HMSO.

17 Secretary of State for Health (2006) *Our Health, Our Care, Our Say: a new direction for community services.* Cm 6737. London: HMSO, para 4.90.

18 *R v Merton, Sutton and Wandsworth Health Authority, ex p Perry* (2001) Lloyd's Rep Med 73, Administrative Division, High Court.

19 'Delay in closing long-stay hospital leaves 93 residents unsure of their future.' *Community Care*, 17–23 August 2006.

20 *Directors Demand More Resources for Services for People with Learning Disabilities.* Press release, 14 October 2005. Association of Directors of Social Services.

Further evidence came in the form of a number of legal cases and local ombudsman investigations. They reflected not only the difficulties faced by local authorities, but also the serious consequences for some people with learning disabilities.

For instance, one investigation revealed that, partly because of concern about costs, a woman with learning disabilities ended up forgotten in a hospital as an informal patient for some ten years, where she suffered abuse at the hands of other patients.[21] In another case, concern from a local authority about the cost of a placement resulted in the person being inappropriately and compulsorily detained on a locked, acute psychiatric ward for over a year.[22] Likewise resources were at the root of a person being inappropriately detained in a psychiatric unit for eight months where he was sedated with drugs.[23] Cases have been reaching the law courts, too, where local authorities have not been going down lawful routes in order to limit their expenditure on placements for people with learning disabilities.[24]

Proposals in Suffolk affecting mental health and learning disability services were prominent. In July 2005, the Suffolk Mental Health Partnership Trust announced it had to save £5 million in a matter of eight months. This would mean 'radical changes' including closing services, stopping developments, reducing teams and saving on management costs.[25] The management speak was fine. But as one mental health user, a former probation officer, of the Bridge House Clubhouse in Ipswich put it at a public meeting:

> I understand about saving money, but what happens to the people?[26]

The logical pattern or progression of shedding of services is sometimes encapsulated at a stroke. The Suffolk Mental Health Partnership NHS Trust proposed in 2005 to close a number of centres, including the Hollies drop-in centre in Ipswich, Bridge House Clubhouse in Ipswich, Old Fox Yard Clubhouse in Stowmarket, the Eastgate Ward in Bury St Edmunds, and a

21 Local Government Ombudsman (2003) *Investigation 01/C/15652: Wakefield Metropolitan District Council.* York: LGO.

22 Local Government Ombudsman (2004) *Investigation 02/C/17068: Bolton Metropolitan Borough Council.* York: LGO.

23 Local Government Ombudsman (2005) *Investigation 04/A/10159: Southend on Sea Borough Council.* London: LGO.

24 *R(A) v Bromley London Borough Council* [2004] EWHC 2108 (Admin); *R(S) v Leicester City Council* [2004] EWHC 533 (Admin).

25 Rebecca Sheppard, '"Radical changes" to save more than £5m.' *East Anglian Daily Times,* 14 July 2005.

26 John Howard, 'People vent anger at NHS public meeting.' *East Anglian Daily Times,* 16 September 2005.

respite centre for people with learning disabilities with complex needs in Newmarket (Healthfields). Also the Pines Occupational Therapy Unit in Ipswich was to close. At a highly charged public meeting, the Chief Executive of the NHS Trust stated that the NHS should not be providing certain types of respite care. In turn, the council's Director of Social Care pointed out that he did not want anybody 'running away' with the wrong idea that the council had resources available to pick up such care.[27]

Such an exchange spoke volumes about the attempts by the NHS to pass people over to local councils, who in turn lacked the resources to cope.

In Suffolk, proposals were duly followed by decisions to close most of the mental health and learning disabilities facilities, together with the horrified reactions of local residents including users of services. Referring to the therapeutic value of these services, and the thousands of people helped to cope with their mental illness, one correspondent explained:

> These are for people who are already vulnerable, who value what they receive from these facilities, and are now having change imposed upon them. They...have no idea what this care will be.[28]

The reactions of patients and their carers, and the expressions used, speak volumes. For instance, on hearing of the closure of a ward for people with dementia in Loughborough, carers said that it was like:

> losing the light at the end of the tunnel.[29]

In Cambridge, the chairwoman of the Friends of Fulbourn Hospital said closure of mental health wards represented 'savage reductions in mental health services' and were an 'absolute scandal'. It was 'letting down people of all ages, who are among the most vulnerable in our society'.[30] Proposals were put in Devon to close a rehabilitation and recovery unit for people with severe and long-term mental illness – because it was costly to run. Patients and their families said the service, at Watcombe Hall in Torquay 'offered a calm haven that aided recovery'.[31] When Morecambe Bay PCT threatened to close two wards for people with mental illness at Westmoreland General

27 'Fury at mental health service cuts.' *East Anglian Daily Times*, 29 July 2005.

28 M. Newell, 'Closures will hit those already vulnerable.' *East Anglian Daily Times*, 7 February 2006.

29 'Ward to close despite opposition.' *News.bbc.co.uk*, 18 July 2006.

30 'Home hospice service and wards face axe.' *Cambridge Evening News*, 27 June 2006.

31 'Mental health unit faces closure.' *News.bbc.co.uk*, 19 July 2006.

Hospital, a mental health charity referred to how frightened people were at losing what they considered to be a 'sanctuary'.[32]

Making the peasants pay: a new poll tax

The discarding of responsibilities by the NHS carries with it not only therapeutic, but also financial, implications for patients.

NHS services are, generally, free of charge. Conversely, local councils charge for the provision of social care services, be they residential or non-residential in nature. The charge can be up to full cost, depending on a person's means. In the case of provision of residential accommodation, there is a duty to charge that can result in the loss of a person's house.

In the case of other, non-residential community care services, there is a power only to charge. That is, councils are not obliged to charge for providing services. Yet it is the one power used to the hilt by local councils. The more the pressure, the greater the use of the power. For instance, in Suffolk in March 2006 the council had announced £24 million savings to be made, of which the greater part would come from the adult social care budget. As a result, it would be looking at introducing charges for community support and day care for people with learning disabilities.[33]

Of course, there has always been tampering at the edges with the principle of not charging. By 1952, an NHS prescription charge of 1s. had been introduced by a Conservative government. In the 1960s, what would now be regarded as an old Labour administration under Harold Wilson in 1965 removed the prescription charge. It was reintroduced in a hurry a short while after. However, New Labour's transferring of health services away from the NHS wholesale – to local councils where people will be charged full cost and may even have to sell their homes – constitutes a significant undermining of one of the three great NHS principles.

The key to New Labour's strategy came in its response to the Royal Commission into long-term care. In opposition, New Labour had expressed itself opposed to people paying for their personal care in their own homes or in care homes, and so – on entering power – had set up a Royal Commission to investigate the issue.[34] By the time the Commission had reported in 2000,

32 'Health chiefs defend ward closures.' *News.bbc.co.uk*, 20 January 2006.

33 Benedict O'Connor, 'Disabled learners set to be hit by cash cuts.' *East Anglian Daily Times*, 7 February 2006.

34 Royal Commission on Long Term Care (1999) (Sir Stewart Sutherland, Chairman) *With Respect to Old Age*. Cm 4192-1. London: HMSO.

the government had altogether changed its tune. This was to such an extent that it dismissed the majority of views of the Commission, even though these views were in accord with New Labour's stance when it had been in opposition.

The underlying but unstated reason was simple. The Commission's recommendations would have meant that social care provided by local authorities in the community should be free, just like health care. But implementation of this would have removed a major plank of the government's plan surreptitiously to re-brand 'health care' for older people and for other vulnerable groups as 'social care' – and then charge people for it. The last line of the following quote arguably gave the game away as to the driver for government policy. Older people must not be seen as a burden. There was however a 'but':

> The fact that people are living longer reflects the achievements of organisations like the National Health Service, social services and the voluntary sector. It is something for society to celebrate and take pride in. Older people are not and must never be seen as a burden on society. They are a vital resource of wisdom, experience and talent. But our ageing society creates new challenges to which we must rise. People aged 65 and over now use almost two thirds of general and acute hospital beds.[35]

The government went on to reject the Commission's recommendations that personal care should be free.

The government's *NHS Plan* had trumpeted the importance of keeping health services free of charge, because charging would be inequitable. This was especially because charges would 'increase the proportion of funding from unhealthy, old and poor compared with the healthy, young and wealthy'. It went on to state that there was a:

> world of difference between the NHS paying to have patients treated, as NHS patients, in a private hospital for free, and what some propose – forcing patients out of the NHS to pay for their own care.

Portentous last words that perversely would come to sum up government policy precisely. For funding long-term care, the government spoke of striking a 'fairer and lasting balance between taxpayers and individuals'. This would be whereby people's health care should be:

35 Secretary of State for Health (2000) *The NHS Plan: the government's response to the Royal Commission on Long Term Care.* Cm 4818-II. London: TSO, para 1.2.

provided squarely in line with NHS principles and they are not forced to sell their homes as soon as they enter residential care.[36]

In fact, the disingenuous policy was going to be that health care, which should have been free altogether, would be improperly passed off as chargeable social care.

Over in the land of adult social care in local councils, government guidance would be issued, ostensibly to make more equitable and consistent the charges made for people receiving 'personal care' in their own homes. In fact the guidance failed to do this and an Age Concern England report found inequity flourishing.[37]

Social workers have traditionally been seen as advocates for their clients. Likewise local councils providing social care services would wish to portray themselves as the caring, compassionate side of the welfare state. Yet in effect they supinely watched as the NHS wrongly categorised thousands of older people as not being in need of continuing NHS health care. This had the consequence that local councils then stepped in and charged those people for the very care that they should have received free from the NHS. This happened wholesale across the country (see Chapter 12). One individual example of the passivity of local councils came to light in an investigation conducted by the local government ombudsman. A social worker had failed to set in motion an application for continuing care funding for a person with Alzheimer's disease. The council was found guilty of maladministration. It and the health authority agreed to reimburse £26,000, equalling the nursing home costs the man's wife had wrongly been forced to pay to the local council.[38]

Local authorities have been given the lead by central government in protecting vulnerable people from abuse, including financial abuse.[39] So it is all the more unfortunate that they should have been so instrumental in taking so much money improperly from so many vulnerable people. Continuing NHS health care was not the only example. Another concerned charging people for after-care under s.117 of the Mental Health Act 1983.

36 Secretary of State for Health (2000) *The NHS Plan: a plan for investment, a plan for reform.* Cm 4818-1. London: HMSO, paras 3.18 and 11.3.

37 Pauline Thompson and Dinah Matthew (2004) *Fair Enough.* London: Age Concern England.

38 Local Government Ombudsman (2003) *Investigation 00/B/16833: Hertfordshire County Council.*

39 *No Secrets.* London: Department of Health, 2000.

Many local authorities charged unlawfully large sums of money for such care for many years.[40] Restitution has been taking place, sometimes amounting to tens of thousands of pounds per person. Some councils resorted to disreputable practices, such as – when a person died – retrospectively attempting to change her legal status and so extract funds from her estate.[41] In a further, almost astonishing case, a council apparently tried to get a woman – who had been detained compulsorily under the Mental Health Act – to agree to waive her rights to free after-care on discharge. Otherwise, the council threatened, she would have to remain in hospital for up to a year.[42]

And yet another example has come when local councils covertly and in some cases unlawfully force families to 'top up' residential care home fees. This is a seemingly widespread practice, about which there is increasing concern.[43]

40 *R v Manchester City Council, ex parte Stennett* [2002] UKHL 34, House of Lords.

41 Local Government Ombudsman (2001) *Investigation 00/B/08307: Leicestershire County Council.* Coventry: LGO.

42 Local Government Ombudsman (2006) *Investigation 04/B/01280: York City Council.* York: LGO.

43 *Government Response to Office of Fair Trading (OFT) Care Homes Study.* London: Department of Trade and Industry, 2005.

12

The Great Hospital and Health Service Clearout

An ever more determined aim of central government has been to clear older people out of hospitals and, once out of hospital, remove them from the ambit of the NHS as far as is practicable. That is, if responsibility for their care – in care homes or in people's own homes – can be shunted over to local councils (who can charge for services), then so much the better. This is amply illustrated by the so-called 'continuing NHS health care' saga, as well as by other policies relating either to hospital discharge or avoidance of hospital admission. The policies are sometimes fuelled by the bandying about of suitably derogatory terms such as 'bed blockers' to refer to, and sometimes virtually to demonise, older people – who may, for example, be taking that bit longer (for both physical and mental reasons) to recover in a hospital bed before discharge is appropriate. Certainly 'bed blocking' is a term that has been used by the Department of Health in the past.

NHS continuing care: putting them out to grass and making them pay

The 'continuing NHS health care' scandal (as many would call it) illustrates most graphically a largely undeclared abandonment of vulnerable, mostly older people by the NHS.

For the wider public, at a national level, the issue became perhaps clearest in a *Panorama* programme shown on BBC television in March 2006. Given an uncompromising title, the 'National homes swindle', it revealed the distress to older people and their families, lack of transparency of government policy and apparently unlawful actions of the NHS encouraged by central government.[1]

The programme harked back to the Labour Party Conference in 1997, when Tony Blair stated that he didn't want children to be 'brought up in a country where the only way pensioners can get long-term care is by selling their home'. However, the programme revealed that not only have thousands of people been forced to sell their homes to pay for such care, but that this compulsion by the NHS and local authorities has been unlawful.

The Chair of the House of Commons Health Select Committee between 1997 and 2005, David Hinchcliffe, was quoted on the programme. He referred to the scandal of older people being forced unlawfully to dispose of their house and what a final and distressing act this is.

At long last, what has been known to some in the health, social care and voluntary fields was put bluntly to the nation by the presenter. A gradual and apparently deliberate policy had been introduced surreptitiously, unsanctioned by Parliament and unannounced.

The reason for all this was because the issue was simply too politically sensitive. The policy had been introduced gradually by stealth and was aimed at the most vulnerable, who didn't know the rules – an ignorance shared it seemed by many NHS staff as well.

By the late 1980s, quietly but steadily with no explicit policy, NHS hospitals began to close significant numbers of beds, with long-stay, older patients being particularly affected, as well as other groups. Typically, by the 1990s, these patients who had once received a free service in NHS premises were being shifted out into private sector nursing homes. There, they might have to pay for their care with their savings and their house. Into the early 1990s, central government (then Conservative) appeared to think that this covert shifting of responsibility might be achieved discreetly and with a minimum of fuss and publicity. After all, it was being perpetrated at the expense – literally – of mostly older, vulnerable people, who would generally be unlikely to complain.

However, despite the best efforts of the Department of Health to avoid publicity, 1994 saw the opening shots in a series of events spanning the next 12 years that would develop into a scandal. It is always tempting to be charitable when things go wrong and to put it down to inadvertence, lack of understanding, or poor decisions made nevertheless in good faith. However, in the case of continuing NHS health care, it is impossible to attribute it to

1 'National homes swindle.' *Panorama*, BBC1, 5 March 2006.

anything other than a wish covertly to save money to the detriment of vulnerable and older people. To have implemented such a policy on the back of proper public debate would have been contentious but at least transparent; to introduce it through the back door was unforgivable.

The health service ombudsman precipitated the first major shots of the campaign in 1994. His report concerned a man who was doubly incontinent, could not eat or drink without assistance, could not communicate – and had a kidney tumour, cataracts in both eyes and occasional epileptic fits. There was no dispute that when he was discharged he did not need active medical treatment but he did need substantial nursing care. The ombudsman was scathing about the failure of Leeds Health Authority to provide him with a free nursing home placement.[2]

The ombudsman has, since then, continued a steady stream of critical investigations, and was eventually forced to publish special reports, so significant had the issue of continuing care become. Apart from one major legal case, the ombudsman was for the most part taking on a seemingly shifty and elusive central government single-handed. Nevertheless, following a major Court of Appeal case in 1999, the Department of Health reissued its guidance in 2001.[3]

In this major legal case the court had found that beyond question the patient concerned qualified for continuing NHS health care. She had been badly injured in a road traffic accident and was described as tetraplegic, doubly incontinent, requiring regular catheterisation, partially paralysed in respiratory function, subject to problems attendant on immobility and also to recurrent headaches caused by an associated neurological condition. She had fairly stable but substantial nursing needs.[4]

In a further significant case, the health service ombudsman had identified that the needs of a person with Alzheimer's Disease living at home, looked after by his wife, also qualified for continuing NHS health care. He was totally reliant on others for his needs to be met, subject to epileptic seizures, muscular spasms, panic attacks, episodes of choking, visual spatial difficulties and hallucinatory experiences. The implications of the ombudsman's findings meant, in this particular case at least, that the services being

2 Health Service Ombudsman (1994) *Investigation E.62/93-94: Leeds Health Authority*. London: HMSO.

3 Health Service Circular 2001/015. *Continuing Care: NHS and local councils' responsibilities*. London: Department of Health, 2001.

4 *R v North and East Devon Health Authority, ex parte Coughlan* (1999) 2 CCLR 285, Court of Appeal.

put into the home had to be provided free of charge by the NHS, rather than supplied by the local council at a charge.[5]

Unfortunately, the new Department of Health guidance issued in 2001 was found by the health service ombudsman to be even less comprehensible than the 1995 guidance it had replaced. The ombudsman's reports had continued, progressing from substantial irritant to increasingly public embarrassment to central government.[6] Forced to act by these reports, but not to concede any failings on its own part, the Department of Health finally threw an offering to the health service ombudsman in 2003. The NHS were to review cases back to 1996 to ensure that people had been correctly assessed against the guidance for continuing care. Where they had not been, reimbursement of money might be necessary. By December 2004, some £180 million had been set aside for repayments to people wrongly charged. However, since the ombudsman had stated that the Department of Health's guidance was deeply flawed, there were always doubts about the effectiveness of such reviews.

A court case in 2006, all too predictably, confirmed that the Department of Health's guidance, coupled with other guidance on 'free nursing care', was seriously flawed.[7] In March 2006, this legal case had forced the Department of Health to instigate a whole new round of reviews, as to whether people had been correctly assessed for continuing NHS health care. Paul Burstow, MP, was now claiming that up to 70,000 people a year were having to sell their home in order to pay for health care that should have been provided free of charge.[8]

Of great concern is not only the effect on patients and their families, but on staff as well – since they too are either in the dark about the rules or forced to play along with their NHS employer's evasions. For instance, evidence to the House of Commons Health Committee was damning. Pauline Thompson of Age Concern England stated:

5 Health Service Ombudsman (2004) *Investigation E.22/02-03: Cambridgeshire Health Authority*. London: Stationary Office.

6 Health Service Ombudsman (2003) *NHS Funding for Long Term Care.* London: TSO; Health Service Ombudsman (2004) *NHS Funding for Long Term Care: follow up report.* London: TSO.

7 *R (Grogan) v Bexley NHS Care Trust* [2006] EWHC 44 (Admin), High Court.

8 Diane Taylor, 'Health criteria strip old and inform of free care.' *Guardian*, 20 March 2006.

> If you ask for continuing care, we find that people are put right off from the very beginning: 'oh, nobody gets it in this area; you have to be nearly dead to get it'.[9]

The *Panorama* programme on continuing care revealed instances of something rather worse than staff ignorance or disinterest. For example, a woman in hospital had given her daughter power of attorney to manage her money. Her daughter believed that her mother qualified for continuing care and so was resisting her mother's discharge to a nursing home, until the NHS would accept full financial responsibility. With access to the mother's money denied by the daughter, discharge to the nursing home was delayed. A hospital consultant then approached the mother to try to persuade her to transfer her power of attorney away from the daughter to the local authority – so she could be discharged to the care home and charged for her care there. The mother refused, a solicitor faxed the hospital, warning it off, and the attempts to change the power of attorney ceased.[10]

A follow-up *Panorama* programme, entitled 'The National Homes Swindle: a Growing Scandal' was shown several months later, because of the unprecedented response to the first programme.[11] It revealed further seemingly extraordinary examples. One such concerned an older woman in a nursing home with advanced dementia and diabetes. She had managed to achieve fully funded continuing health care status. She then developed diabetes-related complications and had first a foot and then a leg amputated. She was now a nursing home resident with advancing dementia and diabetes, and was less one leg. She was reviewed and had her NHS continuing care status removed, presumably on the basis that she was easier to look after because of her reduced mobility. Essentially, she was now legally – and financially of course – deemed to be social care (for which she would be means-tested to pay), with just a small nursing element to be paid by the NHS.

On *Panorama*, the care services minister, Ivan Lewis, attempted to justify government policy of calling such people 'social care' – by referring to how people could be helped to live more independently. Such statements smack of political correctness and of dogma running riot. As CCC, a coalition of commercial, charitable and public service organisations, has pointed out, a census of 15,000 care home residents revealed that 64 per cent were

9 House of Commons Health Committee (2005) *NHS Continuing Care. Sixth Report of Session 2004–05. Volume 1.* HC 399-1. London: HMSO, para 114.

10 'National homes swindle.' *Panorama*, BBC1, 5 March 2006.

11 Shown on BBC1, 23 July 2006.

confused and 27 per cent were immobile *and* incontinent *and* mentally impaired:

> Loss of mental capacity is the single most important factor leading to the need for care in care homes. This and physical dependencies are commonly characterised by complex as well as unpredictable care needs (eg an unpredictable need for toileting assistance around the clock).[12]

To talk of social care and independence in this context is a seeming nonsense. As people's houses and savings continue to disappear, one relative of a nursing home resident put it bluntly on the Panorama programme. For her, it was unfair and meant that people who had worked all their lives, paid taxes, and fought for their country were now being walked all over. It was in effect 'state sanctioned theft'.

Stung into some action, the government did issue policy guidance for consultation in June 2006.[13] Whilst it appeared on the surface to make some of the right noises, very severe doubts must remain about whether the Department of Health at national level, and primary care trusts at local level, have the will or understanding genuinely to rectify matters.

A subterfuge too far: free nursing care

The trick perpetrated by central government via its continuing care guidance can only be understood by juxtaposing it with another set of guidance, to do with free registered nursing care provided in nursing homes.

Put simply, if you are in a care home, are not eligible for continuing NHS health care, but have nursing needs, you will get these paid free by the NHS. This will be up to a maximum of £129 per week for the high band, £80 for the medium band, and £40 for the low band. However, your accommodation, board and personal care costs you will have to pay yourself, and you may have to sell your house. If your money and capital run down to a certain level (about £12,000), the local social services authority (local council) will pay the whole cost.

Free nursing care was introduced in 2001. However, since then, the NHS has systematically attempted to include within 'free nursing care', many people who should have been categorised as continuing NHS health

12 *The best care possible? A CCC policy healthcheck.* London: CCC, p.3.

13 *National framework for NHS continuing healthcare and NHS-funded nursing care in England: consultation document.* London: Department of Health, 2006.

care. In which case, the accommodation, board, personal care and nursing care would all have been provided free. It is likely that virtually all people in the high band of free nursing care and possibly many of those in the medium band should all be receiving continuing NHS health care free of charge. This is on the basis of the legal cases and the ombudsman investigations.

In other words, it is as if central government had deliberately set up free nursing care as a vehicle for systematically removing rights to free NHS health care. It was like offering a crumb in order to take away most of the loaf.

The House of Commons Health Committee had meanwhile identified a perverse incentive resulting in detriment to patients. Nursing homes that failed to provide sufficient nursing inputs to improve health and well-being stood to be paid more. This was because the resulting dependency would mean the resident was assessed as being in a higher band – which would mean more money paid to the nursing home by the NHS. Conversely, if the nursing home successfully achieved rehabilitation and greater independence, then it would be financially penalised because the patient's banding would be reduced by the NHS assessors.[14]

Witch hunting in the hospitals: bed blocking and frequent flying

Adverse labels attached to certain groups of patients can all too easily lead to an atmosphere of discrimination and even vilification.

If continuing care was one way of shifting NHS responsibilities, the Community Care (Delayed Discharges) Act 2003 became another. As usual, part of the declared purpose of the Act was laudable. It is clearly not in people's interests to remain unnecessarily in hospital occupying acute hospital beds. None of us would want to do so. The Act in effect offered both financial carrot and stick.

Although not aimed only at older people on its face, the Act can be taken to have been targeted at older people. After all, they are the main occupiers of hospital beds. They have been perceived by central government to comprise the notorious army of bed blockers. The Act paved the way for NHS hospitals to try to achieve a higher turnover of patients and so better reach statistical targets. The Act imposed fines (described as 'reimbursement') upon local social services authorities (local councils) if they did not make

14 House of Commons Health Committee (2005) *NHS Continuing Care. Sixth Report of Session 2004–05. Volume 1.* HC 399-1. London: HMSO, para 180.

arrangements – sometimes within as little as three days notice – to enable patients to be discharged. The line between ensuring appropriately and inappropriately prompt discharge is a fine one. All too often, such pressures can work to the detriment of patients, particularly older ones with multifactorial problems, physical and mental. Above all they may need time in a stable environment, and it is all too tempting to discharge people prematurely.

In some ways, the *NHS Plan* hinted at the government's attitude. Older people with complex needs made bad statistics, not like the easier throughput patients who could contribute to the magical targets:

> This will not only improve the care of older people and contribute to the elimination of 'bed blocking'. It will also enable the NHS to operate more efficiently by helping to release acute hospital beds. This should enable extra patients to be treated each year, contributing towards the targets on waiting.

The improvements were meant to come in the form of active recovery and rehabilitation services with an extra 5000 intermediate care beds, and a further 1700 intermediate care places as well; of 'rapid response' teams to prevent unnecessary admissions; of more community equipment in people's homes; and of the extension of services for carers.[15]

Yet by 2005, many of these services were quite clearly inadequately funded even to begin to meet the needs of all those who needed them. For instance, in Suffolk, not only were acute hospital beds being cut back in line with this policy, but so too were the intermediate and rehabilitation beds in non-acute settings – from 98 beds (at Sudbury and Newmarket in 2003), down to a proposed 12 non-specialist residential home beds in those two towns in 2006. Rapid discharge from the acute hospital, without the possibility of community hospital beds for those with more complex needs, was a recipe that would appear inevitably to write off certain patients.

More widely, community equipment services, although reorganised, were still struggling in many areas, rapid response teams were of variable effectiveness, and local authorities continued to have little obligation to assist carers directly.

In addition to bed blockers, central government hit, in 2005 and 2006, on a new target – or maybe the same target in different guise. These were people with long-term conditions.

15 Secretary of State for Health (2000) *The NHS Plan: a plan for investment, a plan for reform.* Cm 4818-1. London: HMSO, para 15.14.

On cue, the newspapers picked up the term, running it as a leader entitled: 'GROUNDING FREQUENT FLYERS'. The headlines were as a result of a report from Dr Foster Intelligence, a company set up by the Department of Health and Dr Foster, an independent provider of health-care information.[16]

As ever, there was substance to the window dressing. As government policy stated, it would indeed be better if people were able to have greater control over their own lives, manage their own conditions to the extent that they are able to, and to remain in their own homes where this is practicable and beneficial.

In practice, however, this could easily translate into forcing people (and their informal carers) to fend for themselves – if the policy is regarded as a universal nostrum and inadequately resourced. But it is by no means clear that the money is available, or that anybody really knows the order of resources required. Part of the policy has involved something called 'Evercare', an import from the United States, about which the government has become enthusiastic. However, it has been suggested that any 'success' of this model in the United States has been achieved by restricting provision of services to those patients thought to be profitable. Department of Health commissioned research on Evercare revealed that, even making favourable assumptions, it was unlikely to reduce emergency admissions by more than one per cent. Even if a reduction of up to six per cent were achieved, this would rely on substantial investment in employing advanced nurse practitioners, with an increase of up to 20 to 24 in each PCT.[17]

Thus, the King's Fund warned in 2005 against introducing Evercare without further evidence.[18] Yet even before such a system was tried and tested for cost-effectiveness, the NHS seemed happy to jump in feet first and with eyes closed. As the Community and District Nursing Association put it, while community care might or might not be a 'low cost solution it is not a no cost solution'. Yet Patricia Hewitt was by now, apparently on the basis of little evidence, hoping that unplanned emergency admissions of such

16 'Grounding frequent flyers.' *Guardian*, 13 February 2006. And: Polly Curtis, '"Frequent flyers" costing NHS £2.3bn a year.' *Guardian*, 13 February 2006.

17 *Evercare Evaluation Interim Report.* Manchester: National Primary Care Research Development Centre, 2005.

18 'Evercare needs evaluation of cost effectiveness before it is rolled out further, says Kings Fund.' Press release, 4 February 2005. London: King's Fund.

patients could be reduced by 30 per cent – and that this would save the NHS some £400 million a year.[19]

Despite the flawed evidence, and the limited success even if the flawed evidence was to be believed, some local PCTs needed no second asking. Thus, even accepting that the system, if properly resourced, could avoid some hospital admissions, the Suffolk West PCT simply proposed large scale bed closures before the implementation of any such policy and before the effects could be seen and evaluated. Nor did it apparently identify in any detail the degree and costs of the substantial investment in advanced nurse practitioners that, as the research suggested, would be required.[20]

Pressgang: putting the carers to toil and stress

The shedding of responsibilities by the NHS and local councils, relying on some notion of generally under-funded 'care in the community', can place extreme pressure on informal carers. In a nutshell, 'informal carers might once have plugged gaps in the system of state social provision. Now we are coming to depend on them.'[21]

Realising this, although not admitting in so many words that government policy is contributing to the problem, some legislation has been passed in respect of carers. But many would say that it does not go far enough. For instance, local authority social services departments (local councils) have a duty to assess informal carers (family, friends, etc.). However, they have only a power, but not a duty, actually to provide services. Likewise flimsy is the duty on the NHS to consider requests for assistance from social services in providing for carers. The NHS has a duty to give 'due consideration' to the request, but no duty to act on it (Carers and Disabled Children Act 2000; Carers (Equal Opportunities) Act 2004).

Even Suffolk West PCT's policy on providing rehabilitation and recuperation in people's own homes conceded the relevance of informal carers. The eligibility criteria make clear that if people's needs are such as to require substantial supervision, then they will not be eligible for services in their own home, unless a capable carer is present.[22]

19 Celia Hall, 'Home care will not be cheap, nurses warn.' *Daily Telegraph*, 21 March 2006. And: David Ward, 'Community care could cut deficit, says Hewitt.' *Guardian*, 20 March 2006.

20 *Modernising Health Care in West Suffolk: consultation, 1 August – 31 October 2005*. Bury St Edmunds: Suffolk West PCT, 2005, p.4.

21 K. Brown and E. Matthews (2006) 'Careworn country.' *Community Care*, 6–12 April, p.34.

22 *Modernising Healthcare in West Suffolk: additional information*. Bury St Edmunds: Suffolk West PCT, 2005, p.19.

In any case, it is unnecessary to resort to high-flown policy documents to realise the potential implications for carers of the closure of community hospitals. For instance, in July 2005, letters such as the following began to appear in the local East Anglian Press, spelling out the effect of the closure of community hospital beds. One correspondent wrote about her 83-year-old mother who had fallen and broken her thigh, and the attempts to find a community hospital bed for convalescence and physiotherapy, following an acute hospital stay. She had been:

> told there were no beds available as they were closing them down due to lack of funds. Therefore, she came straight home and I have been looking after her since with no outside help.[23]

When severe cuts to mental health services were announced across Suffolk by the Suffolk Mental Health Partnership Trust, Suffolk Family Carers pointed out the 'huge risk' of families breaking down because there would be no alternative.[24] The same organisation submitted to the Suffolk Health Scrutiny Committee that the PCT proposals presumed that all family carers would be willing and able to care. However:

> many will not be able to because of family commitments, difficult relationships, unsuitable accommodation and personal circumstances. There is a real concern regarding the pressure that will be placed on families to undertake this role in often complex care situations. It must also be recognised that often patients will not allow or cooperate with family members providing rehabilitation or intimate care. We know that paid carers are few and far between in many rural areas.[25]

Likewise, without the local community hospital, one former carer, harking back to her husband's stroke, put it like this:

> with no hospital to take over, I visualise carers like I once was falling down in a heap from sheer exhaustion, with their ailing oldies, hungry and soiled, wailing in distressed confusion when they fail to arise.[26]

23 Sue Abbott, 'Health service money wasted on managers.' Letter. *East Anglian Daily Times*, 9 July 2005.

24 Danielle Nuttall, 'Protestors' fury at mental health cuts.' *East Anglian Daily Times*, 29 July 2005.

25 Jacqui Martin (2005) *Briefing Paper, Submission to Suffolk County Council Health Scrutiny Committee.* H05/18, 5 September 2005.

26 Gwynneth V. West, 'Caring role of small hospitals.' Letter. *East Anglian Daily Times*, 29 July 2005.

13

From Hospital to Homestead: the Great Go-between of Intermediate Care

A major plank of government policy, related both to continuing care and delayed discharge of older people from hospital, is a policy that has become known as 'intermediate care'. It is a policy that on its surface is replete with good intentions and in principle can be effective. However, the practical implementation of the policy sometimes reveals a detrimental underbelly, which both central government and local NHS bodies have not been slow to exploit when financial pressures bite.

Intermediate care is a linchpin. It is fundamental to taking unnecessary pressure off acute NHS hospitals and achieving 'care closer to home'. It aims to ensure timely discharge from hospital as well as to prevent admission in the first place. It could be a useful and even central form of rehabilitation, if applied appropriately and not misused. It straddles also the all-important boundary between health care and social care. Again this is a good thing if the policy is properly implemented, because rehabilitation and recuperation entail both health and social care aspects.

Nevertheless, intermediate care can also become the cover under which vulnerable people with very considerable needs may be denied appropriate and effective health care. It will also be an important component of the 'marketisation' of the NHS. Intermediate care is just the sort of service that the private sector will be looking to take over from local NHS primary care trusts.

This chapter makes some general points about intermediate care. It then goes into some detail as to what went on in West Suffolk. Intermediate care was the central battleground. Across it, a very bitter conflict was prosecuted. The PCT would claim that intermediate care in people's own homes, together with the odd placement in a residential home, would be sufficient to meet all people's non-acute rehabilitation needs. On this basis, scores of acute hospital rehabilitation beds could be closed, together with scores (in fact all) of the community hospital beds in West Suffolk. The PCT argued that it was 'passionate' about this and that it would work. The local community and many clinicians were aghast at such an extreme 'model of care', believing it was being implemented crudely and as a result of financial pressure.

Focusing on what happened in West Suffolk serves also another purpose. When unreasonable, contradictory and instant demands are made on NHS trusts and PCTs, the quality of decision-making can suffer. Such were the demands in West Suffolk for the PCT to make rapid savings that it failed to provide solid evidence for its proposals. Yet, given their drastic nature, evidence was more than ever required. At best, the PCT failed to make out the case on the evidence – both national and general, as well as local and specific. At worst, it appeared to use the evidence highly selectively. Determination it had in plenty, as well as good faith no doubt. But the evidence was rather less. It all seemed to constitute a general, much wider object lesson in how financial and political agendas, both rushed and covert, can undermine the effectiveness of NHS decision-making.

Finally, the chapter provides a number of detailed examples of exactly the type of patient (often but not only older) who, in the eyes of experienced clinicians and patients, stood to suffer serious detriment, were a suitable range of rehabilitation and recuperation not available to them.

Intermediate care: a welcome addition to rehabilitation?

In principle, intermediate care is about taking pressure off acute hospitals, with a view to providing rehabilitation and recuperation closer to people's homes in a non-acute setting. This may be in a person's own home, in a community hospital or sometimes in a specialist care home. It has been generally limited to a period of six weeks, although this does vary. Many of us would indeed prefer to have calmer, more homely rehabilitation and recuperation in, or closer to, our own homes. So far so good.

However, it is not always possible or at least reasonably practicable to have rehabilitation or recuperation in people's own homes. This could be for a number of reasons, including the complexity or intensity of your needs that require too many visits from too many staff, the unsuitability of the home environment (physical layout, family dynamics), too great a degree of medical or nursing instability, the lack of informal carers to provide the care, or the fact that a period longer than six weeks will be required for the rehabilitation – and so on.

In which case people may still need rehabilitation in another setting. This could be a community hospital bed, sometimes (for instance, in case of serious medical instability) in an acute hospital, sometimes in specialist care home units. Indeed, this is what was always envisaged. For instance, following the National Beds Inquiry, implementation of the *NHS Plan* meant that there would be 7000 new beds in total. Of these, 2100 were to be in general and acute wards. There would be 5000 extra intermediate care beds:

> some in community or cottage hospitals, some in specially designated wards in acute hospitals, some in purpose-built new facilities, some in redesigned nursing homes and residential homes.[1]

The original government guidance recognised the need to maintain a balanced approach to rehabilitation, which should continue to be available in a wide range of settings to reflect people's differing needs. Likewise, the Audit Commission warned expressly that intermediate care should not be seen as a universal remedy at the expense of other forms of rehabilitation.[2] Intermediate care was just one type of rehabilitation.

Five years later, published government policy still seems to be saying the right thing. A 2006 White Paper continued to laud the virtues of intermediate care and services closer to people's homes, including community hospitals. It talked also of the importance of people's independence – the key aim of rehabilitation services. Government policy documents had also continued to give good examples. They referred for instance to a range of

1 Health Service Circular 2001/03. *Implementing the NHS Plan: developing services following the National Beds Inquiry*. London: Department of Health, para 7.

2 Audit Commission (2000) *Way to Go Home: rehabilitation and remedial services for older people*. London: Audit Commission, paras 36–37.

integrated rehabilitation services provided in both geriatric and specialist acute hospital wards, as well as in consultant-led community hospital beds.[3]

There is another straightforward reason for steering a balanced, middle way. This involves not putting all the eggs in the intermediate care basket, and instead providing different types of rehabilitation in different settings. The reason is the continuing lack of decisive evidence concerning the effectiveness, and cost-effectiveness, of intermediate care in its various forms. For instance, especially for people with higher needs, it may by no means be cheap.[4] And toward the end of 2005, the *British Medical Journal* stated that the available evidence 'does a little more to clothe the Emperor of intermediate care, but he is still not really fit to be seen out in public'.[5]

Intermediate care: off the leash and going astray?

By 2005, the British Geriatrics Society was reporting that there had been a major reduction in NHS rehabilitation bed numbers, with reprovision being the exception. More than half the respondents to a survey cited finance as the reason. Of these beds, the greater proportion closed were community rehabilitation beds, despite 'being considered to be an excellent setting for intermediate care'. The increase of intermediate care beds in residential homes did not get anywhere near to matching the number of NHS rehabilitation beds closed. Overall, the Society was concerned about the 'diminishing provision of rehabilitation to older people'.[6]

The Society further expressed itself concerned about the move into the community of rehabilitation in the form of intermediate care. There had been a reduction in specialist inpatient rehabilitation beds and thus a reduction in medical input. This was disadvantageous because of the relationship between disease and disability.[7] Thus, practice might be flowing in the wrong direction in a number of ways.

First, instead of being seen additional to other forms of rehabilitation, it seems that intermediate care has too often diverted excessive resources away from other types of rehabilitation. This carries the risk of denying the

3 *Keeping the NHS Local: a new direction of travel.* London: Department of Health, 2003, para 2.3.4.

4 H. Parker and others (2005) *National Evaluation of the Costs and Outcomes of Intermediate Care Services for Older People.* Leicester: Nuffield Community Care Studies Unit, University of Leicester, Summary, para 3.3.

5 'Comment: Intermediate care: policy before evidence.' *British Medical Journal 331*, 320, 6 August 2005.

6 'Rehabilitation bed survey.' *BGS Newsletter Online,* March 2005.

7 *Rehabilitation in the NHS and Social Care.* London: British Geriatrics Society, 2005.

appropriate rehabilitation to people with more complex and difficult needs. This is despite the Audit Commission's explicit warning about this, as well as the import of the original intermediate care guidance.[8] Such a trend would be particularly worrying, given for example the continuing concerns about the treatment of stroke patients, including the provision of post-acute support services and rehabilitation services.[9] Rehabilitation for such patients might typically take a great deal longer than six weeks.

Second, community-based rehabilitation services in the form of intermediate care need more than ever to be resourced properly, given their peripatetic and thus more time-consuming nature. Too often it seems that they are not, with the result that people do not receive the services they require. Waiting lists may grow, denying people the window of rehabilitation they require. This is perverse and anathema to providing rehabilitation at the time it is needed.

Third, many intermediate care services work to a six-week treatment limit. Although some individual patients will be allowed to exceed the six-week limit if necessary, they may not be allowed even to begin to receive intermediate care if their *potential* rehabilitation is judged not to be achievable within six weeks. Concerns have grown that six-week intermediate care does in practice displace slower stream rehabilitation.[10]

Fourth, in the case of some intermediate care teams, the essential balance between health and social care may be lost. This is especially so when the NHS locally decides it cannot afford to fund the requisite number of physiotherapists and occupational therapists. This may then mean that some people do not receive properly planned and supervised rehabilitation. In addition, legally, once the six weeks is up and if services are still provided, then clients and patients may be charged for services still required, insofar as they are 'social care'. This creates another incentive inappropriately to shift the focus of intermediate care over to 'social care' services provided by local councils.

Fifth, the 2006 White Paper explicitly extols the virtues of community hospital beds. They take unnecessary pressure off acute hospitals and can provide both better and more cost-effective rehabilitation and recuperation for older people who cannot return straight home following an acute

8 Health Service Circular 2001/01. *Intermediate Care.* London: Department of Health, para 10.

9 House of Commons Committee of Public Accounts (2006) *Reducing brain damage: faster access to better stroke care.* HC 911. London: Stationery Office, p.6.

10 L. Nazarko, 'Give older people enough time to fully recover.' *Nursing Times,* 31 January 2006. And: M. Cornes and J. Manthorpe, 'Someone to expect each day.' *Community Care,* 8–14 December 2005, p.36.

hospital stay.[11] Subsequent guidance about community hospitals continued to include examples which included NHS rehabilitation and recuperation beds.[12] Likewise in Parliament, Patricia Hewitt, Secretary of State for Health, would refer to Norwich as an example of where a balance had been achieved between care in people's homes and community hospitals. She talked about a reduction in inpatient beds. She did not refer to their complete removal, as Suffolk West PCT and other PCTs – purportedly acting in her name – had been doing.[13]

Yet at the time of the White Paper about 100 community hospitals in England were under threat of either closure or significant reduction in services including many beds. Further signs that rehabilitation was being undermined on the ground came in July 2006. Hundreds of newly trained physiotherapists – key rehabilitation professionals – protested outside Parliament. Why? Because nine out of ten newly qualified physiotherapists had no NHS jobs to go to.[14]

The White Paper did not laud community hospital beds for nothing. There is evidence about their value and cost-effectiveness.[15] And the Commission for Social Care Inspection referred explicitly to the important role which community hospital beds play in enabling people to move nearer to their family before returning home.[16]

The dismantling of rehabilitation in the lanes of West Suffolk

Unfortunately, Suffolk West Primary Care Trust is a classic case in point of how good intentions seemed to be subverted by financial pressures. The subversion was caused by central government which in one breath set out good practice, and in the next ordered (via strategic health authorities and by implication) local NHS bodies to do the opposite. It is worth spelling out the

11 Secretary of State for Health (2006) *Our Health, Our Care, Our Say: a new direction for community services.* Cm 6737. London: HMSO, para 6.40.

12 *Developing community hospitals: models of ownership.* London: Department of Health, 2006.

13 Patricia Hewitt. *Hansard,* 5 July 2006, House of Commons Debates, column 827.

14 Lisa Wilde, 'MPs feel the heat.' *Frontline,* 2 August 2006.

15 John Green and others, 'Effects of locality based community hospital care on independence in older people needing rehabilitation: randomised controlled trial.' *British Medical Journal,* 6 August 2005, 317–322. And: Jacqueline O'Reilly, Karin Lowson, John Young, Anne Forster, John Green and Neil Small. 'A cost effectiveness analysis within a randomised controlled trial of post-acute care of older people in a community hospital.' *British Medical Journal,* July 2006; 333: 228.

16 *Leaving Hospital: the price of delays.* London: Commission for Social Care Inspection, 2004, Executive summary, and para 2.5.

detail, because these arguments are being, and will be, repeated in many other parts of the country.

In line with government policy and indeed good practice, Suffolk West PCT had originally developed an intermediate care strategy, which took a balanced approach to intermediate care and rehabilitation.[17] It translated this strategy into a detailed and carefully argued business case, complete with some acute hospital beds (for the acute stage of rehabilitation), care in people's homes and community hospital beds.[18] Suddenly, within a space of a month, financial restrictions imposed by central government intervened. The PCT promptly redefined what it meant by 'intermediate care' to fit a new strategy that would be consonant with saving money.[19]

The PCT now proposed what many people believed to be an unbalanced, relatively extreme model of rehabilitation that involved the closure of large numbers of both NHS community hospital, and acute hospital, beds. All the eggs would instead be placed precariously in more or less one basket only. Nearly everybody would now receive services in their own homes, or occasionally in a care home. In order to argue this, the PCT found itself having to treat the evidence, both national and local, in a number of highly questionable ways.

The important point about the following paragraphs is not really anything to do with Suffolk West PCT. First the issues are topical and are likely to be relevant to decisions about intermediate care in other parts of the country. Second, Suffolk West PCT is part of the National Health Service. Its decisions are NHS decisions and they therefore tell us something very important and very disturbing about the way in which the NHS is currently being run.

Overall definition of intermediate care

Suffolk West PCT implied erroneously that intermediate care by definition meant closing community hospital beds. The PCT gave the impression to the public that, apart from the occasional care-home placement, intermediate care was about providing rehabilitation and recuperation in people's own homes only. But, as we have already seen, intermediate care policy is all

17 *Intermediate Care: a time of transition.* Bury St Edmunds: Suffolk West PCT, 2003.

18 *Outline Business Case for the development of Sudbury Health and Social Care Centre.* Bury St Edmunds: Suffolk West PCT, March 2005.

19 *Modernising Health Care in West Suffolk: consultation, 1 August–31 October 2005.* Bury St Edmunds: Suffolk West PCT, 2005, p.4.

about taking the pressure off acute hospitals. It is not about closure of community hospital beds – and certainly not about closing them all.

Cost-effectiveness of community hospital beds

Various national evidence, and the government's White Paper, pointed to the cost-effectiveness of community hospital beds. But the PCT would argue that they were too expensive, stating 'hospital care is very expensive'.

The PCT's comparative costings didn't seem to add up. First, it appeared that by mistake the PCT had over-costed the community hospital beds at Walnuttree Hospital, making them appear impossibly expensive (at £244 per day rather than £114). In addition, it had also failed to refer to the cost of beds at the new community hospital (now abandoned), which had been calculated at £123 per day. This compared very favourably with the cost of care home beds (£121) now proposed by the PCT, because community hospital beds can meet a greater range of needs.[20]

The PCT's report prepared for its final decision in April 2006 did not draw this obvious comparison with the new community hospital. Nor did it produce evidence as to why block purchased private care home beds would be more cost-effective than inpatient beds at the new hospital.[21]

Readmissions to acute hospitals

Suffolk West PCT would quite openly admit that patients would be sent home and then reviewed, and 'could be readmitted to [the acute] hospital at any time'.[22] Such a concession seemed more than ever to flow against the whole point of intermediate care. This was to take the pressure off the acute hospital and prevent readmissions known as 'revolving door syndrome'. Frontline workers know this only too well, as Unison representative at Walnutree, Tom Keane, pointed out: 'Some patients are being discharged too early. The conditions they suffer from recur and they are readmitted to hospital.'[23]

In any case, in October 2005, 55 acute hospital beds would also be closed at the acute hospital, to be followed by 30 more in 2006 – thus

20 *Response to Suffolk West Primary Care Trust's Consultation.* Sudbury: Walnuttree Hospital Action Committee, 2005, para 9.2.4.

21 Michael Stonard (2006) *Modernising Health Care in West Suffolk: report for decision, 11th April 2006.* Bury St Edmunds: Suffolk West PCT. See also minutes of decision of 11 April, with amendment to purchase the care home beds by means of block, rather than spot, purchase.

22 Barbara Eeles, 'Cost effective and good for patients, too.' *Suffolk Free Press,* 18 August 2005.

23 Nicki Harvey, 'Anger over health boss's claims.' *Suffolk Free Press,* 25 August 2005.

increasingly closing off the route to greater use (albeit inappropriate) of acute hospital beds.

National evidence for balanced approach to intermediate care

The PCT appeared erroneously to put forward national evidence about intermediate care generally – in order to garner support for its narrow and extreme model in a rural area. The plan for the Sudbury area involved no community hospital beds and six (non-specialist) residential home beds. In fact the evidence cited did no such thing. The evidence in question referred to intermediate care generally – about which there is less controversy (it probably works for some people in some circumstances).

Documents referred to by the PCT included two King's Fund reports: *Intermediate Care: models in practice* and also *Developing Intermediate Care: a guide for health and social services professionals.*[24]

The first of these was far from being filled with examples of intermediate care without inpatient beds (whether or not in rural areas). It described, for instance, a nurse-led unit of inpatient beds in London, a community hospital with 28 beds in Liverpool, a 23-bedded rehabilitation unit for older people in Plymouth, and community-based NHS beds in East Norfolk.

The second pointed out the wide variety of services that could be considered as intermediate care and that the evidence was limited. This was because it was difficult to compare like with like, and large gaps in the evidence still existed.

The PCT stated also that 'most significantly', the Department of Health had published guidance on intermediate care.[25] It referred to these two pieces of guidance in its consultation document under the question about whether there was 'evidence that you don't need community hospital beds' in a rural area. Neither of these two documents had anything to say about this. They certainly did not serve as positive evidence for that proposition; but the PCT nevertheless inferred that they did.[26]

Thus the PCT's claim that such reports and guidance decisively supported its extreme model of care appeared spurious. Indeed, there was a wealth of

24 Barbara Vaughan and Judith Lathlean (1999) *Intermediate Care: models in practice.* London: King's Fund, 1999; Jan Stevenson and Linda Spencer (2002) *Developing Intermediate Care: a guide for health and social services professionals.* London: King's Fund.

25 Health Service Circular 2001/01. *Intermediate Care.* London: Department of Health, para 10. Also: *Intermediate Care: moving forward.* London: Department of Health, 2002.

26 *Modernising Healthcare in West Suffolk: additional information.* Bury St Edmunds: Suffolk West PCT, 2005, p.20.

evidence suggesting that a much more balanced approach to intermediate care was required. The balance would allow for plurality of care in different settings to take account of different needs. The 2006 White Paper referred to the importance of community hospital beds, just as the *NHS Plan* of six years before had done.[27]

Impracticality of rehabilitation for some patients in their own homes

The PCT appeared simply to ignore its own rules concerning the eligibility of patients for intermediate care in their own homes. These rules made clear that, by definition, the PCT's extreme model of care would not meet everybody's needs. There were good reasons for having these rules, since rehabilitation in people's own homes is sometimes impracticable because of people's needs or the home environment. Therefore, the PCT's claims for meeting people's needs without community hospital beds appeared to be a logical contradiction in terms.

The criteria were roughly as follows. Patients excluded from care in their own homes were those with needs that were too complex or too intense (e.g. thay had a need for more than four visits daily or required night-time attendance, or required 24-hour supervision), who did not have an informal carer able and willing to care, who had the wrong home environment (i.e. rehabilitation would have been impracticable or unsafe), who had a degree of medical instability, or who did not have the *potential* to be rehabilitated in six weeks.[28] Even those in residential homes were excluded on grounds of medical or nursing needs greater than would be provided for in their own homes, or of not having the potential for rehabilitation in six weeks. In practice, people with more complex manual handling needs were also excluded from both own home or residential settings.

The consequences of the criteria would clearly rule out significant categories of patient from receiving rehabilitation and recuperation in their own homes or even in residential homes. In addition, the six residential home beds the PCT was prepared to purchase in the Sudbury area (in place of the 68 community hospital beds) would arguably be in breach of standards made under the Care Standards Act 2000. These state that care homes used for intermediate care should have dedicated accommodation, together with

27 Secretary of State for Health (2000) *The NHS Plan: a plan for investment, a plan for reform.* Cm 4818-1. London: HMSO, 2000, para 4.4.

28 *Modernising Healthcare in West Suffolk: additional information.* Bury St Edmunds: Suffolk West PCT, 2005, p.19.

specialist staff, equipment and facilities.[29] None of the care homes in the Sudbury area could boast these. It is notable that the *NHS Plan*, when it referred to extra intermediate care beds, referred to some in community or cottage hospitals, others in specially designated wards in acute hospitals and – crucially – 'some will be in purpose built new facilities or in redesigned private nursing homes'.[30] What the *NHS Plan* did not suggest (for good reason) – but what the PCT now appeared to be advocating – is that ordinary care homes should be used for such rehabilitation and intermediate care.

The PCT, had it only asked itself the question, would have known that its 'new model' of intermediate care would not work for significant groups of people in their own homes or in residential homes in the Sudbury area. Yet there seemed to be a total blind spot in its reasoning, due to the rush with which everything was being done. Its Director of Clinical Services could still state, on the day of the PCT's decision to close all its beds, that: 'There are thousands of beds in West Suffolk: in people's own homes.' This was regarded by the local community as a highly provocative statement.[31] Insofar as it indicated an unduly limited view of rehabilitation and of people's different needs and different home environments, it spoke volumes.

Hasty departure from the PCT's own intermediate care policy

NHS trusts and PCTs, like other public bodies, clearly change their policies from time to time. But if it is done hurriedly and on the hoof, things go wrong. In West Suffolk, the PCT denied changing its policy, even though its new proposals ran contrary to that policy.

It claimed that the extreme model of care it was now proposing was a mere acceleration of an existing strategy. The existing strategy had in fact envisaged community hospital beds and, up to June 2005, had even involved building new ones in Sudbury (see Chapter 10).

Furthermore, the strategy that had envisaged closure of some beds in West Suffolk as community services developed was now in tatters. This was because the report on which the bed closures was based had recommended in 2003 the closure of some 53 beds, if alternative community services were in place. The bed closures that had already occurred since then and were now

29 *Care Homes for Older People: national minimum standards.* London: Department of Health, 2001, standard 6.

30 Secretary of State for Health (2000) *The NHS Plan: a plan for investment, a plan for reform.* Cm 4818-II. London: TSO, para 4.4.

31 'Thousands of beds at home.' *Suffolk Free Press*, 13 April 2006.

proposed were as follows. They were far in excess of what the local policy and locally gathered evidence could possibly underpin.

In summary, the PCT's intermediate care plan stated that it relied substantially on a report it commissioned from a company called Secta. This had recommended that 53 beds could be closed across Walnuttree, Newmarket and West Suffolk Hospitals, if alternatives were provided in the community.[32] By early 2005, before even the PCT's consultation had started, more than this number of beds had been closed. These included 33 beds at West Suffolk (Ward G6) in 2004, 14 beds at Newmarket in 2004, and 36 beds temporarily closed (but never reopened) at Walnuttree in early 2005. This made a total of 83 beds already closed, far in excess of the Secta report's recommendations and the PCT's own intermediate care plan. Now the PCT proposed that a further 55 beds be closed at West Suffolk Hospital, 14 beds at Newmarket and a further 32 beds at Walnuttree.[33] By June 2006, 26 more beds were to be lost at West Suffolk Hospital.[34]

Clearly, these further closures were indeed nothing to do with the existing strategy, which nowhere stated that the ultimate aim was to close all non-acute NHS rehabilitation beds.

Evidence gathering locally

In order to bolster its arguments, the PCT made claims about the needs of its community hospital patients on the basis of seemingly threadbare evidence gathering. In particular, the PCT first appeared to sideline the results of the full and proper analysis carried out by Secta in 2003, which fully recognised the need for community hospital beds. It then substituted the results of an apparently entirely inadequate audit carried out very hurriedly in 2005 by the PCT.

This audit was conducted apparently a) at short notice, ad hoc and in the space of a couple of hours, b) with no involvement of doctors or therapists, and c) without the staff who were involved understanding the methodology and what they were meant to be doing. It appeared also that the PCT had misused some of the data collected to draw misleading conclusions about

32 *Intermediate Care: time of transition.* Bury St Edmunds: Suffolk West PCT, para 2.4.9. And: *Developing New Models of Intermediate Care.* London: Secta.

33 *Response to Suffolk West Primary Care Trust's Consultation.* Sudbury: Walnuttree Hospital Action Committee, 2005.

34 Laurence Cawley, 'Health bosses to axe 26 more beds.' *East Anglian Daily Times,* 15 June 2006.

patient need.[35] Reliably informed about this, the Walnuttree Hospital Action Committee (and, independently, the Newmarket Health Forum) drew this to the attention of the PCT, citing these shortcomings in the audit. In its reply, the PCT chose not to respond one way or another to any of these particular criticisms of the audit.

Thus, the PCT's claims concerning the 'social care' nature of the community hospital bed patients seemed flimsy. Furthermore, the PCT had failed to ask a crucial question in its audit. Even had it turned out that a certain number of patients were inappropriately occupying the beds, it would not have necessarily meant that the beds were not needed. It could have been, as is a well-recognised pattern with some community hospital use, that the PCT was simply misusing the beds, or that referral patterns were amiss. The audit should have considered more widely the needs of the local population and whether there was a requirement for community hospital beds in the future if used properly. The irony of this failure at least to consider the use to which community hospital beds could and should have been put, became clear in January 2006, when the government's own White Paper referred to their importance.

Patient activity in a sub-acute, rehabilitation setting

Apparently lacking evidence of substance, the Suffolk West PCT continued to take what many considered to be an over-simplistic and opportunistic approach to rehabilitation and community hospital beds. For instance, at its decision to close the beds in April 2006, it referred to a visit that the Chief Executive and Director of Clinical Services had made to Walnuttree Hospital the day before.

They had found patients out of bed at what they termed a 'social gathering'. This confirmed, in the PCT's eyes, that not only did those patients not need to be in hospital, but therefore that community hospital beds were simply not required.[36] In fact the patients were at the day hospital or making their way to lunch on foot (some with assistance) or in wheelchairs. As any rehabilitation professional would know, the fact that patients are not in their beds tells you very little about their rehabilitation and other needs, mental and physical, particularly in a 'sub-acute' rehabilitation setting.

35 *Response to Suffolk West Primary Care Trust's Consultation.* Sudbury: Walnuttree Hospital Action Committee, 2005, para 1.5.1.

36 'Thousands of beds at home.' *Suffolk Free Press,* 13 April 2006.

It was left to a hospital porter, Michael Mitchell, to make the obvious point as well as any rehabilitation professional could have:

> Mr Williams said he found patients not in bed but at a 'social gathering'. As he has been a nurse for 25 years he should know that getting the patients away from their beds and walking to a day room and to physio or occupational therapy is all part of their rehab. Secondly, if the patients were at home and he had visited them he would have found some still in bed from the night before in an unfit state; some having already having been put to bed at 5pm that night; most confused and disorientated; most only having ten minutes contact with other people throughout the day. We have many patients who come in to us who just need that little boost to get back to their own homes and these are the people who will suffer from these changes. These changes are all about saving money; if they cost more there wouldn't be any changes proposed.[37]

The comment made by the PCT was unfortunate. It simply confirmed in many minds that the PCT was proceeding on anything but firm evidence and appeared not to understand about rehabilitation. In its blanket dismissiveness, the comment, which was made in public, was perceived to be grossly insulting to both patient and professional alike at the Walnuttree and Newmarket Hospitals.

Rehabilitation and dependency

The Suffolk West PCT's Chief Executive would state a couple of weeks later that his plans would benefit patients and avoid them 'going into an institution with a dependency culture which tends to slow down their progress'.[38] The Chief Executive did not point out that focused use of community hospitals is not about creating dependency. Quite the opposite, as the Commission for Social Care Inspection has pointed out.[39] Indeed, inappropriate discharge of some people to their own homes, where rehabilitation is not possible or practicable, precisely can lead in some cases to 'warehousing' and dependency in people's own homes.

Furthermore, if the PCT was concerned about dependency, it seemed extraordinary that it would end up proposing six residential home beds in

37 Michael Mitchell, 'You're wrong.' Letter. *Suffolk Free Press*, 20 April 2006,

38 Mark Heath, 'Health cuts agreed.' *East Anglian Daily Times*, 28 April 2006.

39 *Leaving Hospital: the price of delays*. London: Commission for Social Care Inspection, 2004, Executive summary, and para 2.5.

the Sudbury area, for those patients whose needs could not be met at home. This is because a) it is well recognised by the Department of Health's own guidance that ordinary care homes may cause dependency,[40] b) there were no specialist care-home rehabilitation units in Sudbury, and c) even the manager at Peterborough, which was cited as a preferred model by the PCT, conceded that there was a dependency (pyjama syndrome) in private residential homes, and she would rather have an NHS set-up.[41] Furthermore, a study by the Commission for Social Care Inspection found that hardly any patients discharged to care homes from hospital returned to their own homes.[42]

Likewise, the PCT's consultation document had referred in blanket fashion, and thus misleadingly, to how difficult it was 'to encourage and develop independence' in hospital. While this is true for some people in some hospital settings, for others it is precisely a community hospital rehabilitation setting that can kick-start and maintain motivation. For example, there is a significant category of person who, isolated in their own homes or because of other home circumstances, may in fact lack or lose motivation and end up dependent. The PCT seemed to be too simplistic and oblivious to plurality of need and plurality of service to meet that need. One setting does not fit all.

Over simple representation of local evidence

The Suffolk West PCT appeared to misrepresent, or at least did not fully explain, local evidence in a number of ways.

For instance, the Chairman of the PCT would claim that it had local evidence for closing all community hospital beds – stating that such a system already was working in Bury St Edmunds and Haverhill. He would also state that 'Beds are not the answer' and conclude that it was important that 'local people know the facts'.[43]

This repeated a claim made by the PCT when it made its final decision.[44] The PCT would also state that it had 'vast and first hand experience of providing this model of care'.[45] These statements were less than helpful.

40 *Intermediate Care: moving forward.* London: Department of Health, 2002, p.11, Appendix 3.

41 *Committee Response to Decisions Taken by NHS Trusts in Suffolk.* H06/6. Ipswich: Suffolk County Council Health Scrutiny Committee, 28 February 2006.

42 *Leaving hospital revisited.* London: CSCI, 2005, p.6.

43 Colin Muge, 'PCT is working on a new model of care.' Letter. *East Anglian Daily Times*, 13 May 2006.

44 Michael Stonard (2006) *Modernising Health Care in West Suffolk: Report for Decision, Suffolk West Primary Care Trust Board, 11th April 2006.* Bury St Edmunds: Suffolk West PCT, para 15.3.

45 Will Grahame-Clark, 'Fear over home plan for care of patients.' *East Anglian Daily Times*, 6 December 2005.

First, any 'success' in Bury and Haverhill – where the specialist care homes were social services led and did not take patients requiring more complex, 'heavy weight' rehabilitation, or rehabilitation that would require more than six weeks – was because:

> more complex patients in those areas end up in the community hospital beds at Newmarket Hospital, Walnuttree Hospital, in Sudbury – or, inappropriately and contrary to Government policy, in acute beds at West Suffolk Hospital. Alternatively they go without. But in future there will be no community hospital beds, and West Suffolk Hospital is anyway running down its beds. Intermediate care will therefore fail older people with more complex needs across West Suffolk.[46]

Thus the PCT did not have experience of operating such a model – because such an extreme model of intermediate care had never been operated in West Suffolk. Community hospital beds had always been relied on.

Extraordinarily, this did not prevent the Chairman of its Professional Executive Committee stating the following after the PCT had voted to close all its beds: 'health services in Newmarket and Sudbury need to catch up with the rest of West Suffolk and it is important we have a consistency of care across the region'.[47] Second, the PCT Chairman's statement was contrary to the government's 2006 White Paper, which had extolled the use of beds because they provide good, cost-effective rehabilitation and recuperation.[48]

Oversimple representation of regional evidence

The PCT thought also to cite other intermediate care operations to justify its proposals. However, the fact that other services operated without community hospital beds was not necessarily 'evidence' that they were successful. The PCT cited no independent evaluations. It anyway turned out that some of the local evidence was far from as straightforward as the PCT claimed.[49] For instance, it cited West Norfolk, but failed to mention that West Norfolk boasted a thriving community hospital at Swaffham, with inpatient beds. It cited also intermediate care in Peterborough. But the PCT did not

46 Walnuttree Hospital Action Committee, 'In response to health chairman's letter.' Letter. *East Anglian Daily Times*, 18 May 2006.

47 Dave Gooderham, 'PCT chiefs defend closure proposals.' *Sudbury Mercury*, 13 April 2006.

48 Secretary of State for Health (2006) *Our Health, Our Care, Our Say: a new direction for community services.* Cm 6737. London: HMSO, para 6.40.

49 *Modernising Healthcare in West Suffolk: additional information.* Bury St Edmunds: Suffolk West PCT, 2005, p.21.

advertise what the Suffolk Health Scrutiny Committee had discovered, casting doubt on the effectiveness of private care-home beds, as opposed to community hospital beds. Talking to the service manager in Peterborough, the Committee's report had noted her view that nursing care in a nursing home was not ideal. Care tended to be provided instead of the rehabilitation that was required; the 'pyjama syndrome' had to be challenged. Instead, she would have preferred to have had all the beds together staffed by NHS nurses.[50]

An NHS community rehabilitation unit

The Walnuttree Hospital Action Committee quoted to the PCT an article written by a consultant in rehabilitation medicine (Rory O'Connor), a professor of rehabilitation medicine (Anne Chamberlain), and a rehabilitation care coordinator (Meriel Best).[51] This raised exactly the same issues which both the Committee and many of the PCT's own clinicians were raising. The PCT did not formally acknowledge, let alone comment on, the Committee's final report and any of the content.

The article is worth referring to in a little detail, because it encapsulates so much of what was at stake in Sudbury, and elsewhere in the country. It refers to rehabilitation in people's own homes and the fact that it is clearly desirable where practicable and effective – which it will not be for everybody, for a variety of reasons.

> It is agreed by all of those who experience disability and who work with disabled people that rehabilitation should be provided as close as possible to an individual's environment. However, the delivery of rehabilitation in an individual's home may not always be easy; the house may be too small or cluttered or the bed may be unsuitable for use in treatment, there may be children or pets, or little privacy.

But outpatient attendance will not necessarily be the answer either:

> Yet attending for outpatient treatments may be unduly tiring for, say, someone with fatigue resulting from multiple sclerosis. Some rehabilitation interventions may be difficult, unpleasant or distressing to the

50 *Committee Response to Decisions Taken by NHS trusts in Suffolk.* H06/6. Ipswich: Suffolk County Council Health Scrutiny Committee, 28 February 2006.

51 Rory O'Connor, Meriel Best and Anne Chamberlain (2006) 'The community rehabilitation unit in Leeds: a resource for people with long-term conditions.' *International Journal of Therapy and Rehabilitation, 13*, March, 3.

> individual if based at home; for example, the early stages of constraint-induced therapy...or bladder retraining.

Sometimes reorientation and adaptation to disability requires intensive encouragement and prompts over a period of time, which would simply not be practicable in a person's own home, and which need to be delivered by skilled staff in a dedicated, integrated unit:

> Other changes, such as those countering maladaptive responses to disability, can only be made where the person has the opportunity to experience another mode of living over sufficient time to produce a change. Some interventions to produce much wanted change require observation, small interventions based on this, followed by repeated observations and repeated changes. Improvements in physical function first achieved in the physiotherapy department can be transferred to practice with the nursing staff in the evenings, and then the person returns home with this new practice consolidated... Families who provide care for the disabled individual may welcome the opportunity of a short respite, while knowing that their relative is benefiting from the stay.

It is for these sorts of reasons that a balanced approach is required offering both support in people's own homes and focused, community inpatient based rehabilitation:

> For these reasons, a flexible goal-oriented rehabilitation programme comprising short periods where patients have the opportunity to stay overnight and access 24-hour nursing support with daily therapy input in a small facility based in the local community, combined with home visits by team members, may provide the optimal solution for some, keeping even those with severe disability living at home for many years.

Sometimes repeated observations and adjustments are required, which logistically are simply not practicable in the home:

> some interventions require repeated observations and adjustments over short periods of time by differing combinations of professionals working together through cycles of assessment, intervention and reassessment, with different team members providing interweaving and parallel treatments. While all of the interventions described in these case reports could have been done in the home by the appropriate professionals, they had not been done before the authors intervened, possibly emphasizing that where situations are complex and

> interconnected, their resolution may be impracticable within most people's domestic arrangements.

Specialised therapy and equipment input may be required in a controlled setting before a task can be achieved safely at home. And cost-effective use of limited resources should also be considered:

> with the present small resources available for rehabilitation, the authors feel that concentrating staff in one area enables them to deliver input more efficiently to more patients than programmes based solely in the individual's home. There is the potential for case management to enhance community rehabilitation, but community matrons will be focused on reducing repeated admissions to general hospitals because of medical problems through development of care plans and liaison with health and social services, rather than promoting rehabilitation goals.

Falling through the net: the excluded ones

The Suffolk West PCT's approach, arguing in effect that one size fits all in people's own homes, would, in the view of many, mean that the most vulnerable patients would suffer. This seemed to be the clear implication of the apparently serious flaws in its approach to intermediate care, pointed out immediately above. This critical view was shared by local general practitioners, senior clinicians within the PCT (who would submit dissenting internal responses to the PCT), and many in the local community. The Walnuttree Hospital Action Committee took expert clinical advice and submitted a detailed report.[52]

Above all, Suffolk West PCT operated criteria that excluded particular categories of patient from intermediate care in their own home or in residential homes. The criteria it operated were not arbitrary. They simply reflected the practical difficulty of delivering care to certain people in particular environments. On the whole, they were therefore entirely reasonable criteria.

But without community hospitals, the only other option was for people to remain in the acute hospital, which a) would often be an inappropriate environment for slower stream rehabilitation, b) was against government policy, and c) was anyway not possible because of all the acute bed closures at the acute hospital. A specialist care home, suitable for rehabilitation, did not

52 *Response to Suffolk West Primary Care Trust's Consultation.* Sudbury: Walnuttree Hospital Action Committee, 2005.

exist in the Sudbury area. Even the dedicated intermediate care facilities (in Bury St Edmunds and Haverhill), which were social services led, did not take more complex patients requiring 'heavier' and maybe slower rehabilitation.

In order to try to debate all this with the PCT, the Walnuttree Hospital submitted a final report to the PCT. It raised the issue of the criteria. It also contained an appendix of 'patient types' whose rehabilitation would appear to be at risk under the PCT's proposals. The PCT never acknowledged or commented on the report or its contents. Separately from its final reports, the Committee had repeatedly raised the issue of the criteria and their implications. By way of answer, the PCT reiterated, seemingly by rote, that the 'new model of care' would work. But when it came down to the awkward detail of patients with complex needs, and explaining how it would work for them, there was silence.

For instance, in November 2004, when closure of Walnuttree Hospital was first threatened, concerned patients made themselves known, including one man who had been recovering from a stroke for three months in Walnuttree, another who had been slowly recovering from pneumonia for five months, and another who had been there for two months. These types of patient would all have been excluded from rehabilitation under the PCT's new proposals and decision, because they did not have the potential to recover within six weeks.[53]

What patients and their relatives know, so too do their general practitioners. Dr Donnelly, a GP in Sudbury, put it simply and straightforwardly:

> A lot of patients can't be cared for at home in any case. For example, one of the patients I recently sent to the Walnuttree Hospital was an elderly man who had had a stroke and had been partially paralysed down one side. As it was, he could cope on his own at home, but then he caught an infection in his good leg. He couldn't get up in the night and he couldn't use a bottle, so I put him into hospital for 10 days to bring the infection under control. In future, he couldn't be cared for at home; he would have to go to the West Suffolk Hospital.[54]

In May 2006, the wife of a Walnuttree patient wrote to the local newspaper. Her husband had had both legs amputated at Addenbrooke's Hospital in Cambridge. She pointed out that although the treatment at Addenbrooke's

53 'MPs welcome bid to save hospital.' *East Anglian Daily Times*, 8 November 2004.

54 Ross Clark, 'Fear in the Community.' *Spectator*, 17 September 2005.

was good, it was as though patients were a 'number and not an individual person'. Whereas at Walnuttree:

> As soon as you enter the wards it does not seem that you are in hospital but a place of friendship and caring.[55]

Indeed, it was just such a patient who would not receive rehabilitation in the West Suffolk of the future. In his own home, it would not be possible because of the space and heavy equipment required; likewise in a care home in the Sudbury area, there are no rehabilitation units. In addition, he would not have the potential for rehabilitation in six weeks – which would rule him out again under the PCT's rules.

At the same time, the NHS-designated 'expert patient' who would seek to take a judicial review case against the PCT explained:

> I had polio 53 years ago and have been diagnosed with post-polio syndrome, a neurological condition... This causes me pain, stiffness and weakness in my joints and muscles... I tire easily and therefore need more time to recover from an injury or illness...my needs are complex now and they will become greater as I grow older. In the future I may not be able to receive rehabilitation at home...and a local nursing home would not have specialist facilities available. Therefore without appropriate treatment, I could become more disabled and be moved permanently to a remote nursing home away from family and friends. I could lose my independence and my home and this would not be care in the community...[56]

During the Suffolk West PCT's consultation process, WHAC spoke to many senior and experienced clinicians about the types of patient who would suffer from the PCT's plans. The WHAC, in its final report, identified patients, or types of patient, who (together with their families) typically might suffer under the PCT's proposals to close all community hospital beds.[57] This would include increased levels of disability, dependence, illness, pain, distress and pressure on informal carers. Such patients' needs would appear not to be met easily if all that is available is acute hospital rehabilitation, intermediate care (as the PCT was proposing it) in their own homes or occasionally in an ordinary care home, or by day hospital attendance. (The

55 C. Ingram, 'Why we need hospital beds.' Letter. *Suffolk Free Press*, 25 May 2006.

56 'Frances, 60, why I'll fight on to save town's hospitals from axe.' *Suffolk Free Press*, 8 June 2006.

57 *Response to Suffolk West Primary Care Trust's Consultation.* Sudbury: Walnuttree Hospital Action Committee, 2005, para 2.4.2.

latter, day hospital attendance, will not work for patients requiring frequent or more continuous rehabilitation activity or assessment, for those who cannot easily – or at all – be transported, or for those for whom the travel is too fatiguing.)

In many ways, the great battle that would be fought over Sudbury's health services centred around patients such as the following. But how their needs will be met in other parts of the country is a pertinent, national issue too, since oversimple approaches by the NHS to rehabilitation will put such patients in jeopardy.

> *1. Man who has had a stroke.* Ernie Shaw (retired storeman, prominent fundraiser and former scoutmaster), a well known Sudbury figure, had a stroke in July. He has received treatment and rehabilitation first at West Suffolk Hospital in Bury St Edmunds and then at Walnuttree Hospital in Sudbury. If the PCT closes Walnuttree, he expressed fears that he would not receive this rehabilitation in future. He is quite right (since the PCT is refusing to allow Sudbury to have any inpatient beds in the new health centre, if it is ever built). He referred to the first class care he had received at Walnuttree and his wife to the wonderful care her husband received there.[58]
>
> In future, he would not receive rehabilitation because it could not be potentially achieved within six weeks (the PCT's rule); in any case, the nature of his rehabilitation needs could not be met at home – always assuming he had carers able to look after him (another PCT rule). Placed in a spot purchased care home bed, he would receive care but not rehabilitation. The acute hospital could not keep him for months and months, a) because it now has insufficient rehabilitation beds and therapists, b) acute hospitals are anyway not the best place to continue non-acute rehabilitation for some patients. Furthermore, an extended stay at the acute hospital would not be care 'closer to home'.
>
> *2. Man with Parkinson's.* Mr Offord-Ryder, 64 years old, suffers from Parkinson's Disease. Following two major operations and subsequent infections at West Suffolk Hospital, he needed rehabilitation. Because of a shortage of beds (in September 2005), the hospital stated that it could not offer him that rehabilitation. Instead the hospital said that he would have to go into a nursing home, where he would not have access to physiotherapy and occupational therapy, both crucial for his rehabil-

58 *Sudbury Mercury*, 2 December 2005.

itation. Fortunately, his wife (a retired nurse), to whom he was newly married, understood the implications of this and wanted him to have rehabilitation in Bury or Sudbury. She spoke out and her husband subsequently received further physiotherapy at the hospital, including passive leg movement to maintain his function until further rehabilitation might be possible.[59]

The important issue in question seemed to have been the need for passive physiotherapy for a month to avoid muscle wastage and contracture. At that point, further rehabilitation potential could be assessed. However, without that continued 'maintenance' for that month, during recovery from two operations, any rehabilitation potential would have been stymied.

In the future, there would be even less chance of such a patient getting the opportunity of rehabilitation. This is because there will be 139 beds less in the system (55 lost at West Suffolk Hospital, 68 at Walnuttree and 16 at Newmarket).

3. Woman with multiple sclerosis. A woman in her early twenties with multiple sclerosis has been in hospital following a serious kidney infection. She is now recovering. However, the enforced bedrest has 'deconditioned' her. She has lost stamina and strength. Abnormal muscle tone has caused the onset of spasticity. She is currently having to use a wheelchair. The acute hospital discharges her to a community hospital.

She is now assessed by a hospital consultant and by therapists. They identify that she could walk again but this will a) not be achieved in six weeks, and b) will require intensive daily rehabilitation and re-education. This will include manual handling by skilled staff, together with adequate space and heavy equipment (including a tilt table). Part of the rehabilitation will also include the wearing of splints that will require close, daily monitoring. After twelve weeks, she is discharged home and does not require the use of a wheelchair.

Under the PCT's future plans (with no community hospital beds), this woman will not receive this rehabilitation. First, she will be excluded under PCT's eligibility criteria, since she did not have the potential for rehabilitation within six weeks. Second, such rehabilitation could not

59 Will Grahame-Clarke, 'Nursing home no good for husband.' *East Anglian Daily Times,* 21 September 2005. And: Will Grahame-Clarke, 'Ex-nurse's victory in battle for hospital bed.' *East Anglian Daily Times,* 23 September 2005.

be carried out in her own home, because of the intensity of specialist input required. Third, nursing homes in the area neither deliver – nor could they deliver – such specialist rehabilitation. Fourth, there will be no community hospital beds.

4. Woman with a hip fracture, heart problem and arthritis. An 81-year-old elderly woman has suffered a hip fracture. She lives alone. She already has a heart problem and arthritis. She is over the acute episode and is more medically stable than she has been. So the acute hospital discharges her to the community hospital.

She is weak, has poor nutritional status, is very frail and is depressed. This continues to threaten her medical stability, and there is the potential for self-neglect if she goes home at this stage. Nevertheless, her records show that she has previously been independent minded, and that there is underlying motivation. Clear rehabilitation potential is identified. It will take some three to four months.

Under the PCT's plans, she would in future, not receive rehabilitation. First, there will be no community hospital beds. Second, placed in a care home, she would be at risk of becoming institutionalized. Third, she has no potential for rehabilitation within six weeks (the PCT's criterion). Fourth, her threatened medical instability – and current lack of motivation and potential self-neglect (through current depression) – would be a problem in her own home. Fifth, she has no 24-hour carer at home (also one of the PCT's criteria).

5. Woman recovering from stroke requires walking rehabilitation and manual handling. A woman has the potential to recover well from a stroke, in particular her ability to walk. However, she has sensory, perceptual and cognitive impairments as well. This brings with it some unpredictability in her behaviour, and a lack of insight into environmental hazards. She wants to get back home, where she lives with her daughter who works long hours.

She has been a month in the acute hospital. However, she is not making progress there because the environment is too busy to allow her to begin an effective process of reorientation. She is discharged to the community hospital, where she is assessed as having clear rehabilitation potential, which will probably take four to six months.

She is in principle motivated, but lacking in confidence. She requires substantial encouragement and reassurance. She is discharged to the community hospital. The physiotherapists have provided intensive rehabilitation involving the use of parallel bars and expert manual handling. The rehabilitation also involves a 24-hour approach to reorientation and re-education.

Under the PCT's plans, her rehabilitation would not be possible. First, she would be excluded from rehabilitation because of the six-week time limit on rehabilitation potential. Second, she could not receive it in her own home, because she lacks insight into personal safety and requires supervision – but there is no carer present all the time (two more PCT rules).

Third, the manual handling required could not be safely carried out in her own home (another PCT rule). The expert manual handling would not be possible in her own home because of lack of space; likewise the use of parallel bars. Even were there space for parallel bars, portable parallel bars would be too unstable for this type of rehabilitation.

Lastly, at home she would lack the motivation and confidence to continue a 24-hour approach. She would be alone for long periods because of her daughter's working hours. If she were placed in a care home in the Sudbury area, she would not get the rehabilitation or the 24-hour encouragement to support the rehabilitation. She would remain disabled and become institutionalised.

6. Medically unstable and confused woman. A 75-year-old woman with a heart condition, chronic obstructive airways disease (emphysema), arthritis and diabetes has suffered a severe chest infection. She lives at home with her older, frail sister.

She was admitted to the acute hospital, but is now being discharged because though still medically unstable to a degree, there is pressure on beds. She is weak and confused – a combination of the residue of the infection, drug toxicity (she is taking a cocktail of drugs) and constipation. Her mobility is threatened.

She is discharged to the community hospital, where a focused, multi-disciplinary medical, nursing and therapy input a) stabilizes her (including the drugs) and removes the confusion, b) maintains physical function during this stabilization, and c) then achieves rehabilitation such that she can return home. She is now sufficiently physically fit to remain at home and has confidence in self-managing and monitoring her drugs and chest condition (including periodic use of oxygen).

Under the PCT's plans, she will in future not be rehabilitated. She would be ruled out from rehabilitation in her own home, under both the PCT's criteria (medical instability, safety, lack of able carer) and as a matter of impracticability (confusion, intensity of input required, re-education etc). Instead, she will be discharged to a nursing home, where she will not recover, become more disabled and become institutionalized.

7. Woman with serious pressure sores. A 70-year-old woman is living at home. She has an intensive need for management of her pressure sores. This is particularly because of the large quantity of fluid discharge, her diabetes and her poor blood circulation. Distracted by the pressure sores, she is failing to manage her diabetes and there is currently a real risk because of this. The intensity of her needs means that it is impracticable for the district nurses to visit sufficiently frequently to ensure acceptable management of the sores. She is admitted to the community hospital where such management is practicable and the sores are dealt with over a period of four weeks. She then returns home.

In future, it is difficult to see how her sores would be managed. District nurses in the community currently sometimes lack the capacity to make frequent visits in complex cases – in which case patients are admitted to Walnuttree. In any case, the PCT's financial projections do not suggest that an adequate number of peripatetic staff will be available in future. And nursing homes will not generally have staff with the necessary expertise in tissue viability.

8. Man with acute arthritis. A 78-year-old man with acute arthritis (polymyalgia rheumatica) is living at home. He has suffered a fall and was admitted to an acute hospital. He now requires a short spell of intensive rehabilitation and re-education. This will enable him in future to prevent further falls and to manage the arthritis by means of drugs and a careful rest-exercise regime. He is discharged from the acute hospital to a community hospital. He receives this intensive rehabilitation and re-education (concerning self-management) over a period of five weeks. He then successfully goes home.

Under the PCT's future plans, he is discharged home from the acute hospital. He does not receive the intensive rehabilitation and re-education that is possible in hospital (it would require too many visits). Relatively isolated, he gets depressed about his inability to manage his own condition. This in turn affects his ability to respond.

He fails to manage his arthritis and falls again – and is readmitted to the acute hospital. The same pattern recurs and he becomes a 'revolving door' acute hospital patient.

9. Obese woman with arthritis, heart problem and diabetes: GP referral for continuous assessment in community hospital. A 51-year-old, 18-stone woman lives at home with her teenage son. Her mobility has become increasingly affected. She is not able to manage the stairs and has been living downstairs. However, recently she has required assistance with transfers. Social services carers have been hoisting her from bed to chair etc.

A social services occupational therapist [OT] now visits and is concerned that the woman has the potential to transfer independently or with the minimum of assistance; and that the daily hoisting is unnecessarily disabling her further. She also recommends a stairlift, because strip washing and use of a commode downstairs is clearly unacceptable.

The OT refers to the GP and requests admission to the community hospital for assessment. In her case, assessment is required over several days, including at night. When this is completed, she then remains at the community hospital for several weeks of intensive rehabilitation. This includes careful walking rehab and some manual handling, carefully managed by a senior physiotherapist.

She is then ready to return home able to transfer herself, without the use of a hoist. The stairlift is not quite ready. But she remains in the community hospital for an extra two weeks, just to ensure that she maintains her level of functioning. Placement in a local care home could have resulted in her beginning to lose function again, because of the model of care [which would not include rehabilitation].

Under the PCT's future plans, this would not happen. The two or three day assessment (including night-time observation) could self-evidently not take place in her own home, nor could the rehabilitation (because of the intensity of it, and the space and heavy equipment required). [I]t would [also] not happen in a care home, because of the impracticality of such an assessment, and because care homes in the locality do not deliver that sort of rehabilitation. She would become more and more disabled.

10. Woman with Parkinson's Disease. A 67-year-old woman with Parkinson's disease is living in her own home. Carers come in regularly. Her drugs are then changed. This alters her behaviour and also her mobility; she suddenly develops transfer and manual handling needs at home. The carers won't manually handle her, because of their lack of training and expertise and the restrictive rules to which they work. Over the next week, she is left in bed for long periods and begins to get weaker. The GP gets her admitted her to the community hospital, where a multi-disciplinary assessment concludes that the drugs should be observed by the consultant neurologist, and that the therapists should work on her mobility. After eight weeks, she successfully returns home.

In the future, she would be admitted to a care home, where she would not receive the rehabilitation, but instead become progressively more disabled.

11. Woman with dementia. A 70-year-old woman lives with her frail husband. He has noticed a deterioration in the woman's self-care abilities. There is also a question about her ability to manage continence. She has now collapsed and her GP has had her admitted for assessment to Walnuttree Hospital. She can't be assessed satisfactorily at Bury [the acute hospital 18 miles away], because her husband is a key player – since he is the only one she trusts and communicates with. He is unable to travel far. The GP is also worried about her ability to manage the drugs she is taking for her heart and arthritis, and the effect they may be having on her. She has become increasingly agitated.

The assessment is conducted over several days. It concludes that she has a degree of dementia, and that her collapse has led to weakened muscles and malnutrition. This has resulted in her sometimes not getting to the lavatory in time.

A stay of three weeks enables a review of her drugs, working out strategies to prolong her self-management abilities, building her strength up, and arranging for a social care package. This could not have been done safely at home, because of her lack of insight into her deterioration, because of her weakened state and because of her agitation.

In future, she would not be assisted to regain this degree of independence. This would not be possible because such continuous assessment of both lost and retained skills could not be done via one-off visits in her own home – nor would a care home be equipped to carry out such an assessment.

12. Patient with terminal cancer. A man with terminal cancer is discharged from the acute hospital. There are no beds in the local hospice. Looking after him at home is felt to be impractical by the Macmillan nurse, the

> man and his family – because of the level of his needs. Arranging palliative care in a care home is impractical for a number of reasons including his intense medical and nursing needs, and the unavailability of an appropriate care home near enough to his home, so that the family can easily visit. He spends his last few weeks of life at the community hospital, close to his home. Under the PCT's plans for the future, this would not be possible.[60]

Thus it was that the Walnuttree Hospital Action Committee – advised by senior clinicians within Suffolk and also in other parts of the country – put forward its detailed concerns to Suffolk West PCT. Concerns that, in the Committee's view, were never dealt with.

60 *Response to Suffolk West Primary Care Trust's Consultation.* Sudbury: Walnuttree Hospital Action Committee, 2005, para 2.4.2.

14

Thresholds and Fencing: Erecting the Social Care Barriers

The gradual, or not so gradual, shedding of responsibilities by the NHS might not matter so much if alternative, comparable statutory provision by local social services authorities (i.e. local councils) were being put in its place for these vulnerable groups of people. However, this is by no means the case.

Even when NHS responsibilities have been shed, and in principle matters fall to local councils, the retreat from meeting people's needs doesn't stop there. In a 2005 Green Paper, the government referred to disabled people and their 'independence, leaving them with control over their lives, and giving them real choice over those lives, including the services they use. Services must recognise the changing world, our changing attitudes and our ageing population.'[1] It also indicated that central government expected services to be delivered by informal and family carers, as well as by a well-trained workforce.

Attractive on its face, such a policy will inevitably be subject to the vicissitudes, messiness and rough edges of implementation. The outcome could all too easily – at least for some people, particularly older people – mean that people will be left to fend for themselves, with a minimum of support, and that the 'choice' refers to provision coming from the private sector.

1 Secretary of State for Health (2005) *Independence, Well-being and Choice: our vision for the future of social care for adults in England.* Cm 6499. London: HMSO, executive summary.

Ultimately, real choice is likely to be exercised only by those who can contribute their own money.

The bare minimum funding provided by local authorities is unlikely, ultimately, to afford people any such choice. This is not idle speculation. It is exactly what has happened in the case of 'choice' that central government introduced in 1992 for people placed in care homes by local councils. The policy started off working reasonably well; it has now descended in many areas into forcing people and their families to pay more (often called 'topping up') for basic care. In many cases this is probably unlawful if it is not the result of genuine choice on the part of the care home resident.

Furthermore, under-funding and the inability of local authorities to pick up patients from the NHS is not new. For example, during the early 1970s, the same issues were around. Shortcomings in community health services – that were meant to replace the long-stay hospital services – looked for a short time as though they would be made up for by the new personal social services departments. However, a few years of rapid growth by social services was halted in the mid-1970s, capital expenditure reduced by 50 per cent. By 1979, for people with mental health problems, only 20 per cent of the required day centre places and 33 per cent of the required residential placements had been provided. For people with learning disabilities, only 33 per cent of the required residential home places and 50 per cent of training centre places were available. In short, both NHS community health services and local authority community care 'failed to develop on anything like the scale required to provide viable substitutes for obsolete institutional services'.[2]

Now, just as then, community care could in principle represent a model of care that would be subscribed to by many people. This would be in and close to people's homes and delivered (or at least commissioned) by, depending on needs, NHS community health services, or local social services and housing authorities. However, the pattern is not a happy one. All too often, neither the NHS, nor local authorities, have the resources to deliver to the standard required, in which case, the burden falls on those vulnerable people themselves, their informal carers, voluntary organisations – and, in terms of knock-on effects, society in general.

In addition, a major part of central government's plans for social care have involved what are called 'direct payments'. Instead of arranging

2 Charles Webster (1998) *The National Health Service: a political history.* Oxford: Oxford University Press, p.126.

services directly, local councils can give the equivalent money to people deemed to be in need. Those people can then purchase their own services from the independent sector. Disappointed at the slow uptake of such payments, government is now advocating an additional avenue. This has been referred to as a system of 'individual budgets'. Basically people will be, against their assessed needs, allocated a notional budget, which they can decide how to spend – with the help of some sort of agent or adviser if necessary. It was all dressed up in the language of empowerment in a White Paper:

> individual budgets offer a radical new approach, giving greater control to the individual, opening up the range and availability of services to match needs, and stimulating the market to new demands from more powerful users of social care.[3]

As ever, in principle, it all sounds marvellous. And direct payments have been effective in giving some disabled people more control and independence. But there is another underlying, practical thrust to these policies. They are a means of running down further public sector provision of services, and of capping the amounts of money made available to individual service users. Already anecdotal evidence of this is emerging in relation to direct payments. They are increasingly it seems being given – some would say forced on – to people inappropriately, sometimes unlawfully, sometimes ineffectively (in terms of meeting people's needs) and with insufficient sums of money attached.

As more people take up, or are forced to accept, direct payments and individual budgets, so the amount paid to each person is likely to reduce, relatively speaking – because of the lack of resources in councils. This will in turn mean that a satisfactory 'market' in relevant services is unlikely to develop. Thus, without denying the potential of direct payments and individual budgets to assist some people very significantly, equally these policies are beginning to take on the shape of a Trojan Horse.

Furthermore, the appealing nature of well-funded 'care in the community' all too easily conceals other agendas, whether perpetrated by the New Labour government, or its predecessor Conservative administration. This was:

3 Secretary of State for Health (2006) *Our Health, Our Care, Our Say*, Cm 6737. London: Stationery Office, para 4.30.

> both to eliminate almost entirely the role of the state in the provision of services for older people and to reduce to a minimum its responsibility for funding them. The aim was to stimulate an active market in the provision of care services...and to transfer the costs of funding care in old age to individuals and their families.[4]

Since the implementation of mainstream community care in 1993, a number of traditional health tasks have shifted over to social care. For instance, the early days were characterised by uncertainty and arguments over whether baths should be regarded as health or social care. The trend was to shift them over to social care. But unable to cope with the implications of people having access to baths or showers, social services authorities have increasingly attempted to reduce their responsibilities.

Local councils now argue all too often, for example, that unless a person is doubly incontinent or terminally ill, then they simply do not need access to a bath or a shower in their own home. Although, in principle, disabled people have a right to access a bath or shower under housing legislation (Housing Grants, Construction and Regeneration Act 1996), nevertheless in practice this right, too, is being undermined because of financial pressures and misunderstanding about the legislation. The 'great unwashed public' is not now an idle term in the context of health and welfare provision.

Placing care on the wrong side of the fence

Simple and wholesale dumping of services and patients onto local councils by the NHS does not work for a number of reasons.

First, local social services authorities have neither the legal remit nor the expertise nor the resources to deliver health care. This may be all important. For instance, people who fail to receive expert health-care rehabilitation at the right time – in the 'window' within which rehabilitation is possible – may remain permanently more disabled than they otherwise would have been. In which case, now requiring care they truly will have become the responsibility of social services, the need for which could have been avoided.

Second, local social services authorities are themselves in serious financial difficulty. They are not in a position simply to mop up the pieces and patients discarded by the NHS. The Association of Directors of Social Services (ADSS) and Local Government Association reported in March

4 Allyson Pollock (2005) *NHS plc: the privatisation of our health care.* London: Verso, p.173.

2006 a 'gaping £1.76 billion black hole in funding for social services'. One of the key reasons given was an ageing population, together with increased life expectancy for younger adults with severe physical and learning disabilities.[5]

In early 2006, the King's Fund published a major report on social care for older people and was emphatic in its finding a) of significant shortfalls in provision of social care, and b) of a need for very much greater investment. It reported also significant unmet needs among older people, which can lead to greater (and more expensive) problems developing; and that the 'proportion of older people receiving home care in England is low by international standards'.[6]

By 2006, all over the country, it was reported that local councils were raising their 'thresholds' of eligibility. Put simply, this means that they were making stricter their test as to who can and cannot receive services. Under government guidance – optimistically but misleadingly named 'fair access to care' – people's needs should be assessed as critical, substantial, moderate or low. Each local authority then sets a threshold or bar, above which needs will be met, below which they will not. For instance, some councils set it below critical and thus will meet only critical needs; others below substantial and will meet both substantial and critical, but not low or moderate, needs. And so on. However, by late 2005 and 2006, the trend was clearly upward.[7]

When the bar is raised, local authorities can lawfully go back to reassess existing users of services and reduce or remove them – even if a person's needs or situation generally have not changed or ameliorated. New service users won't get a look in at all, unless their needs are very high. Local councils were giving a clear message: unwanted by the NHS, you would not be welcomed with open arms by local authorities either. For instance, a correspondent to *The Times* wrote in to describe how his 90-year-old mother had just been reviewed and told within hours that she would lose her entire care package (half-hour daily carer's call and weekly shopping and cleaning), even though she was too frail to use the vacuum cleaner, dared not go out in icy weather, and stood in pain at the sink to wash up. To pay for it privately, she would have to dig deep into her war widow's pension.[8]

5 *Social Services Finance 2005/06: a survey of local authorities.* London: Local Government Association.

6 Derek Wanless (2006) *Securing Good Care for Older People.* London: King's Fund, Summary.

7 *The State of Social Care in England 2004–05: a summary.* London: Commission for Social Care Inspection, 2005, p.10.

8 Michael Patterson, 'Pensions and provision for the elderly.' Letter. *The Times,* 21 March 2006.

Some councils want the best of all worlds, politically and financially. Not prepared to raise the bar because of the political unattractiveness of doing so, they nevertheless attempt to cut people's services anyway. Generally speaking, this approach is likely to lead local authorities into unlawful paths, and many simply hope they will not be caught out.

Third, even within these strict criteria of eligibility, local authorities blithely discriminate against particular groups of service users. For instance, in a significant number of local authorities, rules about the quantity and quality of services available change when people reach their 65th birthday. In some councils, an older person will even see their services reduced automatically on reaching that birthday, even though their needs have in no way changed. In such councils, one nevertheless still finds lip service paid to standard one of the government's National Service Framework for older people – the standard that says there should not be age discrimination.[9]

By 2005, local authority social services overspends (which even in 2001 were £1 billion, almost 9.7 per cent of total social services expenditure) were disproportionately located in children's and learning disability services – not in older people's services. But older people constituted 62 per cent of social service clients. In 2002–3, expenditure on younger adults with learning disabilities rose by 43 per cent, but on older people only 22 per cent. And, in 2004–5, it was projected that overspending was considerably higher on younger adults with learning disabilities (63 per cent), or physical or sensory disabilities (47 per cent) compared with 33 per cent on older people. But it was spending on older people that local authorities were planning most to restrict.[10]

Fourth, these financial pressures on local authorities, together with the exposure of social care to private sector provision (commissioned by local authorities) and the marketplace, has resulted sometimes in the treatment of vulnerable people as movable and removable commodities. This has been illustrated over a number of years by the closure of care homes and forced moves for people who had believed they had a home for life. A veritable string of legal cases has been heard. Although one of the first major ones, involving an NHS unit, was a notable victory for the resident concerned,[11] the courts have by and large failed to protect vulnerable residents from being forced to move from the homes where they have been placed by

9 *National Service Framework for Older People.* London: Department of Health, 2001.

10 *What Price Care in Old Age?* Social Policy on Ageing Information Network (SPAIN), 2005.

11 *R v North and East Devon Health Authority, ex parte Coughlan* (1999) 2 CCLR 285, Court of Appeal.

local councils. Occasionally, though, the courts have come to the rescue and almost savagely exposed the lack of transparency and integrity with which people are sometimes treated by local councils.[12] But such cases are few.

So, stories surface such as the following, brought about by the lack of resources against which local authorities struggle. A couple had not spent a night apart since the Second World War and had been married for 69 years. After one of them had suffered a stroke she was assessed by the council as needing a care home place. Initially, her husband was told he could move in with her and share a double room. Then social services explained that he did not meet the criteria, and he would have to have a care package in his own home instead. For their remaining years, they would thus be separated.[13]

These are not isolated cases. In 2002, an elderly couple in Oxfordshire were told it was too expensive for them to live together in the same nursing home. They were placed 20 miles apart. They had been married for more than 60 years. A couple in Portsmouth, married for 61 years were placed in homes five miles apart because of their different needs. The council promised that an adapted taxi would enable them to see each other five days a week. However, this arrangement broke down when the council needed to save money. When one of them died, the other had not seen his wife for four days.

One in ten people in care homes is still married, often in marriages of 50 years. Adverse publicity in such cases, especially in the national press, often seems to result in councils backing down. But, as Help the Aged has stated, in other (less trumpeted) cases, financial considerations override the rights of older couples to stay together.[14]

Similarly, in July 2006, Wiltshire had denied that there was a bonfire of services and an abandonment of social work values – in its bid to save millions from its social care budget.[15] Yet by August, it was reported that the Council was attempting to place a woman with multiple sclerosis in a care home, rather than continue to provide her with services in her own home – where she had been cared for by her husband for 20 years of their 41-year marriage. The cost of supporting her at home was more expensive than a

12 *R(Goldsmith) v Wandsworth London Borough Council* [2004] EWCA Civ 1170, Court of Appeal.

13 Separated by social services: the loving couple of 69 years.' *Daily Express,* 11 February 2006.

14 Sarah Womack, 'Care home separations "may breach human rights".' *Daily Telegraph,* 4 February 2006.

15 Ian Davey, 'No bonfire in Wiltshire'. Letter. *Community Care,* 27 July – 2 August 2006.

nursing home. So the Council was plumping for the cheaper alternative and proposing to separate the couple.[16]

Striking hard at social care across Suffolk

Not to be outdone by the NHS in cutting services to older people and other vulnerable groups, Suffolk County Council found itself having to move down the same route. By August 2005, it had announced it would be cutting £2.2 million from its adult social care budget. This resulted in a round of reviews of vulnerable service users, including, for instance, withdrawing care from people with multiple sclerosis.

This was barely two months after the Council had assured the people of Suffolk that it would always put people's needs first and implied that people would only lose services if their circumstances had changed. Yet the reported instance – in which a 58-year-old multiple sclerosis sufferer with a dislocated hip lost her domestic assistance – did not involve a change of circumstance. As the Council itself stated, it had reviewed her and decided she did not qualify for help under the new rules it was imposing. This was yet one more example of statutory bodies – whether the NHS or the Council – issuing anodyne statements that say one thing, but then proceeding to do quite another.[17]

The council claimed it could do this because the law meant that by and large it only had to provide help to people who needed personal care. This was not a correct statement of the law and of the national 'fair access to care' criteria.[18] When challenged, the Director of Adult Care accepted this, without explaining why the council had maintained otherwise. However, his restatement of the council's policy was also dubious. He maintained that only exceptionally would people be entitled to help other than personal care.[19] It is by no means clear that this is a correct statement of the law either, as a glance at the fair access to care criteria and the Chronically Sick and Disabled Persons Act 1970 would show. To onlookers, there seemed a real

16 'Cherie Booth backs Wiltshire couple.' *Community Care*, 17–23 August 2006, p.6.

17 David Green, 'Social services cancel help for MS suffer.' *East Anglian Daily Times*, 28 October 2006. And: County council reassures social care service users. Press release, 23 August, 2005. Ipswich: Suffolk County Council.

18 Michael Mandelstam, 'Caution is needed on taking services away.' Letter. *East Anglian Daily Times*, 3 November 2005.

19 Graham Gatehouse, 'We're providing care in accordance with law.' Letter. *East Anglian Daily Times*, 9 November 2005.

danger that the severe cuts proposed by the NHS in Suffolk, coupled with the council's increasing financial problems, would mean:

> that older and disabled people are at real risk of being caught in a cost-saving pincer movement involving both the NHS and social services.[20]

By January 2006, it became clear that much greater cuts would have to be made, perhaps up to £15 million from the adult social care budget, since £24 million had to be saved by the council overall.[21] In March 2006, this was confirmed.[22] Predictably, the Labour opposition in the council would refer to the cuts as 'not a budget for the future – it is the start of a closing down sale'.[23]

The council was in some disarray, a state of affairs that would appear to be exploited by the Suffolk West PCT. Despite the PCT deciding to re-categorise a whole swathe of health care for older people as 'social care', the council's social services department and relevant 'portfolio holder' (i.e. the lead councillor) assured everybody at one point that there would be no overall knock-on effect on the council. On any view, this was a highly questionable claim to make, especially given the cutbacks the council was making.[24]

Questionable, because the lack of rehabilitation that would almost certainly result for some patients under the new plans would mean that they would end up with greater disabilities and require council funding for care home places or services in their own home.[25] In addition, those people who could appropriately receive health-care rehabilitation in their own homes rather in hospital would have a range of other needs, some of which would fall to social services to fund.[26] The councillor who had issued this naive statement seemed to have been badly advised. In displaying such timidity, the social services department arguably appeared to be in denial about

20 Michael Mandelstam, 'Caution is needed on taking services away.' Letter. *East Anglian Daily Times*, 3 November 2005.

21 Graham Dines, 'Council set for £24m cuts.' *East Anglian Daily Times*, 6 January 2006.

22 Benedict O'Connor, 'Disabled learners set to be hit by cash cuts.' *East Anglian Daily Times*, 7 February 2006.

23 Graham Dines, 'Outrage at cutbacks in social care budget.' *East Anglian Daily Times*, 22 February 2006.

24 'County Council Reassures Social Care Service Users.' Press release, 23 August 2005. Ipswich: Suffolk County Council.

25 Nicki Harvey, '100s expected no cuts protest march.' *Suffolk Free Press*, 8 September 2005.

26 Helen Tucker and Peter Morgan (2005) *Modernising Healthcare in West Suffolk: response. Prepared by HTA on behalf of Walnuttree Hospital Action Committee (WHAC).* Helen Tucker Associates.

people's needs, hoping they would simply go away. Correspondence in the regional newspapers put it this way:

> we need plain speaking. There is genuine fear in the community… Bland, ritual reassurance – with no foundation and from those who should know better – merely exacerbates rather than assuages that fear…why is social services not admitting straightforwardly to the cuts it is itself apparently implementing? Lastly, amidst the unforgivable lack of transparency, there is one message emerging loud and clear from both the NHS and social services. In the Suffolk of the future you will be old, sick or disabled at your peril.[27]

There were seemingly discordant voices within the council. Two weeks later, the council leader, Jeremy Pembroke, referred to his enormous concern over the impact on patient care and to the possible total collapse of local health services.[28]

Indeed, even with the community hospital beds still in existence, the local council was already struggling to cope. For instance, in January 2006, it admitted that it could not provide a service for a Walnuttree Hospital patient ready to return home, because it did not have the 'capacity' to meet his needs and restore the service he had previously received before his hospital admission.[29]

Vanishing in the morning mist: social care in Suffolk

During 2006, the financial crisis affecting Suffolk County Council became ever more pronounced, as did its intention to make cutbacks that would have a detrimental effect on vulnerable people. The sort of cutbacks being implementing were by no means peculiar to Suffolk. So the following is not unrepresentative of the way in which councils may act. One day, they may be sanctimonious and scathing about cuts made by the NHS; the next they proceed down the same ignominious route. It is not an edifying picture.

In June 2006, the council announced that it would be reducing and withdrawing day services, and instead encouraging people to take up more social security benefits to which they might be entitled. They could then, as

27 Michael Mandelstam, 'Clear explanation needed on cuts to social services.' Letter. *East Anglian Daily Times*, 16 November 2005.

28 *County Warns of Fears of a Total Collapse of Local Health Services.* Press release, 9 September 2005. Ipswich: Suffolk County Council.

29 Paul Holland, 'Trapped.' *Suffolk Free Press*, 26 January 2006.

the Director of Social Care put it, 'make their own choices because it will give them control over their personal budgeting'. This was part of a general cost saving strategy that involved not filling vacancies, refusing to pay inflation increases to companies and voluntary organisations providing care on the council's behalf – and reviewing the needs of all those currently receiving day care packages.[30]

The council soon followed up with more detail, announcing a wide-ranging review of day services for older people. The overall aim appeared to be to consider possible closure of the 14 day centres operated directly by the Council. Instead people might to go to voluntary and community based centres and activities.[31] The idea lurking behind such plans – that vulnerable people can, en masse, somehow wander around general community facilities – is disturbing. It appears to betray a crude understanding of the complexity and range of people's physical, mental and psychological needs and abilities.

But the Council was not only seemingly desperate to close buildings. It wished also to reduce its staff numbers as well. It had already contracted out most of its personal care services to the private sector. However, it had retained 'in-house' council staff to provide a more specialist service called Home First. This was to provide 12 weeks of support to people, particularly when they had been discharged from hospital.

It was not just a question of providing care, but also to assist people with the process of rehabilitation and reorientation – and thus the regaining of independence. Such a service was of increasing importance, given the determination of the PCTs in Suffolk to shed community hospital beds wholesale. The service was described by the Council as being about 'putting people back on their feet'. The press release – announcing the cutting back of the service – referred to it misleadingly as an assessment service only, and that 12 weeks was not necessary for assessment. As with the NHS, this smacked of a lack of transparency and lack of courage in spelling out the implications of what was afoot.[31]

Yet within a fortnight of the Council deciding that it would be cutting its home care service, it was reported that it did not have enough carers. It transpired that for a month, at least four people in Hadleigh had been left without care. One of them, an 88-year-old man was now being looked after by his registered blind daughter. She had had to cut short her holiday to

30 Graham Dines, 'Fears over new "DIY" day care.' *East Anglian Daily Times*, 14 June 2006.

31 'Council to review provision of adult care.' Press release. Ipswich: Suffolk County Council, 8 August 2006.

come home to look after him. When she rang social services, she explained that 'they just keep saying they have not got enough carers'. The lead councillor for adult social care stated that he sympathised and hoped to find replacement carers 'very soon'.[32]

The threat to people's rehabilitation and independence was clear. But the withdrawal of day services, too, has many ramifications, for both users of those services and their carers. The latter frequently rely on these services to gain crucial respite from their unremitting, daily caring role. One correspondent to the newspapers sensibly questioned whether the county councillors who had made the decision to implement cuts had the 'slightest idea of the stress created for vulnerable people in trying to make new friends' – when their faculties were impaired by age and they had physical and mental problems in addition.[33]

Another writer pointed out that the closure of such services would be catastrophic for some carers. Already sacrificing their own freedoms in order to provide extensive care, they were 'dependent on day services and respite care to prevent them from becoming totally socially excluded'. Such a reduction in day services would lead to carers being unable to cope, and increased care home placement costs for the council.[34] In the case of people with learning disabilities, for instance, such placements can reach far in excess of £100,000 a year.

Thus, a carer spoke out when her husband's hours of attendance at a day centre were halved, and he would now be charged for the transport that took him there. Her husband had Alzheimer's Disease. The effect of this would be on her own health. She had had a heart attack two years before, worn out from caring for her husband – and had to be alert during the night for her husband. Her ability to visit and spend time with her daughter (who was ill with breast cancer) would also be affected. And the annual charge of the transport would amount to £572 for somebody already living on a 'pittance'. In respect of transport to day services, the Council had announced that it was asking 'everyone who needs care to make their own arrangements, or pay for transport…'.[35]

Given that transport is explicitly listed as a service under s.2 of the Chronically Sick and Disabled Persons Act 1970, the council would have to

32 Sarah Gillett, 'Carers crisis hits elderly'. *East Anglian Daily Times*, 19 August 2006.

33 T. Last, 'Money needed for service provision.' Letter. *East Anglian Daily Times*, 29 July 2006.'

34 Duncan Greenwood, 'Care cuts would be devastating.' Letter. *East Anglian Daily Times*, 3 July 2006.

35 'A big mess, says wife of Alzheimer's patient.' *East Anglian Daily Times*, 14 August 2006.

be careful of how it implemented these changes. Similarly, it would have to be careful not to infringe legally the charging rules for such services, designed to protect service users from paying what they cannot reasonably afford. Many other councils, at least, all too often rush into such change and find themselves on the wrong side of the law.

Community resource units (CRUs), providing respite for disabled people – particularly those with learning disabilities – were also under threat. The explanation from Suffolk County Council came in the form of 'care in the community' and more independent living. But, as the parents of adults with severe learning disabilities objected, some people precisely need the structured environment. As one mother explained about her daughter who was:

> 34 years old and has a severe learning disability with a mental age of about two-and-a-half years. She also suffers from autism and other mental health problems. This makes it difficult for her to accept changes in her life, be it carers or surroundings. Therefore a structured service with carers she trusts is a most essential part of her life.[36]

It went on. For instance, the council would come to admit that Suffolk was in a state of crisis also concerning its ability to meet the needs of people with severe dementia. Shortage of beds and trained staff were at the root. As the wife of one dementia sufferer put it:

> All I want is for my husband to be cared for according to his needs and mine. I want him placed once and for all in a nursing home that is suitable for him, so that he isn't constantly shunted from one place to another, that is accessible to me, and somewhere he can end his days in peace and in contact with his family.[37]

Yet this was a time when the NHS, too, was reducing bed numbers drastically – acute beds, and beds used for rehabilitation, recuperation, respite and palliative care. They all were under threat.

36 Dave Gooderham, 'Carer families fear losing centre lifeline.' *East Anglian Daily Times,* 17th July 2006.

37 Laurence Cawley, 'Dementia care hit by "crisis".' *East Anglian Daily Times,* 17 July 2006.

15

The Uprooting of Real Care

Somewhere, amid the welter of targets, indicators, new technology and hard processing of patients on conveyor belts (better and officially known as 'care pathways'), what some would call old-fashioned 'real care' appears to have slipped from sight. This might appear not to matter; after all, if it is old it must be bad. The problem is that so-called 'old-fashioned' real care actually works because it recognises people as individuals, rather than business units or financial bundles.

This is not a lament by the sentimental. In May 2006, the Healthcare Commission, Audit Commission and Commission for Social Care Inspection published a disturbing report, entitled optimistically, *Living Well in Later Life*. Among its findings was evidence of ageism towards older people across all services. This included 'patronising and thoughtless treatment from staff', failure to take needs and aspirations of older people seriously, lack of dignity, lack of respect, and poor standards of care on general hospital wards. The report also found people being repeatedly moved between wards for non-clinical reasons, being cared for in mixed-sex bays or wards, having meals taken away from them before they could eat them due to a lack of assistance – and suffering abuse and neglect. In addition, older people were concerned about access to health in rural areas. And so on.[1]

In July 2006, the Healthcare Commission published a report about events at Stoke Mandeville Hospital that spelt out, albeit in extreme form,

1 *Living Well in Later Life*. London: Healthcare Commission, Audit Commission and Commission for Social Care Inspection, 2006, Summary report.

the logical consequences of putting targets – clinical and financial – before patient care. The Commission referred to events at the hospital as an 'awful tragedy'. In summary, the hospital had suffered two outbreaks of the infection, *Clostridium difficile.*

The first outbreak resulted in some 174 infected patients and 19 deaths. The hospital's infection control team had already expressed concerns that patients were not being adequately isolated. Following the infection, the team made further recommendations. The Board of the Buckinghamshire Hospitals NHS Trust, however, did not act on these. A second outbreak then occurred, resulting in 160 new cases and 19 further deaths. Even then, senior managers at the Trust would not implement the recommendations of the infection control team. It was only after news of the outbreak reached the Department of Health and then received national publicity that the Board acted. These bare facts are highly disturbing. The detailed findings of the Commission are even more so. The following gives a flavour. They reveal the type of shortcut in patient care that is all too common – and should be unacceptable, whether or not an outbreak of infection occurs.

The isolation of patients was not always possible because side rooms that could have been used were ring-fenced to ensure shorter waiting times for non-emergency patients having surgery:

> Managers told the infection control team that the team could not make decisions to isolate patients that led to a breach of the A&E target.

The Trust's determination to meet the government's four-hour target for A&E waits led it to place infected patients with diarrhoea on open wards. The shortage of nurses, due to financial restraints imposed by the Trust, contributed to the spread of infection because they were too rushed to wash their hands, consistently to wear aprons and gloves, to empty commodes promptly and to clean mattresses and equipment properly. This was made worse by the obstruction of access to wash basins by uncollected linen and waste bags. Faeces on bed rails, dirty areas under beds, the same mop used in side wards and the main ward, urine and mop water emptied down a sink on the ward, and urine spillages not cleaned up promptly or properly. Mould was found in shower rooms and cobwebs on ceilings; there were dirty shower seats and hairs in baths. A glove covered in faeces was hanging out of a waste bin on one ward.

The greater the movement of patients between wards, the greater risk of transmission of infection. The proportion of patients moved because of pressure on capacity (as opposed to clinical reasons) during a five-month period in 2005 was around 45 per cent. In one three-month period, 290 patients were moved twice and 112 patients three times. One patient had been moved five times in nine days.

> The review we undertook of case notes of 20 patients with *C. difficile* confirmed that many were moved several times, often at night, and some of the moves did not appear appropriate for the condition of the patient.

Quite apart from infection, such moves are quite simply distressing and detrimental to patients and family alike, especially when it occurs at night. Families were often not informed. Patients were sometimes moved to wards where staff members were not knowledgeable about their condition. Doctors might be unable to find their patients. Clinical notes did not always accompany patients to the new ward.

Low staffing levels had a direct adverse effect. Patients could no longer wait to go the toilet and so had 'accidents' (which are just too awful: morale sapping and acutely embarrassing) because there were no staff members to help. Then, they had to wait still further to have their now soiled sheets changed. Nurses could not complete proper care plans. Dieticians complained that the nursing shortage meant food supplements were not given. Therapists were not given the information they needed to know about patients.[2]

One could add to this also the 'old-fashioned' nursing that would never countenance the development of pressure sores (even without the modern 'high-tech' pressure care paraphernalia). And, likewise, the sensitive and perceptive care that includes taking time to give people baths and hair washes. And the extra bit of assistance – such as reminders, the right environment, a modicum of physical assistance – which enables a person to get to the lavatory instead of too readily being labelled 'incontinent'.

One great irony of the government's attempt to close down the many so-called 'old-fashioned' community hospitals around the country is that it is there, more than anywhere else, that good basic care, respectful of the individual, is likely to be found. One reason for this is the calmer, less pressurised approach to care compared to acute hospitals. Another is often a stable experienced group of staff attuned to humane care, rehabilitation and recuperation. A third is that the staff members are mostly local and thus identify with

2 *Investigation into outbreaks of* Clostridium difficile *at Stoke Mandeville Hospital, Buckinghamshire Hospitals NHS Trust.* London: Healthcare Commission, 2006.

(and indeed may know or know of) patients and their families. The continued undermining and closure of these hospitals renders risible the statements of ministers, such as the new care services minister Ivan Lewis's statement that dignity was not a 'side show' but absolutely 'integral' and 'non-negotiable'.[3]

A survey in 2006 revealed that nearly 46 per cent of nurses felt they had no time to provide comfort to terminally older patients – whereas 60 per cent felt that younger dying patients received better care. As one nurse put it:

> long gone are the days when a nurse would be seen sitting holding the hand of a dying patient and talking to them.[4]

The nurse who runs an acute medical unit at a hospital wrote under a pseudonym about the implications of the constant rush to free up beds and to meet targets:

> Sadly, I have found myself hastening relatives' goodbyes to a deceased loved one as I know that there are seriously ill people waiting to occupy the bedspace. And sometimes I have hissed 'fuck right off' to a bed manager when asked how long it will take me to wipe the excrement and blood from a dead body. The fundamentals of nursing are to ensure that patients are pain-free, clean, comfortable, well-fed, nourished, valued and respected as human beings. We believe passionately in all these things, but they sit at odds with the current belief that this can be all done at superhuman speed.[5]

On 22 February 2006, the National Institute for Clinical Evidence issued guidelines to help tackle the problem of malnutrition in people when they are in the care of the NHS.[6] The Healthcare Commission raised the issue again a mere two months later, its survey of 80,000 patients finding that 18 per cent of patients said they did not receive the assistance they needed to enable them to eat.[7]

And it was all nothing new. The *NHS Plan* in 2000 had referred to the importance of having 'ward housekeepers' to ensure not only the quality, presentation and quantity of meals, but also that 'patients, particularly

3 John Pring, 'New care minister promises "bottom up" approach.' *Disability Now*, August 2006.

4 'No time for dying patients.' News item. *Nursing Times*, 11 April 2006.

5 Karen Moffat (a pseudonym), 'Nurses can't walk away.' *Guardian*, 28 April 2006.

6 'New NICE Guideline Will Help Tackle the Problem of Malnutrition in the NHS.' Press release, 21 February 2006. London: National Institute for Clinical Excellence.

7 *Survey of Patients 2005: services for inpatients*. Briefing note. London: Healthcare Commission, 2006.

elderly people, are able to eat the meals on offer'.[8] But by 2006, rather more progress had been made on the next item listed in the *NHS Plan* – involving bedside televisions and telephones at great expense to patients (as identified by Patient and Public Involvement Forums across England) – than on helping patients stay alive and recover through good nutrition.[9] Ofcom has expressed concern about the level of charges for incoming calls to patients – as has the House of Commons Health Committee, referring to the 'anger and distress' at the cost of such calls, which rise to 49 pence per minute. Even more expense is incurred by having to listen to a recorded message that cannot be skipped.[10]

In Suffolk, the Commission for Health Improvement had reported in 2002 about care at the acute hospital in Bury St Edmunds and the complaints:

> about the treatment of older patients on the wards and the lack of basic nursing care available to them. Concerns were raised about the lack of attention to patients' basic needs in terms of accessing the toilets and help with eating and drinking.[11]

It is all so basic. Perversely, given the hostility shown by some PCTs toward community hospitals, it is the latter that remain outposts of 'real care'. Regular testimony to this appears in local newspapers up and down the country, including Sudbury in West Suffolk:

> My aunt…was moved from West Suffolk Hospital [the acute hospital] to Walnuttree where she feels much calmer, has a better attitude to her food, and acknowledges really caring attention from the staff.[12]

In November 2005, a current hospital patient spoke out from the Walnuttree Hospital, where he was now recuperating, having been discharged from the acute hospital in Bury St Edmunds:

> If I was at West Suffolk I would have been stranded in Bury but here my wife comes to see me every day. The solution for health services in

8 Secretary of State for Health (2000) *The NHS Plan: a plan for investment, a plan for reform.* Cm 4818-1. London: HMSO, para 4.17.

9 *Patients Say: 'Reverse the Charges!'* Birmingham: Commission for Public and Patient Involvement Forums, 2006.

10 House of Commons Health Committee (2006) *NHS Charges.* HC 815-I. London: Stationery Office, para 93. And: *Ofcom own-initiative investigation into the price of making telephone calls to hospital patients.* London: Ofcom.

11 *West Suffolk Hospitals NHS Trust.* London: Commission for Health Improvement, 2002.

12 Letter. *Suffolk Free Press,* 18 November 2004.

> Sudbury is to keep this hospital open. We would be lost without it. The treatment I have received here has been first class and there is nowhere else to go.[13]

A former porter straightforwardly would remind Sudbury of the classic virtues of the Walnuttree and St Leonard's Hospitals: 'the nursing, the caring and the cleanliness is of the highest standard… It has never faltered'.[14] An experienced care worker at the Walnuttree also stated clearly that the convenience and community atmosphere at the hospital was crucial for patients' recovery, since they did not feel isolated as they would at home or on the acute hospital wards:

> Care at home is not enough for many of our elderly patients. Often it is just half-an-hour a day of human contact if they don't have family. Without the right care they will be back in hospital again, which will cost even more.[15]

Similarly, a family wrote in about their mother who had suffered a series of mini strokes, been admitted to the acute West Suffolk Hospital, and now been discharged to Walnuttree when her acute bed was required by somebody else:

> What a transformation in care there was once she was at Walnuttree. It became obvious that she was in the best possible place she could be. The nursing staff were caring, they made time to talk to the patients and relatives. They are giving the patients some dignity in their lives by simple acts such as combing their hair, manicuring fingernails and most of all, smiling and being happy and cheerful in their work. We cannot thank those staff enough… It is going to be a very, very sad day for Sudbury if we lose such a wonderful, caring hospital.[16]

Too easily, these basic care issues are dismissed. They should not be. The following writer referred to the care her mother had received at the Bartlet Hospital in Felixstowe, East Suffolk:

> We sat on the balcony with her, which has wonderful views of the gardens and sea. Also my mother took walks in the garden, stopping to

13 'Nowhere else to go.' *East Anglian Daily Times*, 23 November 2005.

14 Ex-porter. Letter. *Suffolk Free Press*, 13 October 2005.

15 Will Grahame-Clark, 'Fear over home plan for care of patients.' *East Anglian Daily Times*, 6 December 2005.

16 Schwenk family, 'Our caring local hospital.' Letter. *Suffolk Free Press*, 12 January 2006.

> sit in the shelter surrounded at the time by her favourite plant, Lavender. Patients who are gravely ill have their spirits lifted in such an environment. Together with the dedicated care and attention, the Bartlet is a much-needed bridge between hospital and home...is a shining example of aftercare that must not be sacrificed. More luxury flats in Felixstowe, bought by outsiders who sold properties in London are not what are needed.[17]

Local residents speak with sobering common sense. Effective care does not always have to be 'high tech' and delivered at breakneck speed:

> When I was a patient in the Bartlet Hospital, the ward I was in had a good view of the sea. This view had a very soothing effect on me, helped me get better and made me relax and remain calm during my treatment.[18]

Likewise, with her feet on the ground, a local resident at a public meeting responded to Suffolk East PCT's claim that 'old-fashioned services are not the most efficient way of giving best care to patients', when defending the closure of Hartismere Hospital. Her point was simple:

> Old-fashioned care is better than no care at all.[19]

People know. Understanding the loss of community hospital beds, and the vague, unrealistic promises of community health care instead, one marcher through the streets of Newmarket said perceptively and with no hint of exaggeration:

> People will just go home and die. There aren't enough people in intermediate care to take care of them. Those beds in the hospital are full all of the time and they are needed.[20]

The community hospitals generally exercise such an influence because they provide basic good care, that is intuitively recognised by patients, but remains unmeasured and unwanted by NHS managers. For instance, when an 86-year-old states of Hartismere Hospital in Eye that it is a 'lovely place where people are well looked after', and that he would rather 'lie beside the

17 E.A. Bamforth, 'Hospital is a shining example of healthcare.' Letter. *East Anglian Daily Times*, 28 September 2005.

18 A. Yates, 'Hospital closure plan doesn't make sense.' Letter. *East Anglian Daily Times*, 24 November 2005.

19 David Green, 'Will closures be bad for patients?' *East Anglian Daily Times*, 7 October 2005.

20 Will Grahame-Clark, 'Hundreds march to stop bed cuts.' *East Anglian Daily Times*, 31 October 2005.

road' than go back to the acute hospital at Ipswich, this is eloquent testimony.[21] The following speaks volumes, from the East of Yorkshire:

> One visit to Hornsea cottage hospital summed up for me the reason why people love their local hospital. I asked an elderly gentleman what it was like being in Hornsea. He said: 'What's it like? I was eight weeks in Hull Royal [the acute hospital]. When I woke up here I thought I was in bloody heaven.[22]

A local resident who had undergone a major operation for cancer understood the key role of recuperation and convalescence in a community hospital. He had been discharged early from the acute hospital, for his wife to care for his wound at home, although it was infected with MRSA. She could not cope. Fortunately he was found a bed at the Bartlet Hospital, where the:

> relaxed atmosphere quickly restored me to good health and I was able to return home without the worry that my wife would not be able to cope with the situation.[23]

A senior sister, Terena Haukswell, retiring from Sudbury's Walnuttree Hospital after 34 years of service, explained simply:

> We need beds in the town for people to come to before they go home. That bit of breathing space in between leaving West Suffolk Hospital [the acute hospital] and going home will improve their confidence and prepare them for going home.

She said that although she had always wanted to be a nurse, if she had her time over, she would now not become one.[24]

But all this seems to cut little ice with NHS decision-makers. In any case, there are wider issues. The homely community hospitals, nestling in the heart of towns, looking over water meadows, or fronting the sea, are being sold off for housing. It is asset stripping and not in the interests of the patients. For instance, the Walnuttree Hospital sits in the heart of Sudbury, with water meadows on one side, an old mill hotel on another, the great church of St Gregory's on a third. An environment appropriate for a caring

21 David Green, 'War hero eager to help save hospital.' *East Anglian Daily Times*, 6 September 2006.

22 Graham Stuart, MP. *Hansard*, Westminster Hall, 2 November 2005, column 259WH.

23 A. Crawford, 'Convalescence such a key part of health care.' Letter. *East Anglian Daily Times*, 1 May 2006.

24 Nicki Harvey, 'Ward sister's parting shot.' *Suffolk Free Press*, 18 May 2006.

institution, in the heart of its community. Perhaps, as observed by a local historian, it is all too good for patients, whose recovery is assisted by such a setting:

> Today the [Walnuttree] hospital has a reputation second to none with regard to the treatment of its patients... At the time of writing there are plans for a new hospital at Chilton which will replace Walnuttree. Ironically it will probably release land for development with stunning views over the Common Lands which only the rich will be able to afford.[25]

In contrast, the PCT's business plan identified that redevelopment of the hospital would be no more expensive than building a new one on a greenfield site out of town. But redevelopment was never considered, presumably because of the wish to make a killing on the local property market, any proceeds of which would not benefit Sudbury but the NHS generally. Instead, the replacement health centre was to be built out of town (creating traffic, access and transport problems), across fast roads – as local residents are only too aware.[26]

Furthermore, it became clear that on the same site would be three industrial units. The district council unaccountably passed the planning permission required without allowing any amendments, such as to prohibit 24-hour working and to prevent the health centre being used as a rat run for the industrial units. The industrial development would cover more than 30,000 square metres. Even the PCT objected that the developer (Prolog) was 'ignoring the concerns of everyone and making little effort of concessions at all'. Patient care would suffer.[27]

In sum, Suffolk West PCT announced in August 2005 that West Suffolk was providing old-fashioned, ineffective care. Nothing could have been further from the truth. If Suffolk was indeed lagging behind, it was because its community hospitals still tried to provide the human side of real care, rehabilitation, recuperation and sometimes palliative care. It was also because it had not yet sold off its valued local hospitals for 'golf courses, luxury homes and supermarkets', the fate that had already befallen so many NHS hospitals.[28] It seems that patients now come second best to business, property developers, industry and money.

25 Barry Wall (2004) *Sudbury: history and guide.* Stroud: Tempus, p.104.

26 Peter Blackwell, 'What can we expect? Cuts.' Letter. *Suffolk Free Press,* 8 December 2005.

27 Paul Holland, 'Multi-million plans pave way for jobs.' *Suffolk Free Press,* 4 May 2006.

28 Allyson Pollock (2005) *NHS plc: the privatisation of our health care.* London: Verso, p.31.

16

Suffolk Health Services: Gathering Storm Over the Land

In March 2006, a journalist from *Public Finance* came down to Sudbury in West Suffolk to find out what was happening to its health services.

> The pretty Suffolk town of Sudbury is set in the picturesque countryside portrayed by its most famous resident, the painter Thomas Gainsborough. Its timber-framed buildings date back five centuries, ducks quack on the nearby River Stour and the town's ancient common lands are still a haven of tranquillity. Yet appearances can be deceptive, for Sudbury is a battleground. The town's Walnuttree Hospital is threatened with closure, and local residents are up in arms. There have been protests and petitions signed by thousands of locals determined to save the much-loved community hospital and its 30 inpatient beds. Windows sport stickers for the campaign against Suffolk West Primary Care Trust's closure plans.[1]

Appearances certainly can deceive. The writer of this article might also have added that Sudbury and the surrounding area had been identified by Suffolk West PCT itself as requiring a new community hospital with inpatient beds more than anywhere else in Suffolk. This was due to a population of 50,000 and rising, with a large proportion of elderly people, and on the basis of deprivation, mortality rate and rurality.

1 Tash Shifrin, 'Community scare.' *Public Finance*, 17 March 2006.

A further indication of the problems confronting an area like Sudbury, and Suffolk more generally, came with the publication of the region's Health Atlas in 2006. It projected a growth rate – in people aged 85 or over living in the region – of 80 per cent by 2021, with the general population rising at double the national rate. This, it was observed, did not sit easily with the widespread cutbacks to health services being implemented across Suffolk.[2]

The PCT had identified and accepted all this in a previous business case for a new community hospital.[3] In late 2005, the PCT's director of public health confirmed in a new report that Sudbury had the highest mortality ratio for deaths from all causes for those aged under 75 of all the towns in Suffolk.[4]

In 2005 also, the identification of Sudbury as having significant pockets of social deprivation was repeated in a report jointly produced by all the PCTs in Suffolk.[5] And even the strategic health authority for the area had confirmed in December 2005 that the population within its area had a high projected growth rate in older people with greater health and social care needs.[6]

The writer of the article was quite correct. The town had indeed become a battleground. It was a conflict that ran deep, fuelled by fear and anger. Furthermore, the military analogy was by no means confined to this writer. Another well-researched article, focusing on Sudbury but also other parts of the country, carried the headline on the front page of *The Spectator*: 'Labour's war on local hospitals'.[7] Nurses dressed in uniforms from the last world war would take the 'war' to save the hospitals to the streets in Long Melford, adjacent to Sudbury.[8] And an 86-year-old war hero was cited as one of those in Eye, at the Hartismere Hospital, who would fight the 'dictatorship' of the NHS bureaucrats who were trying to close the hospital.[9] He wasn't the only 'old soldier' involved. Ian Lavender, who played Private Pike in the televi-

2 Rebecca Sheppard, 'Health concerns as population grows.' *East Anglian Daily Times*, 4 August 2006.

3 *Outline Business Case for the Development of Sudbury Health and Social Care Centre.* Bury St Edmunds: Suffolk West PCT, March 2005, para 1.32.

4 'Another big health shock for Sudbury.' *Suffolk Free Press*, 22 December 2005.

5 *Suffolk Primary Care Trusts Reconfiguration Options.* Ipswich: Suffolk West PCT, Waveney PCT, Suffolk East PCTs, 2005, para 3.2.

6 *Consultation on New Primary Care Trusts Arrangements in Norfolk, Suffolk and Cambridgeshire.* Cambridge: Norfolk, Suffolk and Cambridgeshire Strategic Health Authority, 2005, p.9.

7 Ross Clark, 'Fear in the Community.' *Spectator*, 17 September 2005.

8 'Nurses take war to streets.' *Suffolk Free Press*, 21 July 2005.

9 David Green, 'War hero eager to save hospital.' *East Anglian Daily Times*, 6 September 2005.

sion series, *Dad's Army*, also weighed in, opposing the cuts to Suffolk health services.[10]

By the time of the general election in May 2005, those people in Suffolk who kept abreast of NHS matters were well aware that the health-care system across the county was in financial difficulty. However, this was nothing new.[11] But central government had tolerated this, wishing, it was supposed, to be re-elected. It appeared also to have accepted that peremptory and drastic debt collection would scarcely be consonant with preserving acceptable levels of patient care.

However, alarm bells were still not ringing unduly. Not only was the debt or deficit – if this was the right word for it – a longstanding issue, but New Labour was the government that had promised improvements in the NHS. Even in a county that returned largely Conservative Members of Parliament, nobody foresaw the sudden and ruthless assault that was to be launched on health services within Suffolk. There were anyway bright spots. In the East of the county, three primary care trusts had merged. This was in recognition of what had been pointed out at the time of their creation – that five PCTs in Suffolk might be too many in number. And Waveney PCT was actually in financial balance and seemed to have struck a balance between hospital and community services.

To the West, Suffolk West PCT had in 2003 adopted a well-thought-through 'intermediate care' policy, which would seek to strike the balance between services provided in the acute hospital, community hospitals and in people's own homes. It was based on several external reviews and reports and had gained broad support from both clinicians and the community alike.

In addition, the West Suffolk Hospitals NHS Trust (an acute hospital trust) was seeking to gain 'foundation status' that would have released it to some extent from the strict financial and other rules laid down by the Department of Health. The Trust saw such freedom as a way of improving patient services. Furthermore, it was reported that general practitioners across the county were performing well by meeting and even exceeding the various targets set by central government.

Although boasting significant areas of denser population in towns such as Ipswich and Bury St Edmunds, Suffolk is a largely rural area. Apart from acute hospitals at Ipswich and Bury St Edmunds, it has a number of

10 Dave Gooderham, 'Hospital gave my life back.' *East Anglian Daily Times*, 6 March 2006.

11 Will Wright, 'Protestors make their voices heard.' *Sudbury Mercury* 22 July 2005.

community hospitals, which are essential in providing services for local people in rural areas. For instance, over in the East, such hospitals were to be found in Aldeburgh, Eye and Felixstowe. In the West, Sudbury boasted two complementary hospitals, and Newmarket one. Suffolk West PCT had recognised the need to replace the two ageing Sudbury hospitals, and build a new community hospital. To this end, the Norfolk, Suffolk and Cambridgeshire Strategic Health Authority had promised in November 2005 that financial problems besetting the PCT would not prevent the building of the new community hospital.

The future looked reasonably bright. Government policy, under the banner of intermediate care, was to relieve unnecessary pressure on acute hospitals. It looked as though the Suffolk PCTs were on course to achieve this through a balanced mix of community services and community hospitals.

The great electoral watershed: the events that flowed from it

Only the cynical suspected that the pre- and post-general election (May 2005) landscapes would look so different; but even they would be shocked by the extent of the storm that was about to break.

People in Suffolk had, in May 2005, a feeling that their health care might be in reasonably safe hands, in the form of a New Labour government and the local primary care trusts and acute NHS trusts. By August 2005, if not before, the overwhelming feeling had turned to fear and anger. By early 2006, it was clear that what was happening in Suffolk reflected a wider national pattern, as 'overspending' or 'deficits' were suddenly reported to be widespread within the NHS.

Evidence of wider problems was, however, of little consolation, especially as Suffolk appeared to be in the vanguard of these unwelcome developments. The situation in the county spawned desperate local campaigns in towns such as Sudbury, Newmarket, Eye, Felixstowe and Aldeburgh to try to turn the tide.

In short, at the end of June 2005, a financial recovery plan was suddenly presented to, and approved by, the Board of the Suffolk West PCT. The Vice-Chairman resigned immediately in protest. Similarly in the East of Suffolk a similar financial recovery plan had been presented to the three combined PCT Boards. Right in the middle of the summer holidays, consultations – containing only one option for financial recovery (closures of certain sets of services) – began in both West and East.

The consultation documents were notable in that the only real detail they contained related to closures, but not to new or replacement services. Community hospital inpatient beds used largely (but not only) by older people requiring rehabilitation and recuperation, day hospitals, respite facilities for people with mental health problems or learning disabilities, and acute hospital beds – all were targeted for reductions or closures.

Originally the PCTs had intended to take their final decisions in late November 2005. Because of protests about the inadequacy of the consultation documents, these decisions were delayed, pending the provision of further information. Nevertheless, in January 2006, the Suffolk East PCTs took the decision to close down a wide range of services. So enormous were the implications that the Suffolk County Council Health Scrutiny Committee referred the proposals to the Secretary of State.

In the West, the PCT's decision was delayed further until April. Nevertheless, undaunted by this delay and the referral to the Secretary of State in the East, the Suffolk West PCT voted for the closure of community hospital beds across West Suffolk. It also tacitly allowed many acute hospital beds to be closed by West Suffolk Hospitals NHS Trust as well. Unaccountably, although the closures in the West were in some ways more aggressive and drastic than in the East, the Health Scrutiny Committee failed to refer to the Secretary of State, as it had done in the East. At this point, several local patients attempted to issue judicial review proceedings against both the PCT and the Scrutiny Committee in May 2006.

As these events unfolded between June 2005 and June 2006, the PCT and local community in Sudbury had in effect been at war, as the latter had sought to defend itself from what it perceived to be the aggressive and uncompromising stance of the PCT.

By August 2006, the campaign against the closures had been running for 12 months. It was now all but lost, although a judicial review legal case was in the offing, as the community prepared to make a last stand. The conflict had during this period turned into a bitter war of words and actions. Across Suffolk and elsewhere, the government's official policy – of NHS primary care trusts working cooperatively with local communities – lay in tatters.

17

Rural Conflagrations and Early Hostilities

There had been signs, even toward the end of 2004, of the cracks that a year later would expose central government policy as at best optimistic, and at worst as seriously misguided.

At this time, the two Sudbury community hospitals had been operated by an acute trust, the West Suffolk Hospitals NHS Trust. In late 2004, the local community had already had a short but bitter fight with the Trust over its attempts to close down Walnuttree Hospital rapidly, on fire safety grounds. However, the Chief Executive creditably changed tack after the fire safety arguments, with which he had been improperly presented, were exposed as overblown (see Chapter 10). Hospital staff and the local community held a party, the proceeds of which went to charity. Nonetheless, the whole episode had been a warning shot from the local NHS. Within six months, it would be back in force in the form of Suffolk West PCT, more determined than ever to close the hospital.

Breaking the machinery of trust: war is declared on Sudbury

The fight for a new community hospital in Sudbury had gone on for some 20 to 30 years. Walnuttree and St Leonards Hospitals were both greatly loved. They provided a wide range of services still, and previously had provided even more.

Nevertheless, it had long been recognised that a new community hospital would eventually be needed. The early days of the campaign for a new hospital began in the 1970s. In 1987, the NHS bought land near the centre of town, known as Harp's Close Meadow (or People's Park), on which to build the hospital. Unfortunately, two local farmers fought a judicial review case to have the land registered as a town green. This legal fight dragged on between 1991 and 1997. During this time, the new community hospital had not progressed. A renewed threat of legal challenge in 2001, following a House of Lords case elsewhere about village greens, prompted the West Suffolk Hospitals NHS Trust to purchase another piece of land further out of town. With even this issue overcome, the decision-making process would remain bogged down in doubts, about-turns and broken promises.

In 2002 and 2003, the strategic health authority had refused an outline business case for a new hospital because of the financial situation of the PCT (which had inherited a deficit on its creation that year). During 2004, the strategic health authority approved the case and then changed its mind, again because of the PCT's finances. At the end of 2004, it promised that the community hospital would go ahead, irrespective of the PCT's finances.[1]

After much work with the local community – including an active steering group with good local representation – the spring of 2005 promised much. The two hospitals were to be closed, but only when the new community hospital was built and operational, together with a wide range of outpatient services and with inpatient beds.

By February, the PCT had 'unveiled a revised multi-million pound plan for a long awaited new hospital – due to open in two years'. It was reported as marking the end of the 30 years of struggle. It would include 32 beds, inpatient and day treatment facilities for physiotherapy and occupational therapy, minor injuries unit, X-ray suite, outpatient consultancy suite, out-of-hours unit, mental health facilities and a base for social workers and community staff. Land would also be left available for an ambulance base, a 50-bed nursing home and a healthy living centre.[2] By April, the PCT had approved the outline business case and the strategic health authority had all but done so. So anticipated was the new development that both staff and steering group were even being taken on coach trips to see how other similar developments were working.

And then came the first ominous signs. The strategic health authority, in considering further more detailed approval in May, raised objections concerning physiotherapy space – inappropriate and disproportionate

1 'Fears grown as new hospital plans delayed.' *East Anglian Daily Times*, 8 November 2004.

2 Patrick Lowman, 'Town's new hospital plan set for boost.' *East Anglian Daily Times*, 23 February 2005.

objections, which were cloaking something altogether more serious. Then the Suffolk West PCT Chief Executive and Director of Finance suddenly departed for seconded posts at the SHA. Their departure was couched in all the customary calming language, on this occasion offered by the Chair of the PCT:

> I am enormously grateful [to them]... Both appointments were made at the beginning of the PCT three years ago, and during that time I think we have made some very good steps forward.[3]

He referred also to the vision and abilities of the departing Chief Executive.[4] The Chief Executive was reported by the SHA as being likely to examine his career options.[5] Removed because of the financial deficits, his departure seemed to spell doom for the health services that he had so well identified as required in Sudbury. Although the SHA would never confess to its exact role, it seems that during late May and early June, it had sent a team to closet itself with the PCT and to dictate what the PCT must do.

Public meeting: a pre-emptive attack is launched

According to government policy, local decisions about NHS services should include full involvement of, and 'ownership' by, the local community.[6] Furthermore, a government code of practice on consultation states that, before formal, written consultation is launched, informal consultation should take place.[7] Up to May 2005, the PCT had actually achieved this, with its original plans for a new community hospital.

However, at a stroke, the PCT showed how apparently worthless such policy and codes of practice are, and how they are apt to be discarded, undermined or ignored at the convenience of the NHS. Accordingly, the next events were rapid and dramatic. A public meeting was called at short notice on 29 June 2005, to be held in St Peter's Church on Market Hill, Sudbury. Despite the short notice, several hundred people attended.

Flanked by other Board members, the Chief Executive spoke. He must simply have been carrying out orders from above. To that extent it was all

3 'Health trust loses senior staff.' *East Anglian Daily Times*, 7 April 2005.

4 'Health chief takes new post.' *Suffolk Free Press*, 7 April 2005.

5 Liz Hearnshaw, 'Ex-chief on secondment could return.' *East Anglian Daily Times*, 30 July 2005.

6 Secretary of State for Health (2006) *Our Health, Our Care, Our Say: a new direction for community services.* Cm 6737. London: HMSO, para 6.59.

7 *Code of Practice on Consultation.* London: Regulatory Unit, Cabinet Office, 2004, para 1.3.

through no fault of his own. Nevertheless his performance revealed the brutal nature of the NHS decision-making that was to engulf Suffolk over the coming year, as well as other parts of the country. With no hint of expressed regret or doubt, he simply stated his proposals for the abandonment of the plan for the new hospital, closure of all community hospital beds, closure of the existing two hospitals, and the relocation of consultant outpatient services away from Sudbury. Replacement services were uncertain in scope and timing. Asked to apologise several times for all the broken promises, he refused, stating that there was nothing to apologise for. This was not the language of consultation but of diktat.

The meeting not only provided the platform for an effective declaration of war on (the health of) the local community, but it in effect turned into the first battle of what was to be a long and bitter campaign. Not helped by a defective amplifier system, the PCT's attitude came over as uncompromising. The PCT managed the considerable feat of exacerbating further the level of hostility, which was already at breaking point even before the meeting had begun.

In terms of winning over the public, the meeting was a public relations disaster for the PCT. Its uncompromising attitude convinced nearly all present at the meeting that only a financially desperate PCT, facing dire threats from its political masters, could behave in such a way. For NHS managers trying to explain and implement sensitive proposals, this public meeting was an object lesson in how not to proceed.

Nevertheless, the same day, a financial recovery plan had already been presented to and approved by the PCT Board. By 1 August 2005, the legally required consultation was launched, with a view to taking decisions to close services by late November, and have the Sudbury hospitals closed by Christmas or soon after. The gloves were off.

Sowing fear and anger in the community

The financial recovery plan, public meeting and consultation document made the community rapidly aware of what was afoot. Sudbury was to lose both hospitals. At some point in the future a new health centre would be built, but this would have a much reduced range of services and no in-patient beds.

The PCT claimed, and continued to claim throughout the period, that its proposals were about modernisation and improvement, and not at root due to financial pressures. It maintained also that they had long been planned –

even though up to May 2005, the PCT had in fact been planning the exact opposite by building a hospital with inpatient beds.

The PCT's financial state was so parlous, and its promises so fragile, that few people believed any of its vague assurances about even the reduced future services that were now promised in the new health centre. In particular, the PCT's assurances about providing a range of health-care services ('intermediate care') in people's own homes were greeted with huge suspicion. This was based on local people's own experience of poorly resourced community health and social care services in a rural area. In sum, the local community could only conclude that this was a savage and rushed assault on local services generally – and in particular on older people, as well as those with mental health needs and learning disabilities.

The PCT claimed it was advocating care in, and for, the community. However, that community was in no doubt that what was being proposed was a removal of care. The anger, fear and consternation excited by the proposals were unprecedented.

18

Setting the Wheels in Motion: the Timetable of War

The reverse suffered by Suffolk West PCT at the public meeting in June 2005 was probably viewed as a mere local misfortune from its point of view. Sudbury, after all, was on the borders of the county and almost in Essex; it constituted a little border trouble.

Back in its stronghold of Bury St Edmunds, in its unprepossessing headquarters of Thingoe House, the PCT lost no time in moving its plan forward. It might have lost the first engagement, but it was aiming to win the war and to do it in record time.

By 1 August 2005, it had rushed out a hurriedly composed consultation document, the consultation period to close on 31 October, and a formal decision, it was hoped, to be taken in late November. Perhaps even closure could begin in December, and be completed early in 2006. This reaction set a pattern throughout the next months. The greater the public opposition to its plans – no matter from which quarter or how well informed – so the more entrenched in its position would the PCT become.

The public meeting had been held on 29 June. Despite the opposition it had faced, and despite central government policy and the code of practice about local involvement in working up proposals, the PCT was moving forward anyway. It had already presented a sweeping financial recovery plan to its Board earlier that same day. The Board members saw financial succour in the form of the new Chief Executive.

The Board was faced with a financial crisis. The former Secretary of State for Health, John Reid, had tolerated this in the pre-general election period up to May 2005. Post-election, his successor, Patricia Hewitt, was not standing for it. The Board members, entirely predictably, gave the financial recovery plan their full support.

Ploughshares into swords: a community revolts

Suffolk West PCT's strategy was to strike quickly and decisively before opposition could be organised. The public meeting, presentation of the financial recovery plan and launching of the consultation took place all within a month. The consultation document was published in the middle of the summer holidays and with such little detail (other than the proposed closures) that the PCT gave the impression of not expecting or wanting serious comment.

A local action committee quickly formed in Sudbury. Known as the Walnuttree Hospital Action Committee (WHAC), it drew on a wide range of interests and expertise. Strikingly, it succeeded in uniting all three main political parties at both local and national level. Its three presidents were Tim Yeo, MP (Conservative), Lord Phillips of Sudbury (Liberal Democrat) and Kevin Craig (prospective Labour candidate at the general election). Local councillors – from county, district, town and parish – were drawn from all three main political parties. Local churches were represented, as were hospital staff (porters, nurses and therapists), general medical practitioners and patients – as well as a range of other expertise. The Town Clerk immediately volunteered administrative support from Sudbury Town Council. The Committee even boasted as its Chairman Colin Spence, the former Vice-Chairman of the PCT.

The Committee would fight a multi-faceted and fierce campaign. Privately, the PCT would admit to both surprise and frustration at such well-organised opposition. The strands of the campaign included:

- postcard and letter-writing to the Secretary of State for Health
- a newsletter
- a weekend of action in Sudbury including a march through the town
- a 24-hour prayer vigil spread across the Sudbury churches (organised by Sudbury Churches Together)
- fundraising events

- raising a petition to the government to intervene
- hiring independent experts to analyse and report on the PCT's proposals
- producing an expert report of its own
- seeking meetings with the PCT and the Secretary of State
- pursuing Freedom of Information Act requests
- a string of detailed letters to the PCT (and copied to the SHA and Secretary of State) questioning it on a large number of clinical, legal and procedural issues
- an internet website to gather support and offer information.

A health campaigner of national prominence, Elisabeth Manero, who saved Edgware Hospital in North London in order to turn it into a model community hospital, referred to the importance of just such a wide arsenal. Weapons should include High Court challenges, prominent media campaigns, support from royal colleges and other eminent bodies, producing evidence, use of council health scrutiny committees and so on.[1]

Across Suffolk (Newmarket, Aldeburgh, Eye, Felixstowe), and indeed across England, a similar pattern would emerge as local campaign groups rapidly emerged to fight the aggressive threat of sudden closures. The churches also became involved in West Suffolk. For example, clergy would meet with local MPs and would comment adversely on the PCT's proposals:

> We don't see how cutting staff is going to improve services – people are going to be in pain. I blame senior management… They have no commitment to patient care – they make the balance sheet look good and then move on.

The PCT responded to the clergy that the comments were 'very disappointing', 'patently not true' and 'offensive'.[2]

More widely in Suffolk, senior clergy launched a multi-denominational campaign against the cuts to health services.[3] It was also the Church that could raise some fundamental points about what 'real care' for people entails. Immediately prior to the decision to close all NHS community hospital beds

1 Mark Gould, 'No closure on campaigns to save community hospitals.' *Health Service Journal*, 23 February 2006.

2 'MPs to meet clergy over NHS crisis.' *East Anglian Daily Times*, 29 December 2005.

3 Benedict O'Connor, 'Clergymen bid to stop health cuts.' *East Anglian Daily Times*, 19 January 2006.

in West Suffolk, Major Betty Jones, a minister at the Newmarket chapel of the Salvation Army, stated that:

> I am deeply concerned and have holy anger that patients' needs – holistic, spiritual, social and psychological – will not be met by these proposals.[4]

The local paper would carry the headline 'Heaven help our hospital', reporting that a 24-hour prayer vigil would take place in Sudbury churches. Richard Titford of Sudbury Churches Together explained that they would simply be praying for Walnuttree Hospital to remain an active hospital in the town and asking for God's guidance on how to achieve it.[5] Even to those members of the community who were not of a religious mind, matters were moving so quickly that divine intervention seemed as good a bet as any.

Battlelines drawn

So the battlelines began to take shape in Sudbury. On the one hand was Suffolk West PCT, Norfolk, Suffolk and Cambridgeshire SHA, the Department of Health and the Secretary of State for Health. On the other side was a lone action committee run essentially by volunteers, backed up by the wider community.

The power imbalance was notable. The NHS bodies held in their hands immense amounts of power in terms of information, money and authority. They literally held the health of whole local communities in their hands. Worse, PCT boards and SHAs do not consist of elected members. Their accountability was limited; to the local community it seemed non-existent. Information and facts are all important, yet were immensely difficult to obtain, even with use of the Freedom of Information Act.

There were of course other forces in the field. It was clear that many clinicians in West Suffolk were appalled at the nature of the proposals, but it was not obvious how far they would speak out. In the event many did, to their immense credit. But those employed by the PCT felt they did so at their peril. Many were frightened of saying publicly what they really believed. Some were warned off in no uncertain terms.

Much was expected of the unions, such as Unison, the Royal College of Nursing and the Chartered Society of Physiotherapy. Although Unison

4 'Staff and patients unite against "nasty medicine".' *East Anglian Daily Times*, 12 April 2006.

5 'Heaven help our hospital.' *Suffolk Free Press*, 18 August 2005.

produced a regional report, *Eastern Promise Broken*, the impact of the unions seemed distinctly muted.[6]

When community health councils were abolished by the government – some said because they were too much of a thorn in holding the NHS locally accountable for decisions – they were replaced in part by Patient and Public Involvement Forms (PPIFs) through the NHS Reform and Health Care Professions Act 2002. Their role broadly is to monitor services and visit NHS premises on behalf of local patients and communities and to report their findings to the NHS – and to report to the Health Scrutiny Committees of councils. Although playing a relatively low key role throughout the period, they did eventually come up with a Suffolk-wide response which condemned the NHS proposals right across the county. No notice was taken; for instance, this opposition was not even mentioned in Suffolk West PCT's final report.

Beyond all these was the Suffolk County Council Health Scrutiny Committee. Such Committees came into being under the Health and Social Care Act 2001. Legally they had the power to refer to the Secretary of State proposals that a) have not been adequately consulted on, or b) 'would not be in the interests of the health service in the area'.[7] In the final analysis, its bite did not quite live up to its bark in the West of Suffolk, but it nevertheless played a significant role.

Last, but by no means least, was the Press. So much would take place behind closed doors that the local community would rely heavily on the Press to investigate and publicise what was going on. In West Suffolk, and in relation to Sudbury in particular, the Press came in the form of the *East Anglian Daily Times*, the *Suffolk Free Press*, the *Sudbury Mercury*, BBC Radio Suffolk, and BBC Look East (television).

Campaigning in the field: an imbalance of power

The great imbalance in power between the NHS decision-makers and a local action committee meant that WHAC had to wage what amounted to a protracted campaign of guerrilla, albeit principled, warfare.

Military metaphor springs to mind because from the outset the PCT gave no suggestion of compromise or even delay. It appeared determined to

6 John Lister (2005) *Eastern Promise Broken.* London: Unison.

7 Statutory instrument 2002/3048. *Local Authority (Overview and Scrutiny Committees Health Scrutiny Functions) Regulations 2002.*

rush through its plans, come what may, and no matter the degree of conflict it provoked. From July 2005 onwards right through to May 2006, the PCT would suffer a number of reverses in both small skirmishes and more major engagements. However, owing to the power it wielded and its lack of accountability, it staggered on, fuelled it seemed by threats from its political masters.

WHAC took a decision at the outset to try to adhere to certain principles in the campaign. These would include attempting to stick to reason, evidence and logic – and avoiding pure emotion, sentiment or personal criticisms. Perhaps WHAC was naive. As the campaign unfolded, it became clear that, on many levels, the local community felt it was up against an apparent ruthlessness and lack of transparency that shocked even the most seasoned of local politicians. From the PCT at local level, through the regional SHA and to the heart of central government, the community felt itself facing an enemy that was forever shifting its ground. It was a game of smoke and mirrors, fuelled it seemed by chaos and desperation in equal measure.

Striking behind the lines

In the early, hot days of July 2005, while the PCT was railroading through its financial recovery plan, the local community, too, acted quickly. By the end of June 2005, it had already organised a postcard campaign aimed at Patricia Hewitt, Secretary of State for Health. Some 20,000 postcards were distributed to homes in Sudbury for people to send.[8] This was because, in an unguarded moment, the PCT had, at the public meeting, pointed the finger at central government. In addition, the local community could not quite believe that a New Labour government, self-appointed defender of the NHS, could countenance its local destruction.

The postcards and letters sent (ultimately 5500 in number) together with a petition (11,500 signatures) submitted in November 2005 (to Patricia Hewitt and Tony Blair) were akin to what would in the past have been a direct request to the monarch for intervention. Given the power wielded by central government and its Ministers, the analogy was perhaps apt.

High-level defections

In these early days, a further blow was suffered by the PCT when an ally came to the local community's aid from an unexpected quarter.

8 Dave Gooderham, 'Health chiefs taken to task over debts.' *East Anglian Daily Times*, 7 July 2005.

The Vice-Chairman of the PCT Board, Colin Spence, learned on his return from holiday about the PCT's decision to abandon the new Sudbury hospital and to close the old. He not only resigned on 1 July 2005, but promptly became Chairman of WHAC. Declaring himself 'shocked and devastated' he stated that the 'community have been extremely let down and I don't want to be part of that collective decision'. Just three weeks earlier, he had been given a detailed presentation of the new community hospital for Sudbury. He felt he had to 'stand with my community'.[9]

His actions stood out even more subsequently, because the rest of the PCT Board's non-executive members – who in principle were meant to speak up for the community – would over the next nine months fall resoundingly silent.

Desultory skirmishes

On a sultry and oppressive July day in 2005, a stormy Sudbury steering group meeting (with both PCT staff and community representatives present) met to discuss the turn events had taken. Members of the local community stated that all trust had been forfeited by the PCT. The meeting was inconclusive. Arguments broke out about the evidence underpinning the PCT's proposals. At one point, the Chief Executive attempted to draw a line under these by referring to an Office of Government Commerce (OGC) document about Sudbury, and stating that the evidence lay within this. Like so many other statements made by the PCT, this tactical mistake would come home to roost at a later date, after a six-month-long battle by the PCT to keep the OGC document secret (see below).

PCT launches consultation in expectation of quick and easy victory

By the beginning of August, the advantage clearly lay with the PCT, despite having run into some unwelcome reverses and having badly misjudged the depth of feeling in the local community. It had launched its consultation document, expecting a quick and easy victory. Word had it that the PCT was in high hopes of pushing through the proposals and of persuading the public of their merits. However, it was perhaps this over-confidence – coupled with the rushed, seemingly superficial and uncompromising nature

9 Benedict O'Connor, 'PCT member reacts on return from holiday.' *East Anglian Daily Times*, 2 July 2005.

of the consultation document – that was soon to prove an Achilles heel for the PCT.

Events were moving with unprecedented haste. In order to try to get to grips with a fast-moving enemy, and to do so constructively, WHAC sought and gained a meeting with the non-executive Board members of the PCT. At a long meeting in early August, question after question was put to them. Scarcely one was answered. This was partly because they had just come to listen, and partly because they didn't know the answers. They promised, however, to seek them out. This was in the first week of August. The information promised was not forthcoming until 17 October, some 11 weeks later, and only shortly before the original closure date of the consultation.

19

The Campaign in Full Flux

As the campaign unfolded, so it was fought on a number of fronts. The Suffolk County Council Health Scrutiny Committee weighed in and delayed the plans of the Suffolk PCTs by demanding that they supply more information. The local community would take to the streets, parks and buses, as well as to Whitehall. Members of the House of Commons and House of Lords would attempt the all but impossible task of eliciting meaningful answers from Ministers in Parliament. The local action committee would ensure that thousands of people responded to the consultation – and the serious and essential business of fundraising to support the campaign was in full swing. As Christmas approached, the Sudbury action committee would devise a board game to be played in the streets and markets of the town. It was called 'Hunt the hospital bed'.

Help from an unexpected quarter

The PCT's headlong, almost euphoric, rush to close down local health services was checked from perhaps an unexpected quarter in early September 2005. The PCT had submitted both the financial recovery plan and consultation document to the Suffolk County Council Health Scrutiny Committee. The PCT must have hoped for the same uncritical acceptance of the proposals by the Scrutiny Committee, as had been given by its own Board back in June. If so, its hopes were to be dashed.

The information presented to the Committee came over as short on detail and betrayed no sign of a thought-through and balanced approach to local health care.[1]

In addition, a number of organisations were invited to give evidence to the Scrutiny Committee; they were very critical.[2] The PCTs had to tread carefully with the Scrutiny Committee. This was because they knew that the Committee had the legal power to derail the proposals – at least for a period – by making a formal referral to the Secretary of State. Accordingly, the Suffolk West PCT had suffered a reverse, and immediately announced that it would after all provide further information shortly, and would also extend the consultation period by six weeks into December.[3]

The extent of the setback became clear when, in October 2005, the Scrutiny Committee published an interim report seriously criticising the PCTs in Suffolk, for a consultation 'extremely poorly handled', for being short on 'honesty about the cost pressures', and for 'rushed and poorly considered cost-cutting proposals'.[4]

Taking to the streets, parks, churches and buses – and to Whitehall

The staff of Walnuttree and St Leonards Hospitals, together with the local community, would decide to take visible action: 'OUT IN FORCE: Walnuttree staff take to the streets', as the front page put it.[5]

By now, a weekend of action had been planned. It included vigils in the churches, and a march through Sudbury. The latter attracted some 500 people, despite the dismal weather on a Saturday in September – including the local MP, the local peer, the mayor, hospital staff and residents.[6] Complete with a 'grim reaper' and local firefighters sounding their sirens, this was of course the local community's day. The PCT could scarcely

1 *Interim Report on Committee Response to NHS Consultations*, 1 November 2005. H05/22. Ipswich: Suffolk County Council Health Scrutiny Committee, para 45.

2 *Select Committee Hearing on Community Hospitals: contributors' notes.* H05/18. Ipswich: Suffolk County Council Health Scrutiny Committee.

3 Dave Gooderham, 'Health consultation gets extra four weeks.' *East Anglian Daily Times*, 20 September 2005.

4 Richard Smith, 'NHS bed cuts face delays.' *East Anglian Daily Times*, 24 October 2005.

5 Benedict O'Connor. *Sudbury Mercury*, 29 July 2005.

6 Will Grahame-Clark, 'Residents: "save our hospitals".' *East Anglian Daily Times*, 12 September 2005.

organise a counter-demonstration. Marches were taking place all over Suffolk as well.

Years before, at the time of the 'poll tax', which Margaret Thatcher had wished to impose, a local historian had sent a photograph of Simon of Sudbury's skull to Number 10 Downing Street. Simon of Sudbury, Archbishop of Canterbury, had been beheaded by the rebels in the Peasants' Revolt of 1382. Now, indicative of the depth of local feeling, a suggestion had now been made that permission be sought to take his skull, complete with axe marks at the neck, from its recess. This was in the vestry at St Gregory's Church, Sudbury, next to Walnuttree Hospital. It could be displayed at the head of the march. Intended of course as a totally non-violent gesture, it was felt it might nevertheless indicate the strength of local feeling. In the event, the suggestion was not pursued in case the gesture were to be misinterpreted and cause undue offence.

The historical analogy with the Peasants' Revolt was fanciful but not quite without interest. Brickwork belonging to Simon of Sudbury's college, dating back to the 1400s, frames one of the disused entrances to the Walnuttree Hospital.[7] Now, as then, local people felt oppressed by an arbitrary and distant power. And just as different sections of the community now opposed the NHS proposals, so then it was not just 'peasants', but also clergy and gentry who were involved. Sudbury was one of the centres of the rebellion. The chief agitator was John Wrawe from Essex, a (former) priest or chaplain, aided and abetted by Geoffrey Parfey, the vicar of All Saints church, Sudbury.[8] One of the first targets of the peasants was the abbey of Bury St Edmunds, which sits adjacent now to Thingoe House, home of the Suffolk West PCT.

Then, Richard II rode out and was trusted by the rebels – only to betray that trust. Now the Secretary of State, Patricia Hewitt, offered up her White Paper as the saviour for community hospitals. But it seems she too flattered to deceive. Many of the community hospitals have indeed been betrayed. There the analogy stops. Violence, sometimes extreme, was perpetrated by the rebels. In East Anglia, the Bishop of Norwich was proportionately vengeful. In Sudbury, it is thought that rebels were rounded up on Market Hill on which St. Peter's Church stood (and stands) – venue of the hot-tempered meeting between hundreds of townspeople and the Suffolk West PCT in June 2005. In the 1930s, workmen found skeletons, many

7 Nicki Harvey, 'You can save Simon's gate.' *Suffolk Free Press*, 23 February 2006.

8 Barry Wall (2004) *Sudbury: history and guide.* Stroud: Tempus, p.38.

headless and thought to be the remains of the rebels, buried against the churchyard wall of St Gregory's Church.

The local community in Sudbury offered no violence to the PCT. (Not, as in 1835, when a Poor Law official came to Sudbury to explain how a new workhouse had to be built – ironically, Walnuttree Hospital in its original form – in line with the unpopular 1834 Poor Law Amendment Act. He was greeted in the Town Hall with such hostility and violence that he had to abandon the meeting.[9])

However, conversely, in the community's view, the PCT was offering harm to local people, albeit not violence. It was in no doubt that the PCT's proposals would directly lead to greater disability, more dependence, distress for both vulnerable people and their carers, and to significantly increased levels of risk. It believed that this could sometimes result in avoidable, premature death – for example, arising from the spiral (sometimes quicker, sometimes slower) of physical and mental decline that can follow from inadequate rehabilitation and recuperation. In addition, the community believed that life and death could be at stake in a more immediate sense as well. The following, anecdotal example, albeit from an area other than Suffolk, is illustrative.

A 90-year-old woman developed a serious chest infection and other potential complications. She needed a period of 'step-up' care, just to manage the infection and get her back on her feet. She was turned away by the local acute hospital. It recognised that clinically she required a bed, but it did not have the capacity to admit her. Likewise, no local nursing home was able to find a space for her at such short notice. She could not have gone to the community hospital, because it had been closed down (despite local protests and warnings about the consequences for local people). She was told that the new 'care in the community' (the fig leaf given at the time for closing the community hospital) would provide three visits a day. She went home. The first visit arrived next morning. By then she had fallen down the stairs and lain there most of the night. She died three days later from the fall and its complications. Her family blames directly the closure of the community hospital.

By early November, a petition consisting of some 11,500 signatures had been delivered to Patricia Hewitt and Tony Blair. This was now the second time in a year that local Sudbury people had gone to London with a petition

9 Phyllis Felton (2006) *Beyond the bricks of Walnuttree Hospital.* Sudbury: private publication. Available from Tourist Information, Sudbury, Suffolk.

to defend the threat to their local health services. This time round, the trip to Downing Street was made by civic leaders, hospital staff and residents not only from Sudbury, but also from other parts of Suffolk including Newmarket, Felixstowe, Eye, Ipswich and Bury St Edmunds.[10] The placard bearing the statement 'The 11th commandment: thou shall not grow old'[11] summed up people's fears.

Although central government made no response to either the petition or the letters, the issue of them both would resurface unexpectedly three months later.

On the bumpy rural buses of West Suffolk

In arguing for the retention of community hospital facilities in Sudbury, the local MP, Tim Yeo, took to the buses. This was to illustrate how difficult it was for people to travel from Sudbury to Bury St Edmunds (to which services were proposed to be withdrawn from Sudbury). He invited the PCT Chief Executive to join him; the invitation was declined.[12] The bus trip, undertaken with a local pensioner who had been at Walnuttree Hospital in Sudbury some three years before with a broken hip, attracted considerable publicity.[13]

The journey took an hour one-way, was a bumpy ride up and down winding lanes, cost £4.80 return and even then the bus did not stop directly at the hospital, leaving people with an uphill walk. On the return trip, people have to cross a busy dual carriageway and wait at a bus stop with no shelter.[14]

Fundraising

Fundraising became a major issue, in order for WHAC to be able to produce publicity to counter the PCT's feelgood but threadbare consultation document. Local fundraising took various forms, including approaches to local businesses who generously donated a range of raffle prizes. These included DVD players, televisions, food hampers, shop vouchers, free restaurant meals, 160-piece tool sets, travel vouchers, beer and wine, watch and necklace sets, stationery sets, beauty treatment vouchers, free MOTs and so on. The businesses who contributed included both chains as well as local,

10 'Strength of feelings drives march.' *East Anglian Daily Times*, 2 November 2005.

11 Dave Gooderham, 'Health workers step up cuts protest.' *East Anglian Daily Times*, 3 November 2005.

12 Nicki Harvey, 'Yeo calls on health chiefs to try the bus.' *Suffolk Free Press*, 14 July 2006.

13 Lisa Cleverdon, 'Hour's bus trip if hospital goes.' *East Anglian Daily Times*, 2 August 2005.

14 Barbara Eeles, 'An hour-long bus trip and a walk uphill.' *Suffolk Free Press*, 4 August 2005.

one-off businesses. Discos, dances, auctions (for example of a signed Chelsea football club shirt) and collection buckets in the market square all played their part.

Hearing local voices

By the middle of October 2005 (as far as most of the public were concerned, two weeks from the originally planned end of the consultation on 31 October), the PCT had received 152 replies to the consultation.[15]

At its own expense – in effect at the local population's expense – WHAC reproduced the consultation document. As the still warm days of early October turned into the wind, wet and cold of November and December, members of the Committee manned a stall outside the Town Hall distributing the consultation document every Saturday and some other days besides. By 12 December, the PCT had received 2589 responses, largely from Sudbury and Newmarket (where a local campaign had also been run). It was not so much the PCT engaging with the public, as the public forcing itself on the PCT.

The PCT subsequently admitted that it had been totally unprepared for such a response. As a consequence, having set a January date for its final decision, it now deferred a decision to 22 February. It also engaged outside help to advise it on how to analyse the volume of response.

As for the roadshows the PCT ran, they remained largely a failure with low turnouts. Except for one in Sudbury, where WHAC had again come to the aid of the PCT, by directing people to the roadshow inside the church on Market Hill.

Taking the fight to central government

The PCT was clearly being propped up by its lack of accountability to the local population, and driven by financial demands from central government.

Consequently, throughout the campaign both MPs and local councillors sought interviews with the Secretary of State. It was a case of trying to talk to the politician general, whose PCTs were running riot in the field. But Patricia Hewitt would simply deny all responsibility for what the PCTs were doing.

15 Benedict O'Connor, '£20m health process not "runaway success".' *East Anglian Daily Times*, 3 October 2005.

WHAC sent a stream of letters to the PCT, the SHA and the Secretary of State. Members of Parliament also kept up a dogged campaign, which included not just visits to the Secretary of State but also Parliamentary questions and speeches.

For instance, in early November, Baroness Ruth Rendell raised, in the House of Lords, the issue of closure of the Sudbury hospitals and the watered down new health centre, with further questions coming from Baroness Gardner of Parkes and Lord Phillips of Sudbury. The reply from the government in the form of Baroness Royall was to the effect that the changes to services were long overdue, were for the benefit of the people of Sudbury and were not being made to effect savings.[16] Nevertheless, true to form, the government did not answer the crucial question from Baroness Rendell as to why the new health centre would not now have the beds that had originally been promised.

Tim Yeo, MP for South Suffolk, in particular harried the Health Secretary at every opportunity. By 24 January he gained time to debate Sudbury and delivered a comprehensive speech.[17]

Hunting for hospital beds in the streets and marketplaces

While pressure mounted in distant Parliament, Christmas approached in Sudbury. A second public meeting of several hundred people, in November 2005, served as continuing evidence about local concerns. Despite the unprecedented local opposition, the PCT showed no signs of being prepared to slacken its pace, to talk, to negotiate or to compromise. For instance, it simply rejected out of hand an interim and independent expert report commissioned by WHAC, without dealing with any of the detailed points it made.[18]

To make matters worse, worrying signs had been emerging from Suffolk County Council. It was badly overspent and had in August announced that it would have to make savings on its social services budget for disabled and older people. Though claiming that it would do so without cutting services to people who needed them, nevertheless the evidence on the ground was less reassuring.

16 Baroness Royall. *Hansard*, House of Lords, 31 October 2005.

17 Tim Yeo, MP. *Hansard*, House of Commons Debates, 24 January 2006, column 1404.

18 Dave Gooderham, 'Health cuts plan "flawed".' *East Anglian Daily Times*, 31 October 2006.

Against this background, and as Christmas drew nearer, WHAC developed a large wooden board game called 'Hunt the Hospital Bed'. Described as an 'NHS game of chance: two turns free at the point of delivery', it gave players a chance to turn up illustrated hospital beds (almost unfindable, worth five chocolates), therapists, nurses or doctors ('rare breeds', worth one chocolate), community hospitals (threatened with loss of habitat) for sale, and numerous NHS managers with clip boards and axes ('common variety', worth no chocolates). WHAC's large Christmas cards featured a photograph of the game and described it as

> A popular game, played and enjoyed by people of all ages in the streets, markets and fairs of Sudbury. Easy to play, difficult to win.

The cards were duly sent to certain members of the PCT, as well as to Patricia Hewitt, Tony Blair and Gordon Brown. Both elderly and young enjoyed the game, the latter for the chocolates, the former for the humorous but grimly accurate note that the game struck.

20

Other Fights in a Changing Landscape

As the campaign entered 2006, the fight continued in other settings. These included the Freedom of Information Act. In addition, an attempt was made to rescue a petition of 11,500 signatures and 5500 letters and postcards, which had been withheld by the Department of Health. This was against a health landscape that in principle at least was meant to be changing in the light of the government's White Paper issued in January 2006.

Fighting for information in the thickets

Away from the frontline of newspaper headlines and letters, market stalls and roadshows, a protracted campaign of cat and mouse had been pursued in the woods and thickets of the Freedom of Information Act 2000 since late July 2005.

Apart from a number of more minor requests, one request in particular threw up a questionable refusal to disclose information. More importantly, it served to expose once again the lack of accountability that seems to bedevil the NHS. Between them, the Department of Health and the Suffolk West PCT both intimated that neither was responsible for the decision not to disclose. In other words it was bad enough that disclosure did not take place; but nobody would even take responsibility for the non-disclosure. This appeared absurd and was yet one more example of the gross lack of accountability pervading the NHS as a whole. Ultimately, the continued non-disclosure became academic after the document in question was leaked.

In July 2005, the PCT Chief Executive had referred in a PCT committee meeting to an Office of Government Commerce report about Sudbury – describing it as containing the evidence for the PCT's proposals to close all community hospital beds.[1]

From August 2005 onward, the PCT refused requests from both Tim Yeo, MP, and WHAC to get sight of the document. The MP would later accuse the NHS generally of 'hiding facts' in its refusal to disclose.[2]

The PCT stated that it was not in the public interest that the document be disclosed. In order to bolster its case, the PCT apparently sought advice from the Department of Health and Department of Constitutional Affairs. In January 2006, the report was leaked to WHAC and the local newspapers. It contained no suggestion that Sudbury should not have inpatient beds. At this point, the PCT appeared to change tack, agreeing that there was no such evidence in the report. It claimed that the Chief Executive's comments at the July meeting, although minuted, had been misunderstood. It also stated that the Chief Executive had been effectively prevented from disclosing by the Department of Health.[3] The PCT maintained that it had 'never been in the power of Suffolk West PCT to make this report available'.[4]

However, it turned out that the published rules concerning these reviews stated that it was for the 'Senior Responsible Officer [in this case the PCT Chief Executive] to determine whether and to whom the report will be released'. Thus, as WHAC put it, 'the PCT need never have sought, let alone blindly followed, advice from the Department of Health'. And blaming the Freedom of Information Act made no sense either, because the Act could justify non-disclosure, but did not, by definition, prevent disclosure. It seemed that the PCT had 'not only failed to exercise its own judgement but sought to find an excuse for non-disclosure and somebody else to blame'.[5]

Whether the PCT had been put in an impossible position by the Department of Health, or the PCT had been deliberately trying to avoid disclosure because of the inconsistency with the July minutes, was in the end irrelevant. What was most concerning was that, between them, the PCT and

1 *Meeting Held 14th July, Confirmed minutes.* Sudbury Health and Social Care Steering Group. Bury St Edmunds: Suffolk West PCT, 2005.

2 Dave Gooderham, 'MP accuses NHS of "hiding facts".' *East Anglian Daily Times,* 11 January 2006.

3 Michael Stonard, 'Hospitals: Trust boss hits back.' Letter. *Suffolk Free Press,* 16 February 2006.

4 Paul Holland, 'Health review secret is out.' *Suffolk Free Press,* 19 January 2006.

5 Walnuttree Hospital Action Committee, 'Hospital: why this secrecy.' Letter. *Suffolk Free Press,* 23 February 2006.

Department of Health had pursued non-disclosure so doggedly – in the name of legislation that was supposed to promote openness and transparency.

Enmities break out

A major plank of WHAC's campaign had been consistent claims that the PCT was providing misleading information. However, it had taken care repeatedly to state that it believed this to be inadvertent and due to haste. Such haste could lead to an overlooking of both facts and logic. Apart from realising that overtly personal criticism would not be productive of any sort of debate, WHAC also believed that the PCT's officers were acting as they were due to the immense political pressure (not always rational) – not in bad faith, but simply because they had lost a degree of judgement and objectivity. WHAC persistently put the problem down to haste and anxiety.[6]

However, the PCT complained bitterly that campaigners, politicians, union representatives (and even the church) were repeatedly exaggerating and distorting facts, thus hindering mature and informed public debate.[7]

The community would respond that to the extent it had made a mistake on outpatient figures, it was a genuine mistake arising because the PCT itself had failed to provide the relevant information. Even the PCT itself had apparently become muddled. On 27 August, it wrote to Tim Yeo, MP, referring to 8000 consultant appointments in Sudbury. On the same day, in an interview, the PCT Chief Executive was referring to 3000 such appointments only.[8]

Clearly exasperated by the concerted opposition, the PCT increasingly began to resort to a degree of personal criticism. Whether this marked fresh, considered tactics or was unintended and misinterpreted, it further alienated large sections of the local community. Such expressions of criticism failed by definition to answer the questions being posed of the PCT. Local people became still more dubious about the competence and good faith of the PCT. By December, the PCT had accused the Mayor and other prominent people in Sudbury of either not having read the relevant

6 Dave Gooderham, 'Campaigner hits at health cuts "rush".' *East Anglian Daily Times*, 29 August 2005.

7 Mike Stonard, 'Health debate hindered by inaccuracies.' Letter. *East Anglian Daily Times*, 27 August 2005.

8 Colin Spence, 'Concerned with tone of health chief's letter.' *East Anglian Daily Times*, 31 August 2005.

documents or of deliberately misleading people – and, in any event, of making local, elderly people 'very worried'.[9]

Confusion escalates and delays final decision

As the final decision approached for Suffolk West PCT, on 22 February 2006, what had appeared to be a brief meeting between the PCT and WHAC took place, to cover a few formalities. Instead it turned into a major fire fight, which would briefly draw in central government to the fray and delay the decision still further. It would also expose yet again the lack of accountability so pervading the NHS.

It turned out that 5500 letters and an 11,500 signature petition, handed to the Department of Health – and all objecting to the plans for Sudbury – had not found their way to the PCT. The PCT stated that it needed to see them. It delayed its decision for six weeks. The Department of Health then refused to hand over the letters and postcards; and it never became clear whether the petition was ever handed over or not. The PCT's Board papers suggested not. The whole episode revealed a sobering lack of interest by the Department of Health in the views of local people, as well as complete lack of accountability (see Chapter 9).

9 Mike Stonard, 'Read the document before you respond.' Letter. *East Anglian Daily Times*, 12 December 2005.

21

Decision-making Day: a Dimming of the Suffolk Light

In the East of Suffolk, the PCTs duly took their decision in January 2006. Despite overwhelming local opposition, the PCTs went ahead anyway with most of their proposals.

The closures approved included the Bartlet Hospital in Felixstowe, Hartismere Hospital in Eye, the Hayward Day Hospital in Ipswich, other day hospitals (older people and mental health) in Kesgrave and Saxmundham and Violet Hill (with Minsmere retained for some functions), the Old Fox Yard clubhouse for people with mental problems, learning disabilities or for substance misusers (Stowmarket), the Hollies employment project at St Clements (with reprovision intended), the Bridge House Clubhouse for people with mental health problems, learning disabilities or for substance misusers (Ipswich) and the Pines adult mental occupational therapy unit at St Clements Hospital. The 32 beds at Aldeburgh were to be reduced to 20; and the 28 beds at Bluebird Lodge, Ipswich, were to be re-designated primarily as step-up, rather than step-down, beds – meaning that people could not be discharged there from the acute hospital, but only as a means of preventing admission to hospital (from their current residence, their own home or a care home).

Not a single vote was cast in opposition.[1] However, the PCTs did modify some of their proposals from the originals; for example, they decided to retain some NHS community hospital beds and slightly lengthen the time of implementation.[2]

In the West of Suffolk, in April 2006, all the recommendations were passed by a vote of 11–0.[3] A long list of closures was involved: 68 beds were to be lost at Walnuttree Hospital (although the PCT referred only to 32, not recognising the existence of the other 36), together with all 16 beds at Newmarket Hospital. At West Suffolk Hospital, the 55 beds originally consulted on had now been closed prematurely anyway. No mention now was made of them. Within a month or so of the meeting, closure of a further 30 was announced.

Changes to the out-of-hours services had already occurred prematurely also. One apparent victory won by the local community concerned the retention of consultant outpatient clinics, which originally had faced relocation away from Sudbury. However, some of these were to be replaced with specialist nurse, GP or therapy clinics. Furthermore, within a day, the PCT had reminded a public meeting in Sudbury that, despite its decision, there was no guarantee that the outpatient services would be reprieved. This was because the forthcoming Suffolk-wide PCT, due to be in place by October 2006, would not be bound by the decision and might choose to do something different.[4]

As it turned out, Sudbury did not have to wait for a new PCT to be formed. Within a few weeks, two outpatient clinics had already been withdrawn, contrary to assurances. A mental health clinic remained open officially, but a decision had apparently been taken to refer no more patients. And a dietetic and nutrition clinic had been withdrawn, ostensibly because of staff shortage, but actually because the West Suffolk NHS Hospital Trust chose not to fill the vacancies. In addition, plans imminently to withdraw the paediatric clinic were leaked to the local newspaper. A future of minimal services in Sudbury was also referred to. This further undermined the local community's confidence in the future of their health services.

1 *Minutes of the Combined Board Meeting, Suffolk East PCTs, 25th January 2006.* Ipswich: Suffolk East PCTs, p.4.

2 Carole Taylor-Brown (2006) *Decisions on Changing for the Better: next steps, 25th January 2006.* Ipswich: Suffolk East PCTs.

3 *Extraordinary Board Meeting in Public, 11th April 2006, confirmed minutes.* Bury St Edmunds: Suffolk West PCT.

4 'It's a question of trust, says health chief.' *Suffolk Free Press,* 13 April 2006.

The Sage Day Hospital was to be closed; the Heathfields Respite Unit for people with learning disabilities was to be saved.

The PCT claimed it had made a further significant amendment. It had originally proposed that it would purchase care-home placements, for people who could not be rehabilitated at home, as and when needed. It now undertook to guarantee six beds purchased at any one time. It made great play of this concession. In reality it was paltry and an example of the PCT attempting to show that it had responded significantly to public concern when it had in fact done no such thing.

First, it might well have had to purchase that number anyway even under the original proposals. Second, the advantage of 'block purchasing' which it was now proposing, with the apparent possibility of creating a 'rehabilitation unit' in a particular home (although this was not made clear), was anyway undermined. It appeared that the PCT would purchase the beds in different care homes. Third, there were no care homes in the Sudbury area with dedicated rehabilitation facilities as demanded by standards made under the Care Standards Act. Fourth, six care-home beds would be an inadequate substitute in both number and function for the 68 community hospital beds being lost.

Nevertheless, the PCT's Chairman would argue that it had 'modified its proposals for the provision of inpatient beds'.[5] This was an example of misleading use of language. There were to be no inpatient beds, only half a dozen residential home beds; the reader would be quite misled into thinking they were hospital inpatient beds. As the response from the Walnuttree Hospital Action Committee made clear: concerning NHS inpatient beds, the PCT 'proposed no beds, and there will be no beds'.[6]

Swaying unsteadily in the Suffolk breeze: the Health Scrutiny Committee

Despite some superficial concessions, designed to keep at bay the Suffolk County Council Health Scrutiny Committee, the latter felt it had no choice but to refer the Suffolk East PCTs' decision to the Secretary of State for Health as not being in local patients' interests. The vote was 10–1 in favour

5 Colin Muge, 'WHAC statements need correcting.' Letter. *East Anglian Daily Times*, 2 June 2006.

6 Peter Clifford, 'PCT questions are in need of answers.' Letter. *East Anglian Daily Times*, 6 June 2006.

of referral.[7] The irony of this process was of course that the PCTs had, all along, only been doing the Secretary of State for Health's bidding.

Nonetheless, some weeks later, in the West an incomprehensible decision was made by the same Committee, when proposals that were more radical and arguably more damaging than in the East were not referred, on a vote of 6–5 against.

Procedural objections were raised, in that only PCT representatives were allowed to speak, and representatives from the local community, including MPs, were not permitted to. One of the members of the Committee resigned immediately in protest. It was seen to be a blow against the democratic process. Tim Yeo, MP for South Suffolk, referred to it as baffling, wrong and incomprehensible. The referral to the Secretary of State:

> was an important part of the consultation process but it has now been thrown away and the people of Sudbury have been badly let down.[8]

He believed it was a breach of natural justice, since the procedure adopted meant that the:

> committee was heavily biased in favour of the PCT proposals and did not give proper consideration to the overwhelming arguments in favour of referral to the Secretary of State.[9]

Local residents easily saw through what had happened, referring to it as constituting 'hardly an example of democracy and natural justice'.[10]

Furthermore, although Suffolk West PCT's presence at the meeting was ostensibly to answer questions, the PCT's Chief Executive had been allowed to make a freestanding statement to the Committee. The Committee's explanation was nonsensical. The Chair stated that the six-month changeover in the West was the crucial difference from the proposals in the East.[11] She omitted to point out that the Suffolk East PCTs had proposed exactly the same time period for changeover as the Suffolk West PCT: six months.[12]

7 Mark Bulstrode, 'It's up to you now, Minister.' *East Anglian Daily Times*, 1 March 2006.

8 Dave Gooderham, 'Hospitals decision "incomprehensible".' *East Anglian Daily Times*, 28 April 2006.

9 Paul Holland, 'MP slams fresh move over hospital closure.' *Suffolk Free Press*, 4 May 2006.

10 R. Anthony Platt, 'PCT's community care plan wasn't convincing.' Letter. *East Anglian Daily Times*, 5 May 2006.

11 Dave Gooderham, 'Row erupts after PCT bosses speak.' *East Anglian Daily Times*, 1 May 2006.

12 *Minutes of the Combined Board Meeeting, 25th January 2006.* Ipswich: Suffolk East PCTs, p.4.

Crucially, the seven points the Committee gave for its referral for the East all applied to the West as well. They were damning and cogent points. In summary:

- The PCT's decisions did not have the support of the local community.
- Neither the Committee nor the local community had confidence that intermediate care without sufficient NHS step-down inpatient beds will meet the health needs of local people.
- The decisions had been rushed through to save money, even with perceived risk to the health of local people.
- Neither the committee nor the local community had confidence that the changes made to the original proposals, to ameliorate the impact of closures, would actually happen.
- The PCT's need to save further money made it even more unlikely that the proposals will be implemented in full.
- The decisions were badly timed because of the imminent reorganisation of the PCTs. This would make it less likely that the amelioration of the original proposal would take place.
- The three PCTs in Suffolk had different approaches to their community hospitals. This would be unsustainable and cast doubt on the implementation of the PCTs' proposals.

The Committee went on to emphasise how the trust of the local community was lost at the outset and never recovered; how the consultation process was rushed during the summer holidays with no prior consultation; and how the overall impression was one of haste and ill-thought-out proposals. The Committee was clear that the proposals were clearly financial in origin and were not 'genuinely based on strategic clinical planning'. All these points applied to the West, perhaps even more so.

On top of all of this, and in relation to the West of Suffolk, the Committee had already referred to the 'much more aggressive move to intermediate care without any NHS beds provided at all'.[13] The Committee's subsequent papers, prepared for its meeting and decision about Suffolk West, noted that:

13 *Referral of the Decisions of Suffolk East PCT*. Letter, 7 March 2006. Ipswich: Suffolk County Council Health Scrutiny Committee.

> unlike in the East of the County, including Waveney, there are to be no NHS beds in the intermediate care system at all. In the East, where there is no NHS provision of beds in Eye, NHS beds are available elsewhere, in Aldeburgh, Felixstowe and Bluebird Lodge, Ipswich. This difference of approach does not appear to be sustainable given that the three Suffolk PCTs are to be merged into one from October 2006.[14]

And, while the Suffolk West PCT viewed residential or nursing home beds as the equivalent of community hospital beds, the Committee had already rejected this contention for the East.[15]

The Committee faced a barrage of criticism and would be threatened with a judicial review legal case. The chair resigned a few weeks after she had presided over the ill-fated decision, on which she had not voted. It was left to a Sudbury patient, who was also a parish councillor, to try to bring a judicial review case against the PCT and the Scrutiny Committee and to sum up:

> But how sad and shameful it is that two elderly and disabled pensioners have to be the ones to put up a fight where others, like the PCT and the scrutiny committee, have failed.[16]

The Scrutiny Committee, under new chairmanship, decided in July to quash its own decision not to refer the Suffolk West PCT to the Secretary of State. It stated that it understood the grounds of the challenge. It undertook to take the decision, whether or not to refer, afresh in September 2006.[17]

However, by this time, the Secretary of State had rejected all but one of the grounds on which the Committee had referred the Suffolk East PCTs' proposals earlier in the year. Nonetheless, she did tell the Suffolk East PCTs to rethink their proposals about Hartismere Hospital – and consider a 'social enterprise' scheme on the site for the future. This would comprise a community venture, typically involving public sector, the local community and the independent sector.[18] Nonetheless, to the dismay of the local community in Eye, the Suffolk East PCTs made it immediately clear – within

14 *Committee Response to Decisions Taken by Suffolk West Primary Care Trust. Prepared for meeting on 27th April 2006.* H06/12. Ipswich: Suffolk County Council Health Scrutiny Committee.

15 *Referral of the decisions of Suffolk East PCT.* Letter, 7 March 2006. Ipswich: Suffolk County Council Health Scrutiny Committee.

16 Dave Gooderham, 'Legal battle to save beds at hospital.' *East Anglian Daily Times,* 6 June 2006.

17 Lisa Cleverdon, 'U-turn on referral of PCT bid to Hewitt.' *East Anglian Daily Times,* 8 July 2006.

18 Mark Bulstrode, 'The axe finally falls on health services.' *East Anglian Daily Times,* 3 August 2006.

days of the Secretary of State's direction – that they still intended imminently to close Hartismere Hospital anyway.

Desperation and a cry for help: looking to the judges

The last desperate throw of the dice for Sudbury residents came with an attempt to launch judicial review proceedings. One of the Sudbury patients bringing the case explained clearly and articulately that her post-polio syndrome meant that:

> I have quite complex medical needs now and will have considerably more problems in future. And for people with these conditions, private beds in care homes are not going to cater for them. I didn't want the matter to have to go to judicial review but we need the right hospital facilities and now is the time to stand up and be counted.[19]

It really was a last desperate throw, because by August, 2006, health (and social care) services in West Suffolk seemed to be in chaos and decline.

The Scrutiny Committee had quashed its own decision about Suffolk West PCT and was having to retake it. Pending this, the judicial review proceedings were stayed, but still hanging over the PCT. Quite apart from this, planning and operational blight had anyway descended, as senior managers and executives scrambled for posts in the reconfigured PCTs that would emerge in October 2006. Intermediate care developments had already been suspended in June.

Development of Sudbury's new health centre – albeit in its watered down form – stood at a standstill. Outpatient clinics appeared to be leaking away from Sudbury, incrementally, by stealth and apparently contrary to promises made as recently as April 2006. Despite reducing its deficit, Suffolk West PCT was still some £11 million overspent, with further cuts to services therefore in prospect.

Up the road, in Bury St Edmunds, the West Suffolk Hospitals NHS Trust, too, still had a serious financial deficit of £12 million hanging round its neck. Concerns had grown that it would be downgraded into a satellite of Addenbrooke's Hospital (nearly an hour's drive away in Cambridge) and become a more modest community hospital. Beds had already closed there by the score, with hundreds of posts being shed as well. Some of its funding was already reported to be drifting north to Cambridge.

19 Will Grahame-Clark, 'Pensioner in legal fight on bed closures.' *Suffolk Free Press*, 20 May 2006.

East of Bury, uncertainty remained at Newmarket Hospital, where 10 out of 16 specialist rehabilitation beds had been closed in December 2005 temporarily but never reopened. The future of the Heathfields centre for people with learning disabilities also remained uncertain. Due to be transferred to Suffolk County Council, this apparently depended on the NHS handing money to the Council to fund its refurbishment – money it was unclear that the NHS had.

As local health services (other perhaps than those directly related to the chosen, government set targets) disintegrated, staff morale plummeted. The staff themselves began to drift away, concerned about their future and their mortgages. The PCT appeared to be waiting in the wings – ready to close Walnuttree Hospital in Sudbury on health and safety grounds because of staff shortages – notwithstanding the judicial review case pending and the PCT's agreement not to implement any changes. But a recruitment freeze, together with the huge uncertainties, meant that vacancies were unlikely to be filled (which situation had accounted for the ten beds already closed prematurely at Newmarket).

And all around this NHS debacle, Suffolk County Council managers and social work staff were a hive of activity too, planning and implementing cost cutting measures. They emerged in swarms to review people's care plans and to remove or reduce services by hook or by crook. All in the thankless cause of making some £15 million savings on the adult social care budget.

Above all, both NHS and social services decision-makers came over as contortionists and illusionists – as they persistently denied that the severe cuts being implemented would adversely affect the people of Suffolk.

22

Conclusions

This book is an account of a system of decision-making that descended into chaos, lack of transparency and lack of accountability – with the potential for highly detrimental consequences for significant groups of vulnerable people as well as the population at large.

A number of lessons emerge. First, the strength of anger and fear generated shows just how important health matters are. Second, the great faults of lack of transparency, trust and accountability associated with the actions of the NHS were profoundly undemocratic. When it is the most vulnerable people who stand to be brushed under the carpet, this becomes a serious matter. And, health care needs can of course rapidly reduce all of us to a greater or lesser state of vulnerability. A lack of transparency hinders or prevents debate; in effect the people affected become invisible and do not officially exist. To harm people is bad enough; not to acknowledge the detriment is unforgivable.

Third, the lack of transparency at both national and local levels appeared inevitable because the government seemed to be implementing a number of concealed agendas. These included a dismantling of the NHS in favour of private sector provision, as well as excluding significant categories of patient from NHS provision – particularly older people with more complex problems and needs, relating to rehabilitation, recuperation and care. In addition, local services more generally – from accident and emergency to maternity – were in retreat in many places.

Fourth, these very faults directly led to local NHS bodies becoming detached and isolated in their decision-making – apparently unable to understand how their actions were perceived in local communities. Even were they acting, according to their own lights, in total good faith, such a situation inevitably led to a situation of conflict. What the NHS came to regard as quite reasonable and transparent in nature, the local community would see as irrational, highly confrontational and secretive. The prevalence and use generally by the NHS of meaningless mantras, euphemism and a form of doublespeak or doublethink made it worse.

Fifth, in turn all this was exacerbated by a systematic lack of accountability that found expression at every level, in terms both of the concealed agendas and the impossibility at times of finding the true decision-maker. The lack of accountability added to the sense that what was taking place was not only highly detrimental to patients and to the NHS as an organisation, but also profoundly undemocratic.

Undemocratic, because the government had no political mandate to implement the scale and type of change it was pushing through. This was evident from the vague nature of its election manifesto, which did not prepare people for what was to come. The impression of this lack of mandate was strengthened by the back door way in which it attempted to shift provision by NHS primary care trusts into the private sector. For instance, the 'Nigel Crisp letter' of July 2005 demanded that primary care trusts shed all services. And, almost a year later, the government placed in the *Official Journal of the European Communities* an advertisement for multi-national companies to take over PCTs. Both letter and advertisement were put out with no announcement and no Parliamentary debate, and in the summer to avoid attention. Were there any doubt about the lack of a political mandate, it would be dispelled by the extent of opposition from local communities up and down the country. And by the way in which central government and local NHS Trusts and PCTs would ruthlessly try to ride roughshod over all this local protest, anger and fear.

Sixth, insofar as decisions are taken that harm vulnerable people, without transparency and without accountability, this is an abuse of power. There was a serious absence of checks and balances to the decision-making that was taking place. That is why in so many ways it appeared to veer off the rails. Excessive, unchecked power by definition leads public bodies and their decision-makers astray, even those with good intentions. The following report about New Labour is telling, referring to the:

> self-belief of the inner circle, who see themselves as valiantly trying to do the right thing in a hostile universe. A leading Blairite was recently at dinner with a friend, and found himself being challenged over the government's activities. Eventually, frustrated by criticism, he leant

> forward and said: 'What you don't seem to understand is that we are good people'.[1]

The late Sir Douglas Black, president of the Royal College of Physicians and author in 1980 of *Inequalities in Health: the Black Report*, was reported as stating the following in terms of large organisations: 'People banded together are capable of follies and excesses beyond what the same people, acting as individuals, would perpetrate on other individuals. Such activities may be termed corporate tyranny'.[2]

Whatever the explanation for what has happened, one thing is overwhelmingly clear. The answers and solutions to running the health service may be elusive. But they will certainly not be found through the lack of transparency and of accountability currently afflicting the way in which the NHS is being run – characteristics that ultimately make things immeasurably worse.

1 Jenni Russell, 'Blair's circle and its ferocious grab for power.' *Guardian*, 6 April 2006.

2 C. Richmond, 'Sir Douglas Black: physician who reported social inequalities in British Health.' Obituary. *Independent*, 8 October 2002.

Index